Implants in Clinical Dentistry

Implants in Clinical Dentistry

Richard M Palmer PhD, BDS, FDS, RCS (Eng), FDS RCS (Ed)
Professor of Implant Dentistry and Periodontology
Guy's, Kings and St Thomas' Hospitals Medical and Dental Schools
London, UK

Brian J Smith BDS, MSc, FDS RCS (Eng)
Consultant in Restorative Dentistry, Unit of Restorative Dentistry
Guy's and St Thomas' Hospitals Trust
London, UK

Leslie C Howe BDS, FDS RCS (Eng)
Consultant in Restorative Dentistry, Guy's and St Thomas' Hospitals Trusts
and Specialist in Restorative Dentistry and Prosthodontics
London, UK

Paul J Palmer BDS, MSc, MRD RCS (Eng)
Specialist in Periodontics and
Postgraduate Tutor in Implant Surgery, Guy's, Kings and St Thomas'
Hospitals Medical and Dental Schools
London, UK

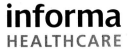

informa
HEALTHCARE

© 2002, 2006 Informa Healthcare, an imprint of Informa UK Limited

First published in the United Kingdom in 2002 by Martin Dunitz Ltd

This edition published by Informa Healthcare, an Imprint of Informa UK Limited,
2 Park Square, Milton Park, Abingdon, Oxon OX14 4RN

Tel: +44 (0)20 7017 6000
Fax: +44 (0)20 7017 6699
Email: info.medicine@tandf.co.uk
Website: www.tandf.co.uk/medicine

Although every effort has been made to ensure that all owners of copyright material
have been acknowledged in this publication, we would be glad to acknowledge in
subsequent reprints or editions any omissions brought to our attention.

Although every effort has been made to ensure that drug doses and other
information are presented accurately in this publication, the ultimate responsibility
rests with the prescribing physician. Neither the publishers nor the authors can be
held responsible for errors or for any consequences arising from the use of
information contained herein. For detailed prescribing information or instructions on
the use of any product or procedure discussed herein, please consult the prescribing
information or instructional material issued by the manufacturer.

A CIP record for this book is available from the British Library.
Library of Congress Cataloging-in-Publication Data

Data available on application

ISBN-10: 1 85317 805 5
ISBN-13: 978 1 85317 805 4

Distributed in the United States and Canada by
Thieme New York
333 Seventh Avenue
New York, NY 10001

Distributed in the rest of the world by
Thomson Publishing Services
Cheriton House
North Way
Andover, Hampshire SP10 5BE, UK
Tel.: +44 (0)1264 332424
E-mail: salesorder.tandf@thomsonpublishingservices.co.uk

Composition by Scribe Design Ltd, Ashford, Kent, UK
Printed and bound in Spain by Grafos SA

CONTENTS

PREFACE

This book is based upon our combined experiences of working together in the treatment of patients with dental implant prostheses at Guy's Hospital and in private practice over the last 10 years. While the chapters are not attributed to specific authors, the surgical chapters are mainly the work of Richard and Paul Palmer; the implant denture chapters, Brian Smith; and the fixed prosthodontics, Leslie Howe. Our initial experiences were with the Brånemark system, which established a benchmark in implant treatment, with high success rates using meticulous techniques. It was immensely valuable to use this system at a time when it rapidly developed to allow sophisticated treatment of the complete clinical spectrum. Working in an academic institute we felt that it was essential to gain experience in other leading implant systems to allow comparison and to educate ourselves and our students. We were thus able to appreciate some of the features of other systems such as single stage implant surgery and the development of implant surfaces which gave the potential for more rapid osseointegration and earlier loading. We were also one of the initial teams to evaluate the Astra Tech ST implant. We believe that the four implant systems (Astra Tech, Brånemark/Nobel Biocare, Frialit and ITI Straumann) described in this book cover most of the important features of modern implant design and that the information contained within this text could apply to many more systems that are available today.

Richard M Palmer
PhD, BDS, FDS RCS(Eng), FDS RCS(Ed)
Brian J Smith
BDS, MSc, FDS RCS(Eng)
Leslie C Howe
BDS, FDS RCS(Eng)
Paul J Palmer
BDS, MSc, MRD RCS(Eng)

ACKNOWLEDGEMENTS

We would like to thank the following people and publishers:

Dr David Radford for producing the scanning electron microscopy images in figures 1.9, 1.10 and 1.11.

Dr Michael Fenlon for help with the case illustrated in figure 5.5.

Dr Claire Morgan for providing figure 15.19.

Dr Paul Robinson for help with the maxillofacial surgical aspects of treatment in the case illustrated in figure 12.14.

The UK subsidiaries of Astra Tech, Frialit, Nobel Biocare and ITI Straumann for providing illustrations of some components illustrated in chapter 1.

Munksgaard International Publishers Ltd, Copenhagen, Denmark, for permission to reproduce figure 1.24 which was taken from Cawood JI and Howell RA, *International Journal of Oral and Maxillofacial Surgery*, **20**:75, 1991.

The British Dental Journal and Macmillan Publishers for permission to reproduce figures 2.1, 2.4, 5.7, 5.20 and 10.1 from *A Clinical Guide to Implants in Dentistry* (ed RM Palmer).

Image Diagnostic Technology, London, UK for Figures 5.8, 5.9 and 5.10.

The highly skilled technical staff at Guy's Hospital, Kedge and Quince London W1 and Brooker and Hamill, London W1.

PART I

Overview

1
Overview of implant dentistry

Introduction

The development of endosseous osseointegrated dental implants has been very rapid over the last two decades and there are now many implant systems available that will provide the clinician with:

- a high degree of predictability in the attainment of osseointegration
- versatile surgical and prosthodontic protocols
- design features that facilitate ease of treatment and aesthetics
- a low complication rate and ease of maintenance
- published papers to support the manufacturers' claims
- a reputable company with good customer support

There is no perfect system and the choice may be bewildering. It is easy for a clinician to be seduced into believing that a new system is better or less expensive. All implant treatment depends upon a high level of clinical training and experience. Much of the cost of treatment is not system dependent but relates to clinical time and laboratory expenses.

There are a number of published versions of what constitutes a successful implant or implant system. For example, Albrektsson *et al.* (1986) proposed the following criteria for minimum success:

1. An individual, unattached implant is immobile when tested clinically.
2. Radiographic examination does not reveal any peri-implant radiolucency.
3. After the first year in function, radiographic vertical bone loss is less than 0.2 mm per annum.

4. The individual implant performance is characterized by an absence of signs and symptoms such as pain, infections, neuropathies, paraesthesia, or violation of the inferior dental canal.
5. As a minimum, the implant should fulfil the above criteria with a success rate of 85% at the end of a 5-year observation period and 80% at the end of a 10-year period.

The most definitive criterion is that the implant is not mobile (criterion 1). By definition, osseointegration produces a direct structural and functional union between the surrounding bone and the surface of the implant. The implant is therefore held rigidly within bone without an intervening fibrous encapsulation (or periodontal ligament) and therefore should not exhibit any mobility or peri-implant radiolucency (criterion 2). However, in order to test the mobility of an implant supporting a fixed bridge reconstruction, the bridge has to be removed. This fact has limited the use of this test in clinical practice and in many long-term studies. Radiographic bone levels are also difficult to assess because they depend upon longitudinal measurements from a specified landmark. The landmark may differ with various designs of implant and is more difficult to visualize in some than others. For example, the flat top of the implant in the Brånemark system is easily defined on a well-aligned radiograph and is used as the landmark to measure bone changes. In most designs of implant, some bone remodelling is expected in the first year of function in response to occlusal forces and establishment of the normal dimensions of the peri-implant soft tissues. Subsequently the bone levels are usually stable on the majority of implants over many years. A small proportion of implants may show some bone loss and account for the mean figures of bone loss that are published in the literature.

Progressive or continuous bone loss is a sign of potential implant failure. However, it is difficult or impossible to establish agreement between researchers/clinicians as to what level of bone destruction constitutes failure, therefore most implants described as failures are those that have been removed from the mouth. Implants that remain in function but do not match the criteria for success are described as 'surviving'.

Implants placed in the mandible (particularly anterior to the mental foramina) enjoy a very high success rate, such that it would be difficult or impossible to show differences between rival systems. In contrast, the more demanding situation of the posterior maxilla, where implants of shorter length are placed in bone of softer quality, may reveal differences between success rates. This remains to be substantiated in comparative clinical trials. Currently there are no comparative data to recommend one system over another, but certain design features may have theoretical advantages (see section on implant design).

Patient factors

There are few contraindications to implant treatment. The main potential problem areas to consider are:

- Age
- Untreated dental disease
- Severe mucosal lesions
- Tobacco smoking, alcohol and drug abuse
- Poor bone quality
- Previous radiotherapy to the jaws
- Poorly controlled systemic disease such as diabetes
- Bleeding disorders

Age

The fact that the implant behaves as an ankylosed unit restricts its use to individuals who have completed their jaw growth. Placement of an osseointegrated implant in a child will result in relative submergence of the implant restoration with growth of the surrounding alveolar process during normal development. It is therefore advisable to delay implant placement until growth is complete, this is generally earlier in females than males, but considerable variation exists. It is usually acceptable to treat patients in their late teens. Although some growth potential may remain in patients in their early twenties, this is less likely to result in an aesthetic problem.

There is no upper age limit to implant treatment provided that the patient is fit enough and willing to be treated. For example, elderly edentulous individuals can experience considerable quality of life and health gain with implant treatment to stabilize complete dentures (see Chapter 6).

Untreated dental disease

The clinician should ensure that all patients are comprehensively examined, diagnosed and treated to deal adequately with concurrent dental disease.

Severe mucosal lesions

Caution should be exercised before treating patients with severe mucosal/gingival lesions such as erosive lichen planus or mucous membrane pemphigoid. When these conditions affect the gingiva they are often more problematic around the natural dentition and the discomfort compromises plaque control, adding to the inflammation. Similar lesions can arise around implants penetrating the mucosa.

Tobacco smoking and drug abuse

It is well established that tobacco smoking is a very important risk factor in periodontitis and that it affects healing. This has been demonstrated extensively in the dental, medical and surgical literature. A few studies have shown that the overall mean failure rate of dental implants in smokers is approximately twice that in non-smokers. Smokers should be warned of this association and encouraged to quit the habit. Protocols have been proposed that recommend smokers to give up for at least two weeks prior to implant placement and for several weeks afterwards. Such recommendations have not been tested adequately in clinical trials and nor has the compliance of the patients. The chance of the quitter relapsing is disappointingly high and some patients will try to hide the fact that they are still smoking. It should also be noted that reported mean implant failure rates are not evenly distributed throughout the patient population. Rather, implant failures are more likely to cluster in certain individuals. In our experience this is more likely in heavy smokers who have a high intake of alcohol. In addition, failure is more likely in those who have poor-quality bone, which is a possible association with tobacco smoking. It should be noted also that smokers followed in longitudinal studies have been shown to have more significant marginal bone loss around their implants than non-smokers. Most of these findings have been reported from studies involving the Brånemark system, probably because it is one of the best-documented and widely used systems to date. More data involving other systems would be useful.

Drug abuse may affect the general health of individuals and their compliance with treatment and may therefore be an important contraindication.

Poor bone quality

This is a term often used to denote regions of bone in which there is low mineralization or poor trabeculation. It is often associated with a thin or absent cortex and is referred to as type 4 bone (see section on bone factors). It is a normal variant of bone quality and is more likely to occur in the posterior maxilla. Osteoporosis is a condition that results in a reduction of the bone mineral density and commonly affects postmenopausal females, having its greatest effect in the spine and pelvis. The commonly used DEXA (Dual Energy X-Ray Absorptiometry) scans for osteoporosis assessment do not generally provide useful clinical measures of the jaws. The effect of osteoporosis on the maxilla and mandible may be of little significance in the majority of patients. Many patients can have type 4 bone quality, particularly in the posterior maxilla, in the absence of any osteoporotic changes.

Previous radiotherapy to the jaws

Radiation for malignant disease of the jaws results in endarteritis, which compromises bone healing and in extreme cases can lead to osteoradionecrosis following trauma/infection. These patients requiring implant treatment should be managed in specialist centres. It can be helpful to optimize timing of implant placement in relation to the radiotherapy and to provide a course of hyperbaric oxygen treatment. The latter may improve implant success particularly in the maxilla. Success rates in the mandible may be acceptable even without hyperbaric oxygen treatment, although more clinical trials are required to establish the effectiveness of the recommended protocols.

Poorly controlled systemic disease such as diabetes

Diabetes has been a commonly quoted factor to consider in implant treatment. It does affect the vasculature, healing and response to infection. Although there is limited evidence to suggest higher failure of implants in well-controlled diabetes, it would be unwise to ignore this factor in poorly controlled patients.

Bleeding disorders

Bleeding disorders are obviously relevant to the surgical delivery of treatment and require advice from the patient's physician.

Osseointegration

Osseointegration is basically a union between bone and the implant surface (Figure 1.1). It is not an absolute phenomenon and can be

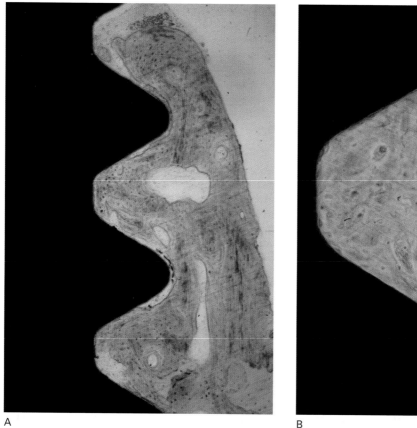
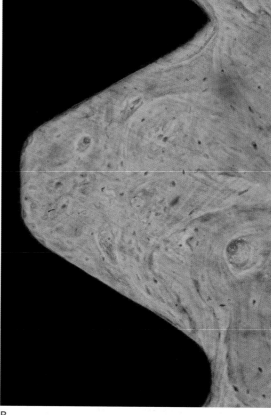

A   B

Figure 1.1

(A) Histological section of osseointegration. At the light microscope level the bone appears to be in intimate contact with the titanium implant surface over a large proportion of the area. Small marrow spaces are visible where bone is not in contact with the implant surface. (B) Higher power micrograph showing almost total bone to implant contact.

measured histologically as the proportion of the total implant surface that is in contact with bone. Greater levels of bone contact occur in cortical bone than in cancellous bone, where marrow spaces are often adjacent to the implant surface. Therefore bone with well-formed cortices and dense trabeculation offers the greatest potential for a high degree of bone to implant contact. The degree of bone contact may increase with time. The precise nature of osseointegration at a molecular level is not fully understood. At the light microscope level there is a very close

adaptation of the bone to the implant surface. At the higher magnifications possible with electron microscopy, there is a gap (approximately 100 nm wide) between the implant surface and the bone. This is occupied by an intervening collagen-rich zone adjacent to the bone and a more amorphous zone adjacent to the implant surface. Bone proteoglycans may be important in the initial attachment of the tissues to the implant surface, which in the case of titanium implants consists of a titanium oxide layer, which is defined as a ceramic.

It has been proposed that the biological process leading to and maintaining osseointegration is dependent upon the following factors, which will be considered in more detail in the subsequent sections:

- Biocompatibility
- Implant design
- Submerged and non-submerged protocols
- Bone factors
- Loading conditions
- Prosthetic loading considerations

Biocompatibility

Most current dental implants (including all systems considered in this book) are made of commercially pure titanium. Titanium has established a benchmark in osseointegration against which few other materials compare. Related materials such as niobium are able to produce a high degree of osseointegration and, in addition, successful clinical results are reported with titanium–aluminium–vanadium alloys. The titanium alloys have the potential disadvantage of ionic leakage of aluminium into the tissues but they have the potential to enhance the physical/mechanical properties of the implants. This would be of greater significance in narrow-diameter implants.

Hydroxyapatite-coated implants have the potential to allow more rapid bone growth on their surfaces and they have been recommended for use in situations of poorer bone quality. The reported disadvantages are delamination of the coating and corrosion with time. More recently, resorbable coatings have been developed that aim to improve the initial rate of bone healing against the implant surface, followed by resorption within a short time frame to allow establishment of a bone to metal contact. Hydroxyapatite-coated implants are not considered within this book because the authors have no experience of them.

All the implant systems used by the authors and illustrated in this book are made from titanium and therefore are highly comparable in this respect. The main differences in the systems are in the design, which is considered in the next section.

Implant design

Implant design usually refers to the design of the intraosseous component (the endosseous dental implant). However, the design of the implant abutment junction and the abutments is extremely important in prosthodontic management and maintenance and will be dealt with in a separate section.

The implant design has a great influence on initial stability and subsequent function in bone.

The main design parameters are:

- Implant length
- Implant diameter
- Implant shape
- Surface characteristics

Implant length

Implants are generally available in lengths from about 6 mm to as much as 20 mm. The most common lengths employed are between 8 and 15 mm, which correspond quite closely to normal root lengths. There has been a tendency to use longer implants in systems such as Brånemark compared with, for example, Straumann. The Brånemark protocol advocated maximizing implant length, where possible, to engage bone cortices apically as well as marginally in order to gain high initial stability. In contrast, the concept with Straumann was to increase the surface area of shorter implants by design features (e.g. hollow cylinders) or surface treatments (see section on surface characteristics).

Implant diameter

Most implants are approximately 4 mm in diameter. A diameter of at least 3.25 mm is recommended to ensure adequate implant strength. Diameters up to 6.5 mm are available, which are considerably stronger and have a much higher surface area. They may also engage lateral bone cortices to enhance initial stability. However, they may not be so widely used because sufficient bone width is not commonly encountered in most patients' jaws.

Implant shape

Various shapes are used by different manufacturers:

- *Brånemark* implants are solid screws (3.3, 3.75, 4, 5 or 5.5 mm in diameter) with a thread pitch of 0.6 mm (Figures 1.2 and 1.3). The implants

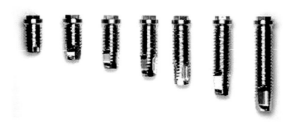

Figure 1.2

The latest design of Nobel Biocare implant (based on the original Brånemark concept) has a self-tapping end. The standard implants are 3.75 mm in diameter and available in a range of lengths from 7 to 20 mm.

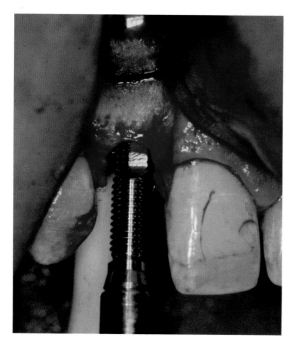

Figure 1.3

A narrow-diameter (3.3 mm) Nobel Biocare implant being installed in a narrow maxillary lateral incisor space.

can be self-tapped owing to the fact that they have a cutting end. The original design of the Brånemark implant was not a self-tapper, and in good-quality bone the implant site needed to be tapped prior to implant insertion. In softer bone (type 4 and possibly type 3) the implant will develop its own thread passage without prior tapping. The original design (and protocol) is preferred by the authors even though it may be slightly more time consuming. This is because the self-tapper design has quite pronounced cutting flutes that do not allow as smooth an entry into the bone site (This feature has been improved in the latest Mark 3 design: Nobel Biocare AB, Göteborg, Sweden; Figure 1.2.) Pre-tapping ensures that the implant will readily seat to the desired level. If self-tapping implants are used in dense bone, the site may have to be made wider with a larger diameter twist drill (or pre-tapped as in the original protocol).

- *AstraTech* implants are parallel-sided self-tapping solid screws (basically 3.5 mm or 4 mm in diameter) with a thread pitch of 0.6 mm (Figure 1.4). To allow for successful seating of the implant, the bone preparation is made with twist drills 0.3 mm less in diameter in normal quality bone and 0.15 mm narrower in hard or dense bone. The single tooth (ST: Astra Meditec AB, Mölndal,

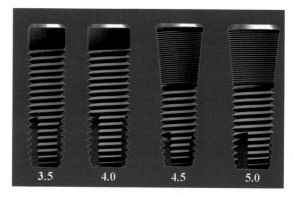

Figure 1.4

AstraTech implants showing the various diameters and designs available. The standard implants of 3.5 and 4.0 mm are on the left and the single tooth (ST) implants on the right. The ST implants have identical bodies to the standard implants but have a microthreaded conical collar that houses an internal anti-rotational double-hexagon element.

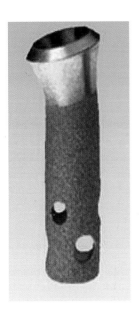

Figure 1.5

An angled hollow-cylinder Straumann implant specifically recommended for anterior maxillary single tooth replacement. This implant has a titanium-plasma-sprayed surface.

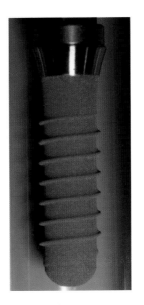

Figure 1.6

A 4.1-mm diameter solid-screw Straumann implant. This particular implant is an aesthetic line implant that has a reduced height of polished collar (1.8 mm, as opposed to 2.8 mm on the standard implant). The surface has been sand-blasted and acid etched. The top of the polished collar expands to a diameter of 4.8 mm.

Sweden) implant has a different design in that the top part has a microthreaded conical collar, which is claimed to distribute stress at the marginal bone more favourably.

- *Straumann* implants used to be available as hollow screws, hollow cylinders or solid screws. The hollow cylinders greatly increase the available surface area for bone contact but are now only available in a pre-angled design

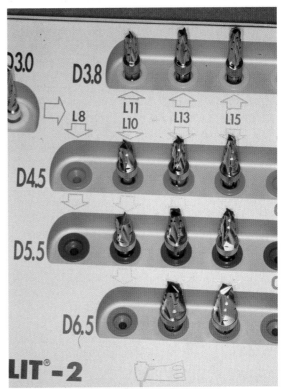

Figure 1.8

The matched drills for the stepped Frialit 2 implants, with lengths of 11, 13 and 15 mm and diameters of 3.8, 4.5, 5.5 and 6.5 mm.

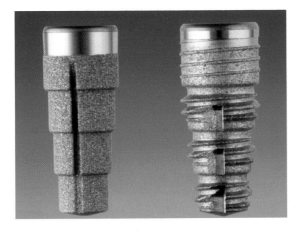

Figure 1.7

The Frialit 2 implants are stepped cylinders and therefore are more like tapered root forms. The implant on the right has threads on each of the steps and is recommended where greater stability at placement is required, such as immediate placement into extraction sockets.

for single anterior tooth replacement (Figure 1.5). Hollow screws are no longer available (a higher rate of fracture was observed in hollow designs). The solid screws are the only design used by the authors (Figure 1.6). They are available in diameters of 3.2, 4.1 and 4.8 mm and have a coarse-thread pitch.

- *Frialit* implants (Figures 1.7 and 1.8) are tapered, stepped cylinders (3.8, 4.5, 5.5 and 6.5 mm diameter at the top). They are therefore more 'root form', with the various diameters designed to replace teeth of corresponding dimensions. Most implants of this design are pushed or tapped into place. An alternative design has self-tapping threads on the steps, which requires that the implant is given three rotations to seat it.

Surface characteristics

The degree of surface roughness varies greatly between different systems. Surfaces that are machined, grit-blasted, plasma sprayed and coated are available:

- *Brånemark* implants have a machined surface as a result of the cutting of the screw thread. This has small ridges when viewed at high magnification (Figure 1.9) and this degree of surface irregularity was claimed to be close to ideal because smoother surfaces fail to osseointegrate and rougher surfaces are more prone to ion release and corrosion. This claim is disputed and the other implants listed below have rougher surfaces that may favour osseointegration. The 3i implants that were based on the Brånemark design are available with an acid-etched surface on the threads apical to the first 2 mm. Brånemark implants are now also available with a treated surface (TiUnite).
- *AstraTech* implants have a roughened surface produced by 'grit blasting', in this case with titanium oxide particles. The resulting surface has approximately 5-μm depressions over the entire intraosseous part of the implant. This surface has been termed 'TiO blasted' (Figure 1.10). Comparative tests in experimental animals have demonstrated a higher degree of bone to implant contact and higher torque removal forces than machined surfaces.

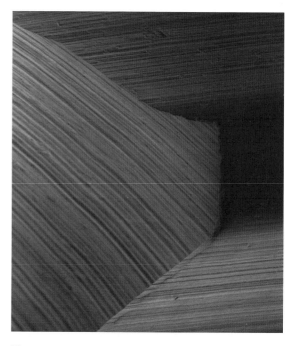

Figure 1.9

Electron micrograph of a 'machined' implant surface. There are ridges and grooves produced during the machining. The macroscopic appearance can be seen in Figures 1.2 and 1.3.

- *Straumann* – surfaces were originally plasma sprayed (Figure 1.11). Molten titanium is sprayed onto the surface of the implant to produce a rougher surface than a blasted one. The available surface area is much larger and this may have advantages in lower quality bone and enhanced performance of short (under 10 mm) implants. Straumann have developed a newer surface called the SLA (Sand blasted–Large grit–Acid etched: Institut Straumann AG, Waldenburg, Switzerland; Figure 1.12). This surface has large irregularities with smaller ones superimposed on top. It is claimed to have an advantage over the plasma-sprayed surface, with a reduction in healing time to achieve osseointegration. All Straumann implants have a highly polished collar (2.8 mm long in the standard implant) to allow soft-tissue adaptation because they were originally designed as a non-submerged system (see section on submerged and non-submerged protocols).

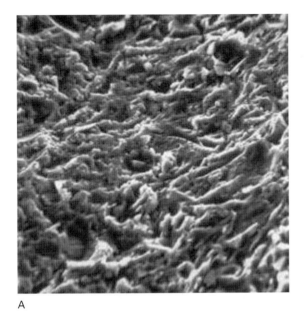

A

Figure 1.10

(A) AstraTech TiO-blasted surface. This scanning electron micrograph shows the numerous pits of approximately 5 μm.

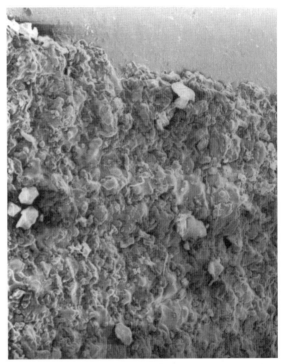

Figure 1.11

Scanning electron micrograph of the Straumann plasma-sprayed surface at the junction with the polished collar (top).

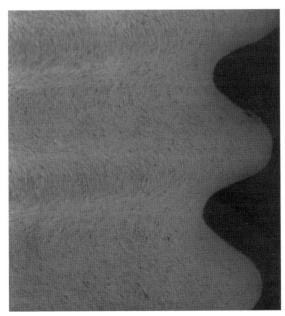

B

Figure 1.10

(B) Lower power view showing the TiO-blasted surface on the thread profiles.

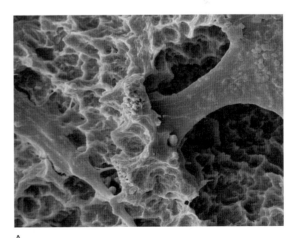

A

Figure 1.12

(A) The Straumann SLA surface produces a complex of large and small pits providing a large area for osseointegration.

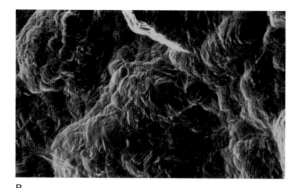

B

Figure 1.12

(B) Scanning electron micrograph of the Frialit grit-blasted and acid-etched surface.

Figure 1.13

Scanning electron micrograph of the acid-etched surface in the Frialit system.

- *Frialit* – implants are available in both plasma-sprayed surfaces and acid-etched and grit-blasted/acid-etched surfaces (Figures 1.12 and 1.13). The top collar is polished to allow soft tissue adaptation.

The optimum surface morphology has yet to be defined, and some may perform better in some circumstances. By increasing the surface roughness there is the potential to increase the surface contact with bone, but this may be at the expense of more ionic exchange and surface corrosion. Bacterial contamination of the implant surface also will be affected by the surface roughness if it becomes exposed within the mouth. The current trend is therefore towards slightly roughened surfaces (blasted/etched).

Implant/abutment design

Most implant systems have a wide range of abutments for various applications (e.g. single tooth, fixed bridge, overdenture) and techniques (e.g. standard manufactured abutments, prepable abutments, cast-to abutments; see Chapters 13 and 14). However, the design of the implant abutment junction varies considerably:

- *Brånemark* – this junction is described as a flat-top external hexagon (Figure 1.14). The hexagon was designed to allow rotation (i.e. screwing-in) of the implant during placement. It is an essential design feature in single tooth (ST) replacement as an anti-rotational device. The design proved to be very useful in the development of direct recording of impressions of the implant head rather than the abutment, thus allowing evaluation and abutment selection in the laboratory (see Chapter 13). The abutment is secured to the implant with an abutment screw. The joint between implant and abutment is precise but does not produce a seal, a feature that does not appear to result in any clinical disadvantage. The hexagon is only 0.6 mm high and it may be difficult for the inexperienced clinician to determine whether the abutment is precisely located on the implant. The fit is therefore normally checked radiographically, which also requires a good paralleling technique for adequate visualization of the joint. Similar designs of external hexagon implants have increased the height of the hexagon to 1 mm, making abutment connection easier. However, newer abutment designs for multiple-connected units (which do not require an anti-rotational property) have abandoned the female part of the hexagon to allow easier connection and avoid problems of malalignment (Nobel Biocare multi-unit abutment). The original design concept was that the weakest component of the system was the small gold screw (prosthetic screw) that secured the prosthesis framework to the abutment, followed by the abutment screw

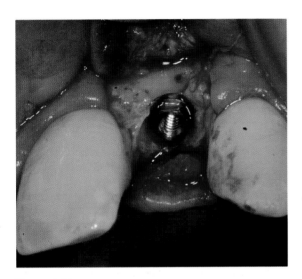

Figure 1.14

The external hexagon at the top of the Brånemark implant shown here immediately after implant placement. The hexagon was originally used to rotate the implant into place, but Nobel Biocare have recently developed a new inserting mechanism within the internal thread.

and then the implant (Figure 1.15). Thus, overloads leading to component failure should be dealt with more readily (see Chapter 16).

- *AstraTech* – this design incorporates a conical abutment fitting into the conical head of the implant, described by the manufacturers as a 'conical seal' (Figure 1.16). The taper of the cone is 11°, which is greater than a morse taper (6°). The abutments self-guide into position and are easily placed even in very difficult locations. It is not usually necessary to check the localization with radiographs. This design produces a very secure, strong union. The standard abutments are solid one-piece components, whereas the ST abutments and customizable abutments are two-piece with an abutment screw. The ST implant and abutments feature an internal hexagon anti-rotation design (Figure 1.17).

- *Straumann* – this implant has a transmucosal collar, a feature that many of the other systems incorporate in the abutment design. The abutment/implant junction is therefore often supramucosal and the connection and check-

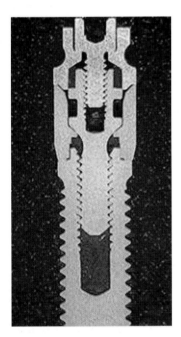

Figure 1.15

A section through the 'original' Brånemark implant stack. At the top, a small gold screw secures the prosthetic gold cylinder to the abutment screw, which in turn holds the abutment onto the implant.

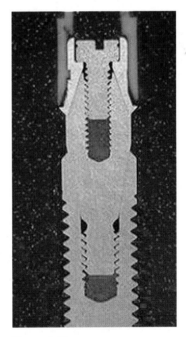

Figure 1.16

Section through an AstraTech stack showing a very good fit between the abutment and the implant. The interface is an internal cone with an angle of 11°.

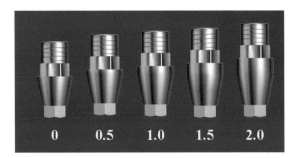

Figure 1.17

A selection of AstraTech single tooth (ST) abutments of various lengths. The lower part shows the anti-rotational hexagon which fits within the collar of the ST implant. The conical sides of the abutment fit within the internal cone of the implant head. The top part has an octagonal anti-rotation design to accept the ST crown.

ing of the fit of the components are easier than most systems. The aesthetic line implant has a shorter collar (1.8 mm) to allow submucosal placement of the abutment/prosthesis union but the connection is still easy due to the internal tapered conical design with an angle of 8° (Figure 1.18).

- *Frialit* – this has some of the features of the previously described systems. Basically, the abutment fits within the implant head but is parallel sided (Figures 1.19 and 1.20). It features an internal hexagon anti-rotational system and an abutment screw, which also secures the prosthesis in screw-retained fixed bridge designs. The junction seal is improved with a silicone washer within the assembly (not to be confused with the intra-mobile element of the IMZ system, which is not considered in this book).

Submerged and non-submerged protocols

The terms submerged and non-submerged implant protocols were at one time clearly applicable to different implant systems. The classic submerged system was the original protocol as described by Brånemark. Implants were installed with the head of the implant (and cover-screw) level with the crestal bone and the muco-

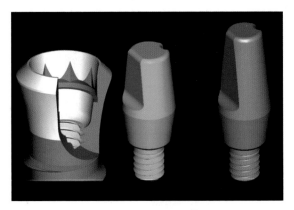

Figure 1.18

The left 'cut-away' picture shows the head of the standard solid-screw Straumann implant, featuring an internal conical design (and anti-rotational grooves) that allows a very precise fit with the solid abutments shown on the right.

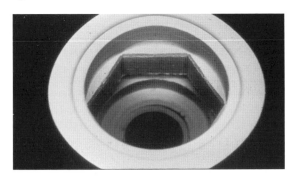

Figure 1.19

The internal hexagon of the Frialit 2 (Friatec AG, Mannheim, Germany) implant. The abutments are shown in Figure 1.20.

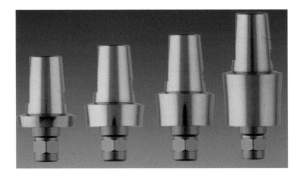

Figure 1.20

Frialit 2 abutments showing the hexagons that engage the 'hex' in the implant head.

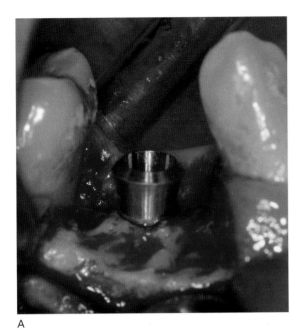
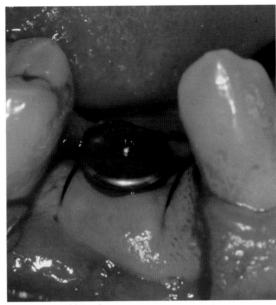

A

B

Figure 1.21

(A) A 4.1 mm standard Straumann solid-screw implant has been placed so that the polished collar is above the crest of the bone. (B) A closure screw has been placed on top of the implant and the flaps sutured around the collar to leave the implant exposed. This implant was designed to be used in this 'non-submerged' fashion.

periosteal flaps closed over the implants and left to heal for several months (Figure 1.14). This had several theoretical advantages:

1. Bone healing to the implant surface occurred in an environment free of potential bacterial colonization and inflammation.
2. Epithelialization of the implant–bone interface was prevented.
3. The implants were protected from loading and micromovement, which could lead to failure of osseointegration and fibrous tissue encapsulation.

The submerged system requires a second surgical procedure after a period of bone healing to expose the implant and attach a transmucosal abutment. The initial soft-tissue healing phase would then take a further period of approximately 2–4 weeks. Abutment selection would take into account the thickness of the mucosa and the type of restoration.

The best example of a non-submerged system

is the Straumann implant. In this case the implant is designed with an integral smooth collar that protrudes through the mucosa, allowing the implant to remain exposed from the time of insertion (Figures 1.21). The most obvious advantage is the avoidance of a second surgical procedure and more time for maturation of the soft-tissue collar at the same time as the bone healing is occurring. Although this protocol does not comply with the three theoretical advantages enumerated above, the results are equally successful.

However, clinical development and commercial competition have lead to many systems being used in either a submerged or non-submerged fashion even though they were primarily designed for one or the other. This can, therefore, be somewhat confusing and there may be some advantage in using a system in the manner for which it was originally devised, i.e. if you wish to use a non-submerged protocol why not choose a system that was designed for this purpose?

Another difference between systems designed for these protocols is the level of the implant/abutment junction in relation to the bone. Brånemark, AstraTech and Frialit implants (all primarily submerged systems) are placed with the head of the implant at the level of the bone. At the time of abutment connection the interface with the implant is at the same level.

Brånemark implants

During the first year of loading, the bone level in the Brånemark system recedes to the level of the first thread where it should stabilize (Figure 1.22). Three possible reasons for this have been proposed:

1. The threads of the implant provide a better distribution of forces to the surrounding bone than the parallel-sided head of the implant.
2. The establishment of a biological width for the investing soft tissues. The junctional epithelium is relocated on the implant and not on the abutment.
3. The interface between the abutment and implant is the apposition of two flat surfaces (flat-top implant) that are held together by an abutment screw. This arrangement does not form a perfect seal and may allow leakage of bacteria or bacterial products from within the abutment/restoration, thereby promoting a small inflammatory lesion that may affect the apical location of the epithelial attachment.

AstraTech implants

In the AstraTech system the bone margin recedes slightly apically in the first year in much the same way as it does with the Brånemark system. However, in other cases, and particularly with the AstraTech ST implant, the bone may remain at the level of the implant head (Figure 1.23). The biological implication of this is that the junctional epithelium must be superficial to this and therefore located on the abutment. The possible reasons for this arrangement in contrast to the explanations given above for the loss of marginal bone are:

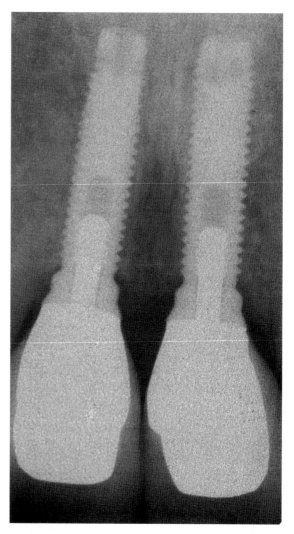

Figure 1.22

Radiograph of two Brånemark implants after 1 year in function, showing the bone level to be at the first thread of the implants.

1. The surface of the implant maintains bone height more effectively in the collar region. This may be due to the blasted surface (TiO blast) or the presence of microthreading (a similar machined conical head in an old Brånemark design loses bone to the first thread).
2. The implant/abutment junction is a conical junction – a cone fitting within a cone – that

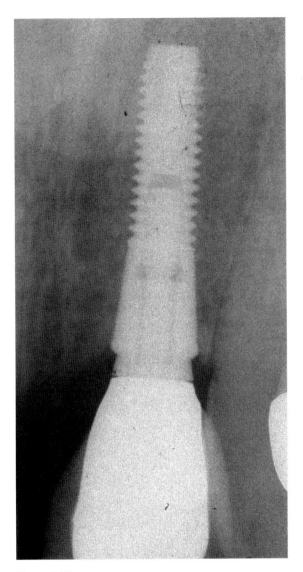

Figure 1.23

Radiograph of an AstraTech ST implant after 1 year in function, showing the bone crest at the level of the top of the microthreaded collar.

provides a tighter seal, thereby eliminating microbial contamination/leakage at the interface and also producing a more mechanically sound union with no chance of micromovement. The stability of the junction may facilitate positional stability of the junctional epithelium.

Straumann implants

The Straumann implant/abutment interface is conceptually different to those described above. The integral smooth transmucosal collar of the implant is either 2.8 mm (with the standard implant) or 1.8 mm (with the aesthetic line plus implant) in length. The implant/abutment junction may be submucosal or supramucosal, depending upon the length of the transmucosal collar, the thickness of the mucosa and the depth to which the implant has been placed. The end of the smooth collar coincides with the start of the roughened endosseous portion, which is designed to be located at the level of the bone at the implant placement. There is, therefore, potential space for location of the junctional epithelium and connective tissue zone on the collar or neck of the implant at a level apical to the abutment implant junction. Moreover, the implant/ abutment junction is a highly effective conical seal. This should prevent any movement between the components and the interface, which would prevent bacterial ingress.

The preceding considerations of the different implant systems reveal a number of basic differences:

1. The designed level of the implant/abutment interface.
2. The design characteristics at the implant abutment interface in terms of mechanical stability and seal.
3. The macroscopic features of the implant and its surface characteristics.
4. The level of transition of the surface characteristics on the implant surface.

This multitude of features has an impact on the level of the bone crest and the position of the junctional epithelium/connective tissue zone. Despite what appears to be a large and fundamental difference, the bone level comparison between the systems is clinically and radiographically very small (less than 1 mm at baseline values) and the maintenance of bone levels thereafter is very similar, with all systems reporting highly effective long-term maintenance of bone levels. The differences reported in longitudinal trials are not sufficient to recommend one system over another.

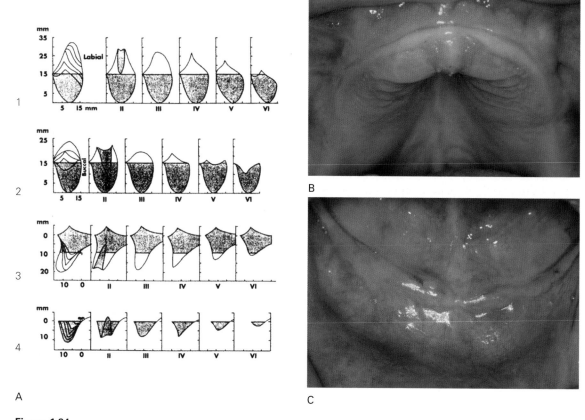

Figure 1.24

(A) Classification of jaw resorption as described by Cawood and Howell (1991), showing cross-sectional profiles through different regions: 1 = anterior mandible; 2 = posterior mandible; 3 = anterior maxilla; 4 = posterior maxilla. (B) Example of an edentulous maxilla that would be clinically classified as class III in both the anterior and posterior regions. Although the ridges appear broad, there may be little bone in the posterior region due to extension of the maxillary air sinuses. (C) Example of a severely resorbed edentulous mandible that would be classified as class V or VI. Confirmation would require radiographic examination.

Bone factors

When an implant is first placed in the bone there should be a close fit to ensure stability. The space between implant and bone is initially filled with a blood clot and serum/bone proteins. Although great care is taken to avoid damaging the bone, the initial response to the surgical trauma is resorption, which is then followed by bone deposition. There is a critical period in the healing process at approximately 2 weeks post-implant insertion when bone resorption will result in a lower degree of implant stability than that achieved initially.

Subsequent bone formation will result in an increase in the level of bone contact and stability. The stability of the implant at the time of placement is very important and is dependent upon bone quantity and quality as well as the implant design features considered above. The edentulous ridge can be classified in terms of shape (bone quantity) and bone quality. Following the loss of a tooth, the alveolar bone resorbs in width and height (Figure 1.24).

In extreme cases, bone resorption proceeds to a level that is beyond the normal extent of the alveolar process and well within the basal bone of the jaws. Determination of bone quantity is considered in the clinical and radiographic sections of the treatment planning chapters (Chapters 2–6). Assessing bone quality is rather more difficult. Plain radiographs can be misleading and sectional tomograms provide a better indication of medullary bone density (see Chapter 2). In many cases the bone quality can be confirmed only at surgical preparation of the site. Bone quality can be assessed by measuring the cutting torque during preparation of the implant site. The initial stability (and subsequent stability) of the implant can be quantified using resonance frequency analysis, which to date has been used mainly in experimental trials.

The simplest categorization of bone quality is that described by Lekholm and Zarb (1985) as types 1–4. Type 1 bone is predominantly cortical and may offer good initial stability at implant placement but is more easily damaged by overheating during the drilling process, especially with sites over 10 mm in depth. Types 2 and 3 are the most favourable quality of jaw bone for implant treatment. These types have a well-formed cortex and densely trabeculated medullary spaces (type 2 has more cortex/denser trabeculation than type 3). Type 4 bone has a thin or absent cortical layer and sparse trabeculation, it offers poor initial implant stability and fewer cells with good osteogenic potential to promote osseointegration, and therefore has been associated with higher rates of implant failure.

Healing resulting in osseointegration is highly dependent upon a surgical technique that avoids heating the bone. Slow drilling speeds, the use of successive incrementally larger sharp drills and copious saline irrigation aim to keep the temperature below that at which bone tissue damage occurs (approximately 47°C for 1 min). Further refinements include cooling the irrigant and using internally irrigated drills. Methods by which these factors are controlled are considered in more detail in the surgical sections (Chapters 7–11). Factors that compromise bone quality are infection, irradiation and heavy smoking, which have been dealt with earlier in this chapter.

Loading conditions

Osseointegrated implants lack the viscoelastic damping system and proprioceptive mecha-

nisms of the periodontal ligament, which effectively dissipate and control forces. However, proprioceptive mechanisms may operate within bone and associated oral structures. Forces distributed directly to the bone are usually concentrated in certain areas, particularly around the neck of the implant. Excessive forces applied to the implant may result in remodelling of the marginal bone, i.e. apical movement of the bone margin with loss of osseointegration. The exact mechanism of how this occurs is not entirely clear but it has been suggested that microfractures may propagate within the adjacent bone. Bone loss caused by excessive loading may be slowly progressive. In rare cases it may reach a point where there is catastrophic failure of the remaining osseointegration or fracture of the implant. Excessive forces may be detected prior to this stage through radiographic marginal bone loss or mechanical failure of the prosthodontic superstructure and/or abutments (see Chapter 16).

It has been shown that normal/well-controlled forces result in increases in the degree of bone to implant contact and remodelling of adjacent trabecular structures to dissipate the forces. Adaptation is therefore possible, although osseointegration does not permit movement of the implant in the way that a tooth may be orthodontically repositioned. Therefore, the osseointegrated implant has proved itself to be a very effective anchorage system for difficult orthodontic cases.

Loading protocols

Loading protocols, i.e. the duration of time between implant insertion and functional loading, have been largely empirical. The time allowed for adequate bone healing should be based upon clinical trials that test the effects of factors such as bone quality, loading factors, implant type, etc. However, there are very limited data on the effects of these complex variables and currently there is no accurate measure that precisely determines the optimum period of healing before loading can commence. This has not limited the variety of protocols advocated, including:

- Delayed loading (for 3–6 months)
- Early loading (e.g. at 6 weeks)
- Immediate loading

Delayed loading

This has been the traditional approach and has much to commend it because it is tried, tested and predictable. Following installation of an implant, all loading is avoided during the early healing phase. Movement of the implant within the bone at this stage may result in fibrous tissue encapsulation rather than osseointegration. In partially dentate subjects it may be desirable to provide temporary/provisional prostheses that are tooth supported. However, in patients who wear mucosally supported dentures it has been recommended that they should not be worn over the implant area for 1–2 weeks. In the edentulous maxilla we would normally advise that a denture is not worn for 1 week, and in the mandible for 2 weeks, because of the poorer stability of the soft-tissue wound and smaller denture-bearing surface. The original Brånemark protocol then advised leaving implants unloaded and buried beneath the mucosa for approximately 6 months in the maxilla and 3 months in the mandible, due mainly to differences in bone quality. There are many data to support the cautious approach advocated by Brånemark in ensuring a high level of predictable implant success. However, the original Straumann protocol did not differentiate between upper and lower jaw, a 3–month healing period being recommended for both.

Early loading

A number of systems now advocate a healing period of just 6 weeks before loading. This has been tested by 3i with an implant that has an acid-etched surface (and with a design based upon the Brånemark implant) and by Straumann with their SLA surface-treated implants. Some caution is recommended in that the implants should be placed in good-quality bone in situations that are not subjected to high loads. In these favourable circumstances the results are good.

Immediate loading

It has been demonstrated also that immediate loading is compatible with subsequent success-ful osseointegration, provided that the bone quality is good and the functional forces can be controlled adequately. In studies on ST restorations, the crowns are usually kept out of contact in intercuspal and lateral excursions, thereby almost eliminating functional loading until a definitive crown is provided. In contrast, fixed bridgework allows connection of multiple implants, providing good splinting and stabilization, and therefore has been tested in immediate loading protocols, with some success. However, the clinician should have a good reason to adopt the early/immediate loading protocols particularly as they are likely to be less predictable.

The long-term functional loading of the implant-supported prosthesis is a further important consideration that will be dealt with in the following section.

Prosthetic loading considerations

Carefully planned functional occlusal loading will result in maintenance of osseointegration and possibly increased bone to implant contact. In contrast, excessive loading may lead to bone loss and/or component failure. Clinical loading conditions are largely dependent upon the factors described below, which are dealt with in more detail in Chapters 13–15.

The type of prosthetic reconstruction

This can vary from an ST replacement in the partially dentate case to a full arch reconstruction in the edentulous individual. Implants that support dentures may present particular problems with control of loading because they may be largely mucosal supported, entirely implant supported or a combination of the two.

The occlusal scheme

The lack of mobility in implant-supported fixed prostheses requires the provision of shallow cuspal inclines and careful distribution of loads in lateral excursions. With ST implant restorations it is important to develop initial tooth contacts on the natural dentition and to avoid guidance in lateral excursions on the implant restoration. Loading will also depend upon the opposing dentition, which could be natural teeth, another implant-supported prosthesis or a conventional removable prosthesis. Surprisingly high forces can be generated through removable prostheses.

The number, distribution, orientation and design of implants

The distribution of load to the supporting bone can be spread by increasing the number and dimensions (diameter, surface topography, length) of the implants. The spacing and three-dimensional arrangement of the individual implants will also be very important, and is dealt with in detail in Chapter 5.

The design and properties of implant connectors

Multiple implants are usually joined by a rigid framework. This provides good splinting and distribution of loads between implants. It is equally important that the framework has a passive fit on the implant abutments so that stresses are not set up within the prosthetic construction.

Dimensions and location of cantilever extensions

Some implant reconstructions are designed with cantilever extensions to provide function (and appearance) in areas where provision of additional implants is difficult. This may be due to practical or financial considerations. Cantilever extensions have the potential to create high loads, particularly on the implant adjacent to the cantilever. The extent of the leverage of any cantilever should be considered in relation to the anteroposterior distance

between implants at the extreme ends of the reconstruction. This topic is dealt with in more detail in Chapter 5.

Patient parafunctional activities

Great caution should be exercised in treating patients with known parafunctional activities.

Choice of an implant system

In routine cases it may not matter which system is chosen; this is particularly the case with treatment in the anterior mandible. However, in our experience the choice of a system in any particular case depends upon:

- The aesthetic requirements
- The available bone height, width and quality (including whether the site has been grafted)
- Perceived restorative difficulties
- Desired surgical protocol

Therefore, we would suggest the following:

- In the aesthetic zone, choose an implant where the crown contour can achieve good emergence from the soft tissue with a readily maintainable healthy submucosal margin.
- Choose an implant of the appropriate length and width for the existing crestal morphology. Ensure that choice of a reduced width implant does not compromise strength in the particular situation.
- If the site will only accommodate a short implant or if the bone quality is poor or grafted, then choose an implant with a roughened surface rather than a machined surface.
- If there are likely to be difficulties with prosthodontic construction due to difficult angulation of the implants, choose a system that is versatile enough to cope with these difficulties, i.e. has a good range of solutions/components.
- If you wish to use a submerged or non-submerged protocol, then choose a system that has a proven published record with that particular protocol.

Bibliography

Adell R, Lekholm U, Rockler B, Brånemark PI (1981). A 15 year study of osseointegrated implants in the treatment of the edentulous jaw. *Int J Oral Surgery* **10**: 387–416.

Adell R, Eriksson B, Lekholm U, Brånemark PI, Jemt T (1990). A long-term follow-up study of osseointegrated implants in the treatment of totally edentulous jaws. *Int J Oral Maxillofac Implants* **5**: 347–59.

Albrektsson T, Sennerby L (1991). State of the art in oral implants. *J Clin Periodontol* **18**: 474–81.

Albrektsson T, Zarb GA, Worthington DP, Eriksson R (1986). The long-term efficacy of currently used dental implants. A review and proposed criteria of success. *Int J Oral Maxillofac Implants* **1**: 11–25.

Ali A, Patton DWP, El Sharkawi AMM, Davies J (1997). Implant rehabilitation of irradiated jaws—a preliminary report. *Int J Oral Maxillofac Implants* **12**: 523–6.

Astrand P (1993). Current implant systems. *J Swed Dent Assoc* **85**: 651–63.

Bain CA (1996). Smoking and implant failure—benefit of a smoking cessation protocol. *Int J Oral Maxillofac Implants* **11**: 756–9.

Bain CA, Moy PK (1993). The association between the failure of dental implants and cigarette smoking. *Int J Oral Maxillofac Implants* **8**: 609–15.

Brånemark PI, Zarb GA, Albrektsson T (1985). *Osseointegration in Clinical Dentistry*. Chicago: Quintessence Publishing.

Brown D (1997). All you wanted to know about titanium, but were afraid to ask. *Br Dent J* **182**: 393–4.

Buser D, Weber HP, Bragger U, Balsiger C (1991). Tissue integration of one-stage ITI implants: 3-year results of a longitudinal study with hollow cylinder and hollow screw implants. *Int J Oral Maxillofac Implants* **6**: 405–12.

Buser D, Belser UC, Lang NP (1998). The original one stage dental implant system and its clinical application. *Periodontol 2000* **17**: 106–18.

Cawood JI, Howell RA (1988). A classification of the edentulous jaws. *Int J Oral Maxillofac Surgery* **1**: 232–6.

Cawood JI, Howell RA (1991). Reconstructive preprosthetic surgery. I. Anatomical considerations. *Int J Oral Maxillofac Surg* **20**: 75–82.

De Bruyn H, Collaert B (1994). The effect of smoking on early implant failure. *Clin Oral Implants Res* **5**: 260–4.

Ericsson I, Johansson CB, Bystedt H, Norton MR (1994). A histomorphometric evaluation of bone-to-implant contact on machine-prepared and roughened titanium dental implants. *Clin Oral Implants Res* **5**: 202–6.

Gotfredsen K, Nimb L, Hjorting-Hansen E, Jensen JS, Holmen A (1992). Histomorphometric and removal torque analysis for TiO_2-blasted titanium implants. *Clin Oral Implants Res* **3**: 77–84.

Humphris GM, Healey T, Howell RA, Cawood J (1995). The psychological impact of implant-retained prostheses: a cross-sectional study. *Int J Oral Maxillofac Implants* **10**: 437–44.

Johansson CB, Albrektsson T (1991). A removal torque and histomorphometric study of commercially pure niobium and titanium implants in rabbit bone. *Clin Oral Implants Res* **2**: 24–9.

Lang NP, Karring T, Lindhe J (1999). Proceedings of the 3rd European *Workshop on Periodontology: Implant Dentistry*. Berlin: Quintessence Publishing.

Lazzara R, Siddiqui AA, Binon P, Feldman SA, Wener R, Phillips R, Gonshor A (1996). Retrospective multicenter analysis of 3i endosseous dental implants placed over a 5 year period. *Clin Oral Implants Res* **7**: 73–83.

Lekholm U, Zarb GA (1985). Patient selection and preparation. In Brånemark PI, Zarb GA, ALbrektsson T, eds, *Tissue integrated prostheses*, pp 199–209. Chicago: Quintessence Publishing Co.

Listgarten MA, Lang NP, Shroeder HE, Schroeder A (1991). Periodontal tissues and their counterparts around endosseous implants. *Clin Oral Implants Res* **2**: 1–19.

Norton M (1998). Marginal bone levels at single tooth implants with conical fixture design. The influence of surface macro- and microstructure. *Clin Oral Implants Res* **9**: 91–9.

Schenk RK, Buser D (1998). Osseointegration: a reality. *Periodontol 2000* **17**: 22–35.

Schnitman P, Wohrle PS, Rubenstein JE, DaSilva JD, Wang NH (1997). Ten year results for Brånemark implants immediately loaded with fixed bridge prostheses at implant placement. *Int J Oral Maxillofac Implants* **12**: 495–503.

Schulte W, d'Hoedt B, Axmann D, Gomez G (1992). The first 15 years of the Tuebingen Implant and its further development to the Frialit-2 system. *Zeitschrift für Zahnarztliche Implantologie* **8**: 77–96.

Sennerby L, Ericsson LE, Thomsen P, Lekholm U, Astrand P (1991). Structure of the bone–titanium interface in retrieved clinical oral implants. *Clin Oral Implants Res* **2**: 103–11.

Smith DE, Zarb GA (1989). Criteria for success of osseointegrated endosseous implants. *J Prosth Dent* **62**: 567–72.

Smith RA, Berger R, Dodson TB (1992). Risk factors associated with dental implants in healthy and medically compromised patients. *Int J Oral Maxillofac Implants* **7**: 367–72.

Steinemann SG (1998). Titanium—the material of choice? *Periodontol 2000* **17**: 22–35.

Von Wowern N (1977). Variations in structure within the trabecular bone of the mandible. *Scand J Dent Res* **85**: 478–85.

Von Wowern N (1977). Variations in the bone mass within the cortices of the mandible. *Scand J Dent Res* **85**: 444–5.

Weber HP, Buser D, Donath K, Fiorellini JP, Doppalapudi V, Paquette DW, Williams RC (1996). Comparison of healed tissues adjacent to submerged and non-submerged unloaded titanium dental implants. *Clin Oral Implants Res* **7**: 11–19.

Wennerberg A, Albrektsson T, Andersson B (1993). Design and surface characteristics of 13 commercially available oral implant systems. *Int J Oral Maxillofac Implants* **8**: 622–33.

Westwood RM, Duncan JM (1996). Implants in adolescents: a review and case reports. *Int J Oral Maxillofac Implants* **11**: 750–5.

PART II

Planning

2
Treatment planning: general considerations

Introduction

This chapter provides an overall view of treatment planning. The reader should consult the chapters on planning for single tooth restorations, fixed bridges and implant dentures for more detailed considerations. The treatment plan should begin with a clear idea of the desired end result of treatment, which should fulfil the functional and aesthetic requirements of the patient. It is important that these treatment goals are realistic, predictable and readily maintainable: realistic means that the end result can be readily achieved and is not unduly optimistic; predictable means that there is a very high chance of success of achieving the end result and that the prosthesis will function satisfactorily in the long term; and readily maintainable means that the prosthesis does not compromise the patient's oral hygiene and that the 'servicing' implications for the patient and the dentist are acceptable.

In this chapter it will be assumed that treatment options other than implant-retained restorations have been considered and there are no relevant contraindications (see Chapter 1). Evaluation begins with a patient consultation and assessment of the aesthetic and functional

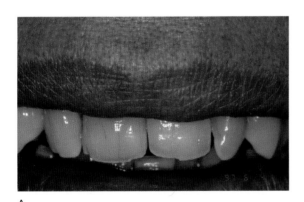

A

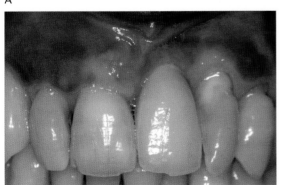

C

B

Figure 2.1

(A) In normal function this patient reveals the incisal half of the anterior teeth. (B) The same patient smiling reveals most of the crowns of the teeth, but not the gingival margin. (C) The patient with the lips retracted showing a gross discrepancy of the gingival margins that is not visible in normal function and smiling.

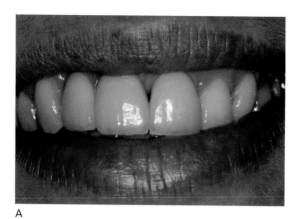
A

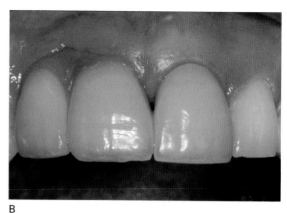
B

Figure 2.2

(A) A patient smiling who just reveals the gingival margins and is therefore aesthetically more demanding than the patient in Figure 2.1. (B) The same patient with the lips retracted. The upper right central and lateral incisors are implant-retained restorations. The interdental papilla between the two implants has been replaced with prosthetic 'gum work' because the soft-tissue deficiency was impossible to correct surgically. The aesthetics is satisfactory and the patient is able to adequately clean the area.

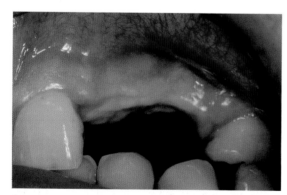
A

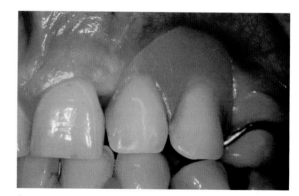
B

Figure 2.3

(A) A patient with missing maxillary lateral incisor, canine and premolar teeth. The ridge has resorbed in a vertical direction and towards the palate, resulting in loss of normal arch form. (B) The existing prosthesis reveals that the apparently large space only accommodates two teeth, and prosthetic gum work is required to make good the ridge deficiency. (C) The ridge form at surgery prior to grafting shows the vertical loss of bone. The ridge is quite broad but palatally located.

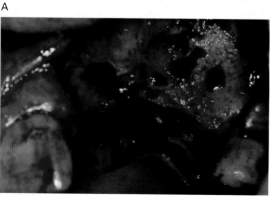
C

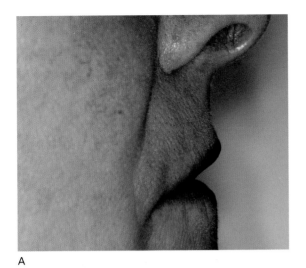
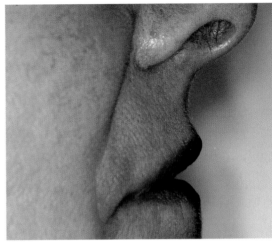

A   B

Figure 2.4

(A) Profile of a patient wearing a removable denture with a labial flange to provide lip support. (B) Profile of the same patient showing poorer lip support following removal of the labial flange.

requirements, and proceeds to more detailed planning with intraoral examination, diagnostic set-ups and appropriate radiographic examination. At all stages in this process it is important to establish and maintain good communication (verbal and written) with the patients to ensure that they understand the proposed treatment plan and the alternatives.

Aesthetic considerations assume great importance in most patients with missing anterior teeth. This is an increasing challenge for the clinician and is related to:

1. the degree of coverage of the anterior teeth (and gingivae) by the lips during normal function and smiling (Figures 2.1 and 2.2)
2. the degree of ridge resorption, both vertically and horizontally (Figure 2.3)
3. provision of adequate lip support (Figure 2.4)

The appearance of the planned restoration can be judged by producing a diagnostic set-up on study casts or providing a provisional diagnostic prosthesis. The latter usually proves to be more informative for patients because they can judge the appearance in their own mouths and even wear the prosthesis for extended periods of time

to adequately assess it. Both diagnostic casts and provisional prosthesis can serve as a model for the fabrication of:

1. a radiographic stent to assess tooth position in relation to the underlying ridge profile (Figure 2.5)
2. a surgical stent (or guide) to assist the surgeon in the optimal placement of the implants (Figure 2.6)
3. a transitional restoration during the treatment programme

Ideally, patients should be examined with and without their current or diagnostic prosthesis (Figure 2.7) to assess:

• facial contours
• lip support
• tooth position
• how much of the prosthesis is revealed during function
• occlusal relationships

The diagnostic set-up should then be adjusted, if necessary. to fulfil the requirements of the desired end result before proceeding with treatment.

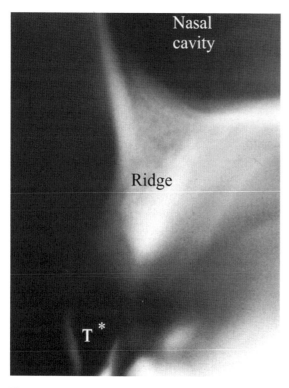

Figure 2.5

A sectional tomogram taken on a Scanora™ (Soredex Orion, Helsinki, Finland), showing the ridge profile in relation to a radiographic outline of the proposed tooth position (T*) from a radiopaque stent that the patient was wearing.

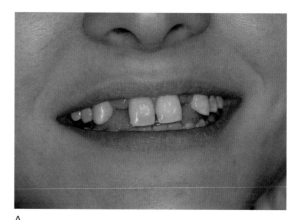

A

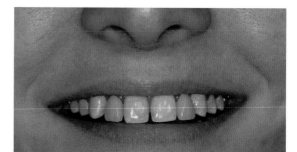

B

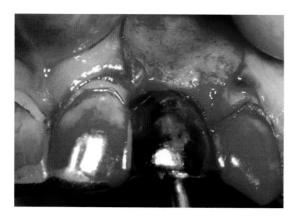

Figure 2.6

A surgical stent being used to guide the surgeon during the implant surgery. This stent is a rigid plastic blow-down made on a duplicate cast of the diagnostic wax-up. It fits on the adjacent teeth and reproduces the labial contour of the tooth that is to be replaced.

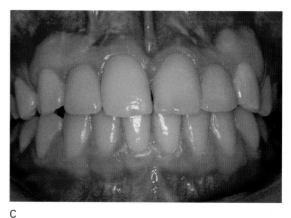

C

Figure 2.7

(A) A young patient with developmentally missing maxillary lateral incisors. (B) The same patient wearing an existing partial denture allows assessment of the aesthetics and tooth position. (C) The completed result with two single tooth implants replacing the lateral incisors.

Reduced or insufficient function is a common complaint for patients who have removable dentures or who have lost many molar teeth. Functional inadequacy is often a perceived problem of the patient and is assessed by interview rather than any specific clinical measure. The variation between individuals with regard to how they perceive this problem is large. A shortened dental arch extending to the first molar or second premolar may provide adequate function and appearance for some patients. However, missing maxillary premolars (and occasionally first molars) often presents an aesthetic problem.

Provisional dentures can be used to clarify these needs.

Initial clinical examination

Thorough extraoral and intraoral clinical examinations should be carried out on all patients to ensure the diagnosis of all existing dental and oral disease. The diagnosis and management of caries, periodontal disease and endodontic problems is not the remit of this book and the reader is referred to other more relevant texts. Factors of more specific relevance to implant treatment are dealt with here and in the related more detailed chapters on single teeth, fixed bridges and implant dentures (Chapters 3–6).

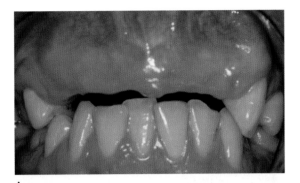

A

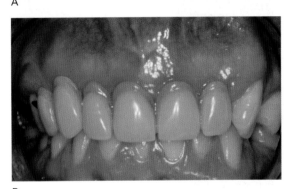

B

Figure 2.8

(A) A patient with missing maxillary anterior teeth in whom the lower incisors nearly touch the soft-tissue ridge in centric occlusion. The space available for implant components will also depend upon the level of placement of the implant heads in the underlying bone. (B) The same patient with their existing partial denture. The prosthetic teeth have been ridge lapped and no labial flange has been provided. This provides further evidence that there has been minimal ridge resorption since loss of the teeth.

Evaluation of the edentulous space or ridge

The height, width and contour of the edentulous ridge can be assessed visually and carefully palpated. The presence of concavities/depressions (especially on the labial aspects) is usually readily detected. However, accurate assessment of the underlying bone width is difficult, especially where the overlying tissue is thick and fibrous. This occurs particularly on the palate, where the tissue may be very thick, and can result in a very false impression of the bone profile. The thickness of the soft tissue can be measured by puncturing the soft tissue with a calibrated probe after administering local anaesthetic (ridge mapping).

The profile/angulation of the ridge and its relation to the opposing dentition are also important. The distance between the edentulous ridge and the opposing dentition should be measured to ensure that there is adequate room for the prosthodontic components (Figure 2.8). Proclined ridge forms will tend to lead to proclined placement of the implants, which could affect loading and aesthetics. Large horizontal or vertical discrepancies (Figure 2.9) between the jaws must be recognized and management appropriately planned.

The clinical examination of the ridge also allows assessment of the soft-tissue thickness, which is

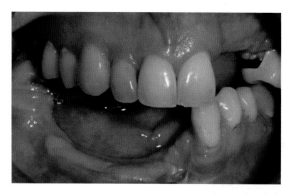

Figure 2.9

This patient has suffered extensive loss of mandibular bone following a road traffic accident that resulted in a fractured mandible and osteomyelitis. There is now a marked vertical and horizontal discrepancy between the jaws.

important for the attainment of good aesthetics. Keratinized tissue that is attached to the edentulous ridge will also generally provide a better peri-implant soft tissue than non-keratinized mobile mucosa. The length of the edentulous ridge can be measured to give an indication of the possible number of implants that could be accommodated. This is best done with callipers and a millimetre rule. The space should be measured between the tips of the crowns, the maximum contour of the crowns and at the level of the edentulous ridge. However, this also requires reference to:

1. radiographs, to allow a correlation with available bone
2. the diagnostic set-up for the proposed tooth location
3. the edentulous ridges bound by the teeth; the available space will also be affected by angulation of adjacent tooth roots, which may be palpated and assessed radiographically

Initial radiographic screening

A screening radiograph should give the clinician an indication of:

1. overall anatomy of the maxilla and mandible and potential vertical height of available bone

2. anatomical anomalies or pathological lesions
3. sites where it may be possible to place implants without grafting, and sites that would require grafting
4. restorative and periodontal status of remaining teeth

In most instances the dental panoramic tomograph (DPT) is the radiograph of choice (Figure 2.10). It provides an image within a pre-defined focal trough of both upper and lower jaws that gives a reasonable approximation of bone height, the position of the inferior dental neurovascular bundle, the size and position of the maxillary antra and any pathological conditions that may be present. It is therefore an ideal view for initial treatment planning and for providing patient information, because it presents the image in a way that many patients are able to understand. Some areas may not be imaged particularly well, but this can be minimized by ensuring that the patient is positioned correctly in the machine and that the appropriate programme is selected. It provides more information about associated anatomical structures than periapical radiographs but with less fine-detail of the teeth. It should be remembered that all DPTs are magnified images (at approximately ×1.3). Distortion also occurs in the anteroposterior dimension, reducing their usefulness when planning implant spacing/numbers. The initial screening radiograph allows selection of the most appropriate radiographic examination for definitive planning (see Chapters 3–6 for single teeth, fixed bridgework and implant dentures).

Study casts and diagnostic set-ups

Articulated study casts allow measurements of many of the factors considered in the previous section. The proposed replacement teeth can be positioned on the casts using either denture teeth or teeth carved in wax (Figure 2.11). The former have the advantage that they can be converted into a temporary restoration that can be evaluated in the mouth by clinician and patient. The diagnostic set-up therefore determines the number and position of the teeth to

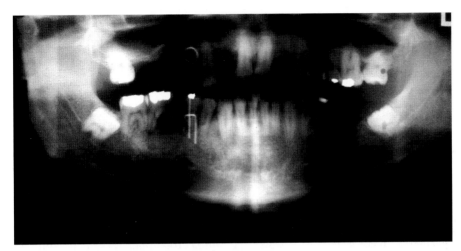

Figure 2.10

A dental panoramic tomogram provides a very good screening radiograph to show the major anatomical features of the jaws in relation to the existing teeth. This patient has large maxillary air sinuses, resorption of some molar teeth, periodontitis and impacted lower third molars. He requires a great deal of preparatory work before implants can be considered.

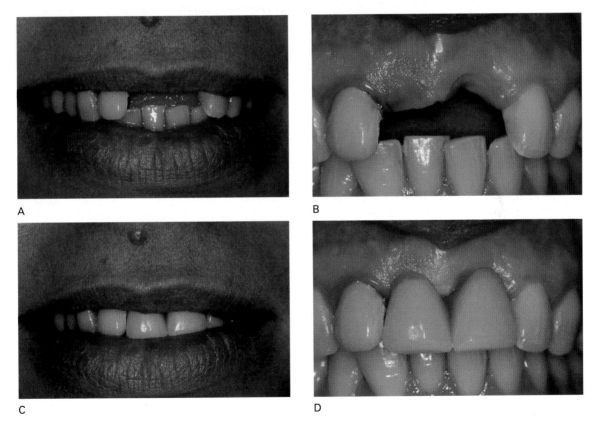

Figure 2.11

(A) A patient with missing maxillary central incisors following loss of a bridge that had extended from tooth 12 to tooth 21. The bridge was sectioned at tooth 12 and tooth 21 was extracted. (B) The intraoral view showing good ridge height at tooth 11 but loss of vertical height at tooth 21, which was extracted following an endodontic infection. (C) The patient with a diagnostic denture in place with the lips at rest. (D) The intraoral appearance of the diagnostic denture. There is no labial flange and the discrepancy in ridge height between teeth 11 and 21 is less obvious. This patient was treated without ridge augmentation.

be replaced and their occlusal relationship with the opposing dentition.

Once the diagnostic set-up has been agreed by the patient and clinician, it can be used to construct a stent (or guide) for radiographic imaging and surgical placement of the implants. The stent/guide can be positioned on the original cast and, with reference to the radiographs, the clinician can decide upon the optimum location, number and type of implants (see Chapter 5).

Basic treatment order

Deciding on the treatment order may be very straightforward in some circumstances and in others extremely difficult, particularly for those cases involving transitional restorations.

A traditional plan may include the following:

1. Examination – clinical and initial radiographic.
2. Diagnostic set-up, provisional restoration and specialized radiographs, if required.
3. Discussion of treatment options with the patient and decision on final restoration.
4. Completion of any necessary dental treatment, including:
   • Extraction of hopeless teeth
   • Periodontal treatment
   • Restorative treatment, new restorations and/or endodontics as required.
5. Construction of provisional or transitional restorations, if required.
6. Construction of surgical guide or stent.
7. Surgical placement of implants.
8. Allow adequate time for healing/osseointegration according to protocol, bone quality and functional demands.
9. Prosthodontic phase.

Conclusion

It is imperative to consider all treatment options with the patient, and during detailed planning it may become apparent that an alternative solution is preferred. In all cases the implant treatment should be part of an overall plan to ensure the health of any remaining teeth and soft tissues. Once the goal or end point has been agreed, it should be possible to work back to formulate the treatment sequence. The cost of the proposed treatment plan is also of great relevance. The greater the number of implants placed, the higher will be the cost, and this may therefore place limits on treatment options. In difficult cases it is better to place additional implants to the minimum number required, to take account of possible failure and improved predictability and biomechanics.

Bibliography

Budtz-Jorgensen E (1996). Restoration of the partially edentulous mouth—a comparison of overdentures, removable partial dentures, fixed partial dentures and implant treatment. *J Dent* **24**: 237–44.

Ekestubbe A (1993). Reliability of spiral tomography with the Scanora technique for dental implant planning. *Clin Oral Implants Res* **4**: 195–202.

Garber DA (1996). The esthetic implant: letting restoration be the guide. *J Am Dent Assoc* **126**: 319–25.

Grondahl K, Lekholm U (1997). The predictive value of radiographic diagnosis of implant instability. *Int J Oral Maxillofac Implants* **12**: 59–64.

Kent G, Johns R (1994). Effects of osseointegrated implants on psychological and social well-being: a comparison with replacement removable prostheses. *Int J Oral Maxillofac Implants* **9**: 103–6.

McAlarney ME, Stavropoulos DN (1996). Determination of cantilever length to anterior–posterior spread ratio assuming failure criteria to be the compromise of the prosthesis retaining screw–prosthesis joint. *Int J Oral Maxillofac Implants* **11**: 331–9.

Oikarinen K, Raustia AM, Hartikainen M (1995). General and local contraindications for endosseal implants—an epidemiological panoramic radiograph study in 65 year old subjects. *Commun Dent Oral Epidemiol* **23**: 114–18.

Wennstrom J, Bengazi F, Lekholm U (1994). The influence of the masticatory mucosa on the peri-implant soft-tissue condition. *Clin Oral Implants Res* **5**: 1–8.

Wise M (1995). *Failure in the Restored Dentition: Management and Treatment*. Chicago: Quintessence Publishing.

3
Single tooth planning in the anterior region

Introduction

Single tooth restorations are often thought to be the most demanding implant restorations, particularly from the aesthetic viewpoint. Achievement of an ideal result is dependent upon:

1. the status of the adjacent teeth
2. the ridge and soft-tissue profile
3. planning and precise implant placement
4. sympathetic surgical handling of the soft tissue
5. a high standard of prosthetics

The assessment and planning is dealt with in this chapter and surgical and prosthodontic factors in subsequent chapters.

Clinical examination

Examination should start with an extraoral assessment of the lips and the amount of tooth or gingiva that is exposed when the patient smiles (Figure 3.1A). A high smile line exposing a lot of gingiva is the most demanding aesthetically with both conventional and implant prosthodontics. The appearance of the soft tissue and particularly the height and quality of the gingival papillae on the proximal surfaces of the teeth adjacent to the missing tooth are particularly important in these cases (Figure 3.1B). If there has been gingival recession this should be noted. Exposure of root surface on the adjacent teeth labial surfaces may be correctable with periodontal mucogingival plastic surgery procedures, but recession on proximal surfaces is not usually correctable. The patient needs to be made aware of the limitations (which are the

same as those that apply to tooth-supported fixed bridgework). It is always easier to judge the aesthetic problems if the patient has an existing replacement, preferably one without prosthetic replacement of soft tissue. A simple 'gum-fitted' removable partial denture that has a satisfactory appearance is very helpful (Figure 3.1C). The height of the edentulous ridge and its width and profile should be assessed by careful palpation. Large ridge concavities are usually readily detected. Ridge mapping is advocated by some clinicians. In this technique the area under investigation is given local anaesthesia and the thickness of the soft tissue is measured by puncturing it to the bone, using either a graduated periodontal probe or specially designed callipers. The information is transferred to a cast of the jaw that is sectioned through the ridge. This method gives a better indication of bone profile than simple palpation but is still prone to error. Whenever the clinician is in doubt about the bone width and contour, it is advisable to request a radiographic examination to achieve this (see section on sectional tomography).

One of the most important assessments is measurement of the tooth space at the level of the crown, at the soft-tissue margin and between the roots. The first is important for the aesthetics and is best judged by measuring the width of the crown in comparison to the contralateral natural tooth, if present. The available width at the root level determines whether an implant and abutment can be accommodated without compromising the adjacent tooth roots and soft tissue. A commonly quoted minimal dimension is 6 mm, both in the mesiodistal and buccolingual plane. This allows for an average implant of 4 mm in diameter to have a margin of 1 mm of bone surrounding it. The mesiodistal dimension is commonly compromised in the maxillary

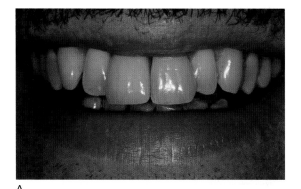

A

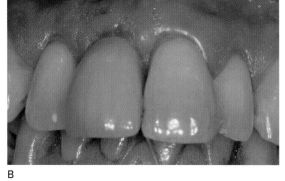

B

Figure 3.1

(A) This patient, who has tooth 11 replaced with a single tooth implant, does not expose any gingival tissue when he smiles. (B) An intraoral view of the single tooth implant at position 11. Note that the adjacent incisors have small amounts of gingival recession on the labial and proximal aspects, which was present before treatment. This loss of attachment on the proximal surfaces affects papillary height and is very difficult or impossible to regain. (C) The same patient before treatment, confirming the position of the gingival margins on the natural teeth. The prosthesis is a simple 'gum-fitted spoon denture', which provides acceptable aesthetics but poor function. It is a useful diagnostic aid.

C

lateral incisor region and the lower incisor region, where the natural teeth are small (Figures 3.2 and 3.3). In the case of young patients with developmentally missing maxillary incisors, it is advisable to liaise with the treating orthodontists to agree space requirements and to check that adequate space has been achieved before removal of the orthodontic appliance. The adjacent root alignment can sometimes be palpated but usually requires verification radiographically. Spaces that are 5 mm wide mesiodistally may be amenable to treatment with a narrow-diameter implant/abutment (e.g. 3.3 mm rather than 4 mm in diameter) provided that the forces it is subjected to are not too high. For example, utilization of narrow implants would be contraindicated in a patient with a parafunctional activity such as bruxism.

On the other hand, patients with a spaced dentition have excess mesiodistal space. Provided that the ridge has an adequate bucco-lingual width, the clinician could plan to place a wider diameter implant that more closely matches the root of the tooth that is being replaced (Figures 3.4 and 3.5). The selection of the most appropriate implant diameter has a great bearing on the aesthetics and surgery. This is dealt with in more detail in the surgical section (Chapter 9), which also compares some of the implant systems available.

Examination of the occlusion

This usually can be accomplished by simple clinical examination. The adjacent tooth contacts (and that of the pre-existing prosthetic replacement if available) should be examined in centric occlusion, retruded contact and protrusive and lateral excursions. Occlusal contacts on the single tooth implant restoration should be designed such that contacts occur first on adjacent teeth. This takes account of the normal physiological mobility of

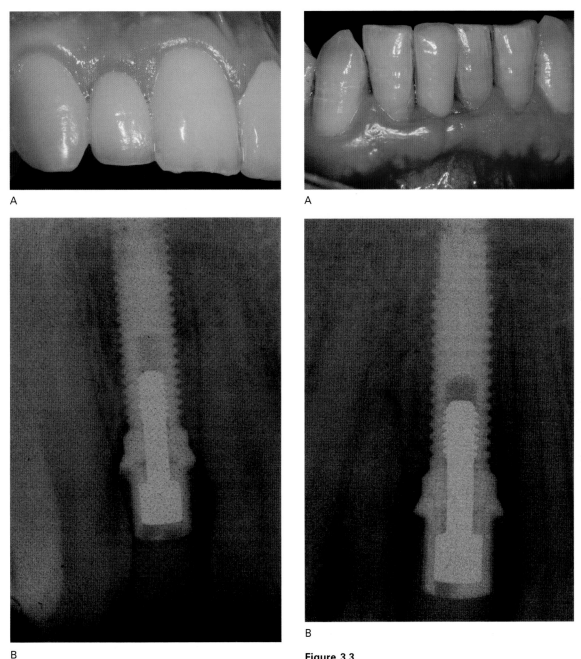

A

B

Figure 3.2

(A) Replacement of a small upper lateral incisor with a single tooth implant showing good soft-tissue form and aesthetics. (B) Radiograph of the single tooth implant which in this case is a narrow-diameter (3.3 mm) Nobel Biocare (Brånemark design) implant. This is a good choice for narrow spaces and low load situations.

A

B

Figure 3.3

(A) Replacement of lower incisors (in this case the lower right central incisor) can be particularly challenging because of the limited space available. (B) Radiograph of the narrow-diameter (3.3 mm) Nobel Biocare implant replacing the lower central incisor. A standard abutment has been used, which further compromises the available space. A customized narrower abutment could have been used.

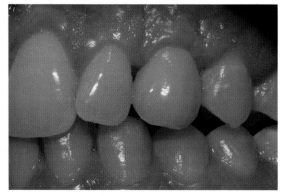

A

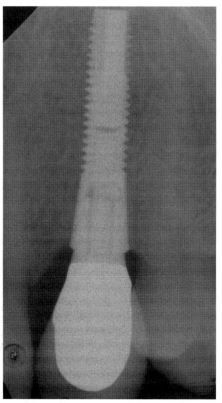

B

Figure 3.4

(A) The maxillary canine has been replaced by an AstraTech single tooth (ST) implant, which has a 4.5-mm or 5.5-mm diameter top. The latter is the more suitable for a canine replacement. (B) Radiograph of the AstraTech ST implant with the bone margin at the top of the implant. The implant/abutment junction is an internal cone that gives considerable strength and stability, both of which are important requirements for canine replacements.

the teeth compared with the rigid osseointegrated implant. Difficulties can arise when replacing canines in a canine-guided occlusion. Under these circumstances attempts should be made to achieve group function and light contacts on the implant restoration. Similar precautions are required with central and lateral incisor replacements in Class 2 Divison 2 incisor relationships with deep overbites (Figure 3.6).

Radiographic examination

Radiography for single tooth replacement in individuals with little bone loss normally can be accomplished by intraoral radiographs taken with a long cone paralleling technique. However, it must be remembered that an overall evaluation of the mouth should be made for a full assessment of treatment needs. Image quality is of the utmost importance and the clinician should ensure that all relevant anatomical structures are shown on the image being used and that any allowances for distortion of the image are made. It can be surprisingly difficult to obtain accurate radiographic mesiodistal measurements of spaces at sites in the arch such as the maxillary lateral incisors/canines and the mandibular canines. This is due to the curvature of the arch and the difficulty of achieving parallel film alignment with the space. The clinical measures can be checked against the radiographic measures to obtain a more accurate estimate.

Sectional tomography

Although some clinicians use computed tomography (CT) scans for single tooth planning, we would consider this to be in excess of what is normally required. The CT scans, however, may be very important aids with more complex cases and they are therefore dealt with in the chapter on fixed bridge planning (see Chapter 5). Many modern dental panoramic tomograph (DPT) machines now offer sectional tomography for implant planning (see below).

In order to optimize the information provided by these more advanced radiographic techniques, it is advisable to provide information

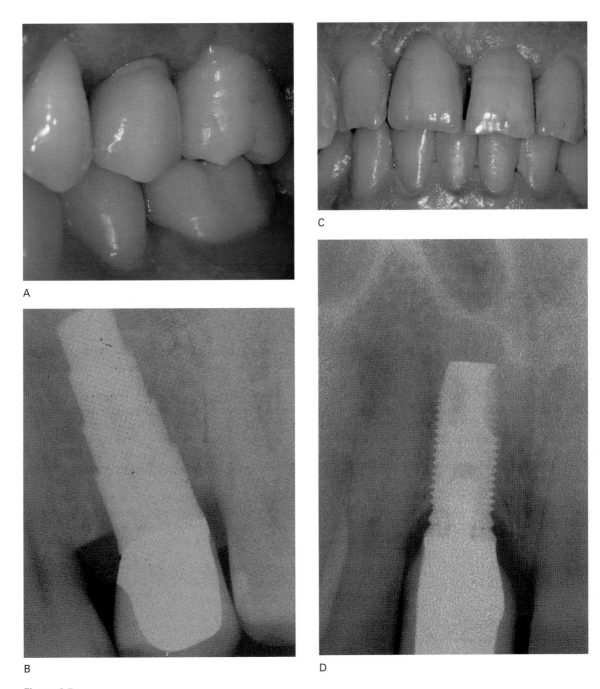

Figure 3.5

(A) The second bicuspid has been replaced with a 4.5-mm diameter Frialit 2 implant. (B) Radiograph of the Frialit 2 implant (push-fit, stepped cylinder design), which shows a very good match between the size of the crown and the diameter of the implant. (C) The upper right central incisor has been replaced with a 5-mm diameter Nobel Biocare implant. (D) Radiograph of the wide-diameter implant, which more closely matches the diameter of the natural tooth root and crown. However, in many cases there is insufficient bone width buccolingually in the incisor region to accommodate wide implants, therefore implants of about 4 mm diameter are more commonly used.

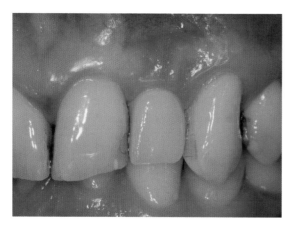

Figure 3.6

The upper lateral incisor has been replaced by an AstraTech single implant tooth 6 years before this photograph. There has been complete stability and no complications despite the difficult Class 2 Division 2 incisor relationship.

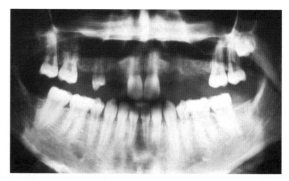

A

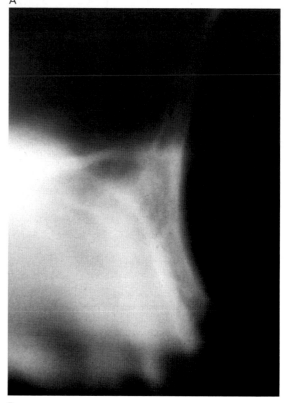

B

Figure 3.7

(A) Dental pantomogram taken on a Scanora at ×1.7 magnification. The young patient has a large number of developmentally missing teeth, including maxillary lateral incisors and canines. (B) Sectional tomogram of the anterior ridge, which is angled labially and is thin.

about the planned final restoration. A suitable existing partial denture or a customized stent that mimics the desired tooth set-up is constructed and radiographic markers incorporated. The radiopaque marker can be placed in the cingulum area of the tooth if a screw-retained crown is planned, to indicate the access hole for the screw. Alternatively, the labial surface of the stent can be painted with a radiopaque varnish to show the labial profile and cervical margin of the planned crown in relation to the underlying bone ridge (Figure 3.7). Simpler types of stent involve placing radiopaque markers (e.g. ball bearings of various diameters or twisted wire shapes) into a baseplate, designed to help determine mesiodistal distortion and location.

Scanora™ (Soredex Orion, Helsinki, Finland) is an example of the new generation of tomographic machines with facilities to generate high-quality sectional images. In contrast to CT scanning, where the sectional images are software generated, the Scanora produces a tomographic image directly onto film. It uses complex broad-beam spiral tomography and is able to scan in multiple planes. The scans are computer controlled with automatic execution. They rely on good patient positioning and experience in using the machine. The patient's head is carefully aligned within the device and this position is recorded with skin markers and light beams. A conventional DPT image is

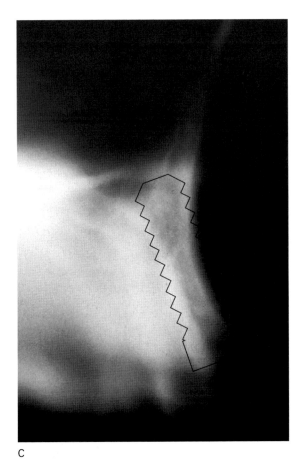

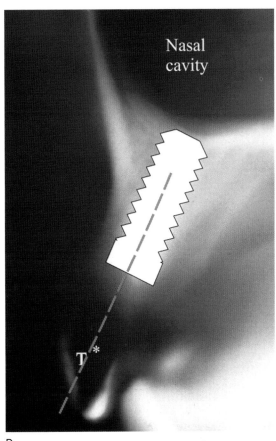

C

D

(C) A transparent overlay of a 4-mm diameter implant has been superimposed on the ridge profile. There is insufficient width of bone to accommodate this implant, and not even a 3.3-mm diameter implant. This site needs to be made wider. (D) The sectional profile of the tooth (T*) to be replaced can be visualized by coating the radiographic stent with radiopaque varnish. The Scanora section of this wider ridge profile has been assessed using a transparent overlay of the appropriate implant design, which can be accommodated within the available bone volume. The red dashed line shows that the angle of the implant would pass through the labial face just apical to the incisal tip. A cemented restoration would be satisfactory.

produced and the sites that require sectional tomographs are determined. The patient is repositioned in exactly the same alignment and the appropriate tomographic programme is selected for the chosen region of the jaw.

The Scanora magnification is ×1.3 or ×1.7 for routine DPTs but is ×1.7 for all sectional images. Tomographic sections are normally 2 or 4 mm in thickness. As with all tomograms, the image

produced includes adjacent structures that are not within the focal trough, which therefore appear blurred and out of focus.

In order to facilitate planning using images at different magnifications, transparent overlays depicting implants of various lengths and diameters at the corresponding magnifications can be superimposed directly on the radiograph. These provide a simple method of assessing implant

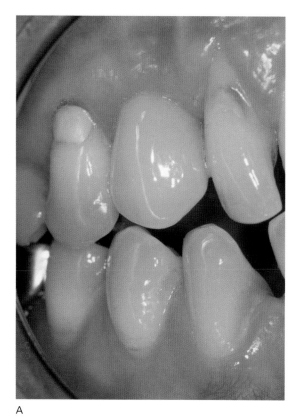
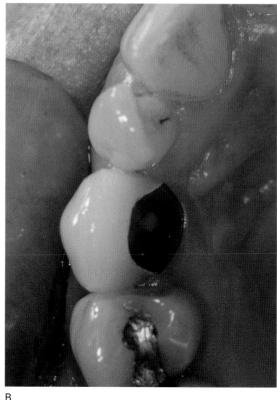

A   B

Figure 3.8

(A) The upper right canine has been replaced by a single tooth implant in an ideal position giving a very good buccal emergence profile. (B) The palatal view of the crown at the upper right canine shows that it is a cemented crown with a very nice contour. The angle of the implant was close to the long axis, passing close to the cusp tip.

sites and implant placement at different angulations.

Diagnostic set-ups

Patients with aesthetically acceptable provisional restorations may not require diagnostic wax-ups. There are considerable advantages in using the pre-existing prosthesis or a new provisional restoration that can be worn by the patient to provide a realistic potential end result. This can be agreed upon between patient and clinician and recorded. Wax-ups are difficult for the patient to judge and computer-manipulated images may not be entirely realistic or achiev-

able. We routinely use simple acrylic removable prostheses for this purpose (see section on removable partial dentures). The set-up should establish the emergence profile of the crown and estimate the level of emergence from the soft-tissue at the planned cervical/gingival margin.

Cemented or screw-retained crowns

The preceding information should provide the clinician with sufficient information to indicate whether it is possible and/or desirable to provide a cemented or screw-retained crown. This is dealt

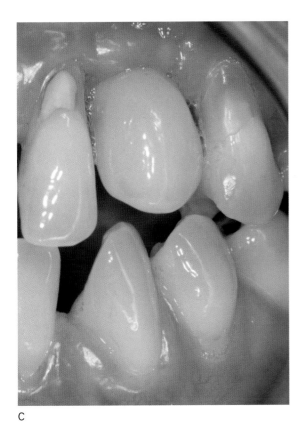

C

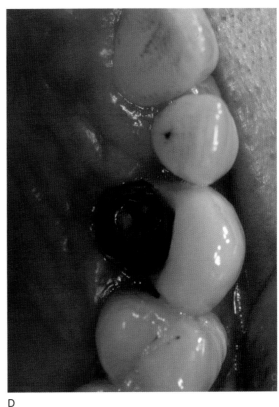

D

(C) In contrast, the single tooth implant replacing the canine on the patient's left side has a more ridge-lapped buccal profile. (D) The palatal view shows the cemented crown with a much more bulbous palatal contour because the implant is palatally placed and the angle of the implant goes through the cingulum area.

with in some detail in the surgical chapter on single teeth (Chapter 9), but needs to be considered here. Nowadays, most anterior single tooth crowns are cemented. This produces very good aesthetics without a visible screw hole on the palatal surface, even though this can be restored carefully with tooth-coloured restorative material. An optimum labial contour and emergence profile is achieved with an implant that is angled with its long axis passing through the incisal tip or slightly labial to it. This restoration cannot be screw-retained (Figure 3.8). However, in cases where there has been fairly extensive ridge resorption that has not been corrected by bone grafting, the position and angle of the implant may be more palatal. This allows screw retention through the palatal surface,

permits full retrievability of the crown and would make it possible to retighten a loose abutment should it occur. The disadvantage is that it is usually associated with a ridge-lap labial margin (Figure 3.9). The above mainly applies to the upper incisors and canines. In the premolar zone the implant is normally in the long axis of the crown, allowing either cementation or screw retention, according to the clinician's preference.

Provisional restorations

In the majority of treatment plans the provisional restoration is an essential component. It helps to establish the design of the final reconstruction and

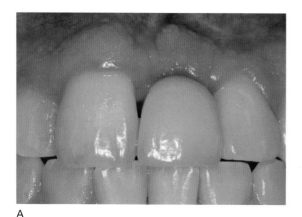
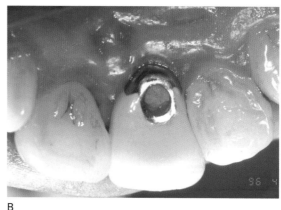

A   B

Figure 3.9

(A) The single tooth implant replacing the upper left central incisor is very palatally placed, resulting in a marked ridge-lap of the crown. (B) A palatal view of the restoration shows that there is a hole in the cingulum that gives direct access to the abutment screw (i.e. the long axis of the implant), making the restoration retrievable (although the crown is cemented to the abutment).

is used by the patient throughout the treatment stages. The following provisional restorations are most commonly used for single tooth restorations.

Removable partial dentures

Although it has been suggested that dentures should not be worn for 1 or 2 weeks following implant surgery, this does not usually apply to the single tooth cases. Single tooth or short-span dentures usually can be worn immediately after surgery. The denture can be adjusted so that little or no pressure is transmitted at the site of the implant. Acrylic dentures are simple and inexpensive to construct and allow easy adjustment to accommodate any changes in tissue profile following implant placement and the transmucosal abutments when they are fitted. When used as an immediate replacement following tooth extraction the shape of the gum-fitted pontic can be adjusted to develop a good emergence profile and soft-tissue contour.

Adhesive bridgework

Many patients prefer the idea of a fixed provisional restoration. Adhesive bridgework is normally retained by a single adjacent retainer that should permit removal by the clinician. Therefore, the Rochette design is recommended as drilling out the composite lugs within the framework holes should allow removal. However, this occasionally proves to be more difficult than one might expect and the removal and replacement of adhesive bridges considerably adds to the treatment time, particularly in the restorative phase. It is worth making the prosthetic tooth from acrylic or composite, to allow more rapid adjustment when the bridge is recemented over a protruding abutment. The fixed restoration has considerable advantages in cases where it is important to avoid any loading of the ridge/mucosa, e.g. where grafting or regenerative techniques have been used (Chapter 12).

Treatment schedules

The treatment schedule for single tooth replacement in most cases should be relatively simple:

1. Initial consultation, clinical evaluation and radiographic examination
2. Agreement of aesthetic/functional demands

using existing prosthesis or diagnostic set-up/new provisional prosthesis

3. Treatment of related dental problems that could compromise implant treatment
4. Surgical placement of the implant and provision of temporary prosthesis
5. Healing phase to allow osseointegration according to established protocol
6. Abutment choice and connection
7. Prosthodontic treatment

However, there are a number of situations that will need modification:

1. Immediate replacement following extraction (see Chapter 11)
2. Soft tissue or bone augmentation prior to implant placement (see Chapter 12).
3. Early loading or immediate loading protocols. Provided that bone quality and implant stability are good, early loading (e.g. 6 weeks following implant placement) should not compromise success. Promising results have been shown with immediate loading, but failure rates can be higher, particularly where loading is difficult to control (see Chapter 1).

Conclusion

This chapter has dealt with most of the basic planning issues of anterior single tooth replacement. However, many of the more detailed issues are best considered in the surgical chapter (Chapter 9) and the prosthodontic chapter (Chapter 13).

Bibliography

Andersson B, Odman P, Carlsson GE (1995). A study of 184 consecutive patients referred for single tooth replacement. *Clin Oral Implants Res* **6**: 232–7.

Engquist B, Nilson H, Astrand P (1995). Single tooth replacement by osseointegrated Brånemark implants. *Clin Oral Implants Res* **6**: 238–45.

Hess D, Buser D, Dietschi D, Grossen G, Schonberger A, Belser U (1998). Esthetic single-tooth replacement with implants: a team approach. *Quintessence Int* **29**: 77–86.

Kemppainen P, Eskola S, Ylipaavalniemi P (1997). A comparative prospective clinical study of two single-tooth implants: a preliminary report of 102 implants. *J Prosth Dent* **77**: 382–7.

Millar BJ, Taylor NG (1995). Lateral thinking: the management of missing upper lateral incisors. *Br Dent J* **179**: 99–106.

4
Single tooth planning for molar replacements

Introduction

The considerations for replacement of single molars are not primarily aesthetic as in the preceding chapter on anterior teeth, but the mechanical considerations are far more important. It is not generally recommended to replace a molar by a single implant of 4 mm diameter or less because of the potentially large cantilever forces that it could be subjected to (Figure 4.1), resulting in biomechanical failure. The basic alternatives are therefore placement of two standard implants or a single wide-diameter implant. The space requirements and potential costs are quite different.

Two-implant solutions

Molar spaces of 11 mm mesiodistal width can, theoretically, be treated by placement of two 4-mm diameter implants. This requires extreme care and skill to avoid damage to adjacent tooth roots. Also, the space between the two implants may prove to be too small to allow a properly contoured restoration and an adequate bone and soft-tissue zone (Figure 4.2).

In most cases the space should be at least 13 mm to allow the two-implant solution (Figure 4.3). The space has to be measured at the level of the crestal bone and the adjacent tooth roots must not converge within the space.

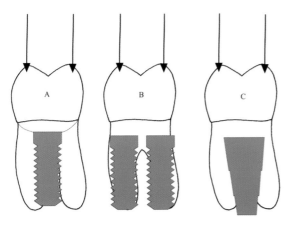

Figure 4.1

Alternative implant solutions for a single molar. The size discrepancy between a single 4-mm implant (A) and the normal occlusal table of a molar may subject it to leverage forces that are too high and biomechanical failure. The situation is considerably improved by using two implants (B) or a single wide implant (C).

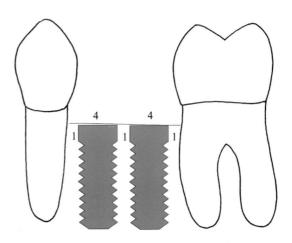

Figure 4.2

An 11-mm space at the level of the crestal bone could theoretically accommodate two 4-mm diameter implants and allow a space of 1 mm between them and the adjacent teeth.

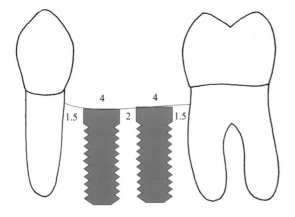

Figure 4.3

A 13-mm space at crestal level allows placement of two 4-mm diameter implants. A safer margin between implants and teeth (1.5 mm) is provided and a minimum of 2 mm between implants.

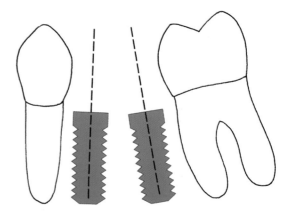

Figure 4.4

The space at the level of the occlusal surface is reduced due to tilting of the distal molar, although there is more bone width available apically. The surgery may be easier but the prosthodontics could be compromised or, in severe cases, made impossible.

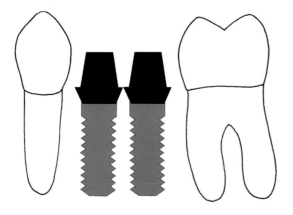

Figure 4.5

Two 4-mm diameter implants have been placed with wider margins between them and the adjacent teeth. The abutments that flare to a wider diameter may touch or leave insufficient space for a healthy soft-tissue collar. This could be improved by using narrower abutments.

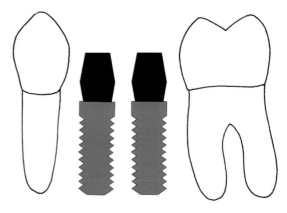

Figure 4.6

When space is limited the selection of an alternative implant system can help enormously. This figure illustrates placement of two AstraTech implants. Selection of the 3.5-mm diameter implant rather than the 4-mm implant would provide an additional saving of 1 mm. The AstraTech abutments are narrower than the implant heads and provide space saving for the superstructure and soft tissue.

It is important also to measure the space available at the occlusal plane, particularly if there is tilting of the adjacent teeth. Under these circumstances an unfavourable path of insertion of prosthodontic components may prevent the reconstruction, or the implant abutments may touch. The choice of implant diameter, implant system and implant abutment will have a marked impact on the available space as illustrated in Figures 4.4–4.7.

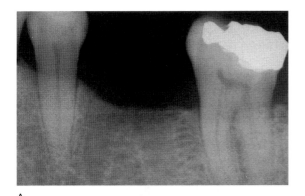

A

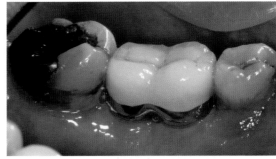

E

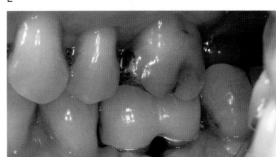

F

B

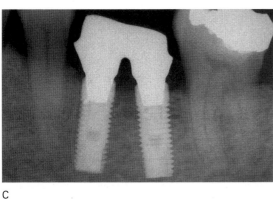

C

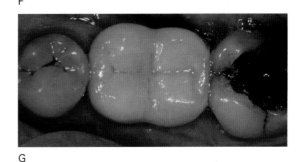

G

Figure 4.7

(A) Radiograph of a mandibular molar space, suggesting adequate room for two implants. (B) Radiograph with transparent overlay of two standard diameter implants, confirming adequate mesiodistal space. The implants are no longer than the adjacent natural roots and are above the inferior dental canal. (C) Radiograph of two AstraTech 4-mm standard implants used to replace the mandibular first molar. The two implants have been joined together with a gold casting fabricated on two cast-to abutments. The abutments are narrower than the implants at the level of the implant head and the shape of the casting facilitates soft-tissue contour and plaque control. (D) Occlusal view of the screw-retained casting on the two implants. (E) Lingual clinical mirror view of the completed restoration. A porcelain-fused-to-metal crown has been cemented onto the gold substructure. (F) Buccal view of the completed restoration. The space between the implants has been contoured to facilitate oral hygiene with a bottle brush. (G) Occlusal view of the completed cemented crown without access to the abutment screws.

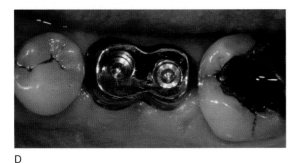

D

Single implant solutions with wide-diameter implants

Many molar spaces are less than 12 mm, and economic considerations often indicate the use of single implant replacements. Wider diameter implants are available in most systems, and in all the systems described in this book (Table 4.1).

The mechanical advantages of a wide-diameter implant for molar replacement are:

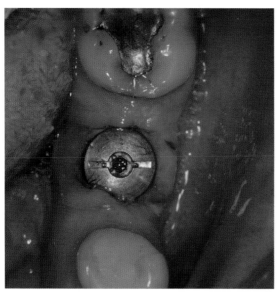

A

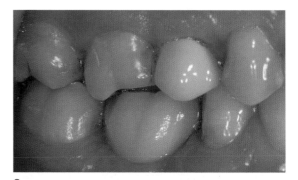

C

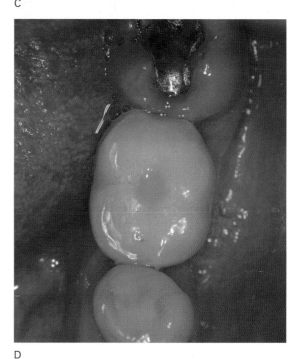

B

D

Figure 4.8

(A) A mandibular molar space showing a single tooth implant healing abutment with good soft-tissue width both mesially and distally. (B) Radiograph of the mandibular molar replaced by a 10-mm long Nobel Biocare 5-mm diameter wide-platform implant. There would have been adequate space for two 4-mm implants but at much greater cost. (C) Clinical photograph of the mandibular first molar replaced by a single wide-diameter implant. The appearance and soft-tissue contours are good. (D) Occlusal view of the completed restoration. The crown has been cemented to a standard abutment. However, an access hole (filled with composite) has been fabricated to allow the crown to be retrievable. This allows tightening of the abutment screw if it should become loose due to the considerable occlusal forces in the molar region.

Table 4.1 Examples of wider diameter implants available from various companies

Make	Type	Diameter
AstraTech	Single tooth (ST)	5 mm
Nobel Biocare	Brånemark regular and wide platform	5 and 5.5 mm
Frialit	Frialit 2 stepped cylinder	5.5 and 6.5 mm
ITI/Straumann	Wide body, solid screw and wide neck	4.8 and 6.5 mm
3i	Brånemark type	5 and 6 mm

3i: Implant Innovations, West Palm Beach, FL, USA
AstraTech: Astra Meditec AB, Mölndal, Sweden
Nobel Biocare: Nobel Biocare AB, Göteborg, Sweden
Frialit: Friatec AG, Mannheim, Germany
ITI/Straumann: Institut Straumann AG, Waldenburg, Switzerland

1. Better force distribution with reduction of leverage forces because implant diameter more closely matches that of the crown.
2. The implant is stronger and less likely to fracture.
3. The abutments and abutment screws are usually bigger and stronger.
4. The surface area of the abutment is usually larger and will provide more retention.

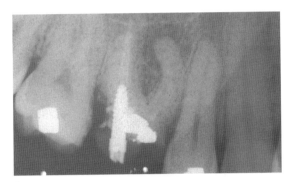

A

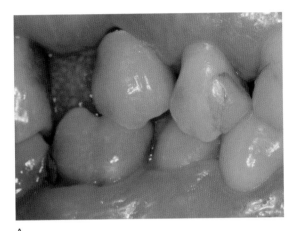

A

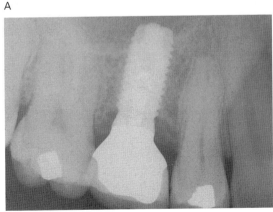

B

Figure 4.9

(A) Radiograph of a maxillary first molar with failed endodontic treatment and a broken-down crown. The adjacent teeth have small restorations. (B) The first molar has been replaced by a single tooth implant: a 5-mm diameter wide platform Nobel Biocare. The implant is 10 mm in length and extends just into the maxillary sinus. Insufficient mesiodistal space was available for a two-implant option.

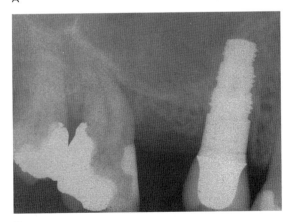

B

Figure 4.10

(A) The maxillary molar is missing. The maxillary second premolar is a single tooth implant. (B) Radiograph showing that the second premolar has been replaced by a Frialit 2 implant (4.5-mm diameter screw design). The maxillary sinus has extended into the molar space, making implant placement impossible without sinus grafting. The second molar has a questionable prognosis. If this tooth is lost, a sinus graft would allow replacement of both molars.

The mesiodistal molar width should always provide sufficient space for a wide-diameter implant (Figure 4.8 and 4.9). However, this is not always the case in the buccolingual dimension. Narrow ridges occur in both posterior maxilla and mandible, often only allowing placement of normal-diameter implants without recourse to grafting. In many cases (particularly shortly after loss of the molar) there is sufficient buccolingual width and the wide-diameter implant should be ideal. The increased surface area that it provides also has a distinct advantage in the molar regions, where bone height is often limited by expansion of the maxillary sinus and the position of the inferior alveolar nerve (Figure 4.10). The minimal length of implant recommended would be 8 mm, although 10 mm would be preferred in most cases. The selection of an implant with a surface that has been treated to increase further its area and improve the rate and quality of osseointegration is preferred in these circumstances. Unfortunately, there are no large-scale longitudinal trials of molar replacements to substantiate these opinions.

Conclusions

If space and economics allow, choose the two-implant option. In other cases ensure that the buccolingual width will accommodate a wide-diameter implant (assuming that the mesiodistal space is adequate). Caution should be exercised in patients with bone height less than 10 mm, poor bone quality or high functional demands.

Bibliography

Andersson B, Odman P, Carlsson GE (1995). A study of 184 consecutive patients referred for single tooth replacement. *Clin Oral Implants Res* **6**: 232–7.

Bahat O, Handelsman M (1996). Use of wide implants and double implants in the posterior jaw: a clinical report. *Int J Oral Maxillofac Implants* **11**: 379–86.

Balshi TJ, Hernandez RE, Pryszlak MC, Rangert B (1996). A comparative study of one implant versus two replacing a single molar. *Int J Oral Maxillofac Implants* **11**: 372–8.

Becker W, Becker BE (1995). Replacement of maxillary and mandibular molars with single endosseous implant restorations. *J Prosth Dent* **74**: 51–5.

Langer B, Langer L, Herrmann I, Jorneus L (1993). The wide fixture: a solution for special bone situations and a rescue for the compromised implant. *Int J Oral Maxillofac Implants* **8**: 400–8.

5
Fixed bridge planning

Introduction

Planning for implant-supported fixed bridges follows the lines described in the previous chapters. The chapter on single tooth replacement in the anterior region (Chapter 3) dealt with the aesthetic demands and the chapter on molar replacements (Chapter 4) with some of the loading and spacing considerations. Extensive bridgework in partially dentate and edentulous jaws involves planning for placement of multiple implants in sites that may be more demanding surgically (see Chapters 10 and 12). The number and distribution of implants is a complex variable and is dealt with below.

Clinical examination and diagnostic set-ups

Patients requiring extensive fixed bridgework often need more detailed examination and consideration of treatment alternatives than those requiring more simple restorations.

In partially dentate patients the following should be evaluated:

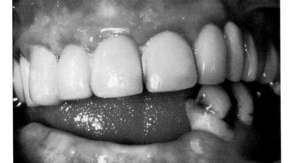

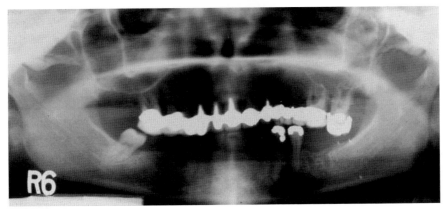

Figure 5.1

(A) Clinical appearance of a patient who has an extensive maxillary bridge and very few mandibular teeth. The mandibular arch appears to be ideally suited to implant treatment. (B) Radiograph of the same patient showing good bone height in the anterior mandible. However, the maxillary teeth have a poor prognosis and are affected by advanced untreated periodontal disease, endodontic lesions and caries. Loss of all the maxillary teeth places a different perspective on the management of the lower jaw.

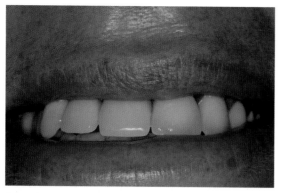

A

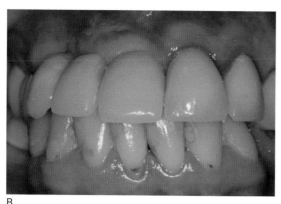

B

Figure 5.2

(A) Patient with lips at rest, showing less lip support on the right than on the left. (B) Intraoral view of the same patient who has been provided with a diagnostic partial acrylic removable denture without a labial flange. The cervical aspects of teeth 13, 12 and 11 are more palatally placed because of extensive resorption of the labial bone. This results in the incisal tips being cantilevered forward, to establish a relationship with the opposing teeth. This set-up may be unfavourable mechanically and aesthetically for implant treatment, and grafting should be considered.

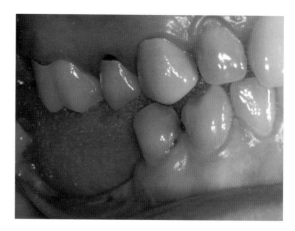

Figure 5.3

A patient with missing lower molars and moderate resorption of the ridge. The interocclusal space is increased and the prosthesis would require long crowns. The amount of bone height above the inferior dental canal is often limited, and implant lengths of about 10 mm are commonly used. Shorter implants may produce very unfavourable implant/crown ratios and an onlay graft may be indicated to provide enough bone for longer implants and to reduce the interocclusal space.

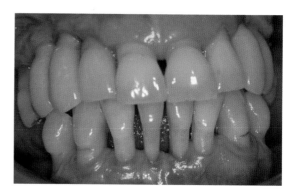

Figure 5.4

A patient who has been treated with implant-supported bridges on both sides of the maxilla distal to the central incisors. The bridges have long crowns because of the extensive vertical resorption of bone following tooth loss. Sufficient bone was present to provide implants of 10 and 13 mm in length. The lip coverage was favourable and the teeth have been treated for periodontal disease.

1. Examination of the restorative, endodontic and periodontal status of the remaining teeth. This should reveal treatment needs and an idea of the prognosis of the teeth (Figure 5.1). This is extremely important because the implant restoration should have a good long-term prognosis and adjacent teeth or opposing teeth should, for the most part, offer a comparable prognosis. This is not always the case and the patient should be made aware of the potential prognosis of the natural dentition and the possibilities for future replacement, should this become necessary. A good example would be replacement of first and

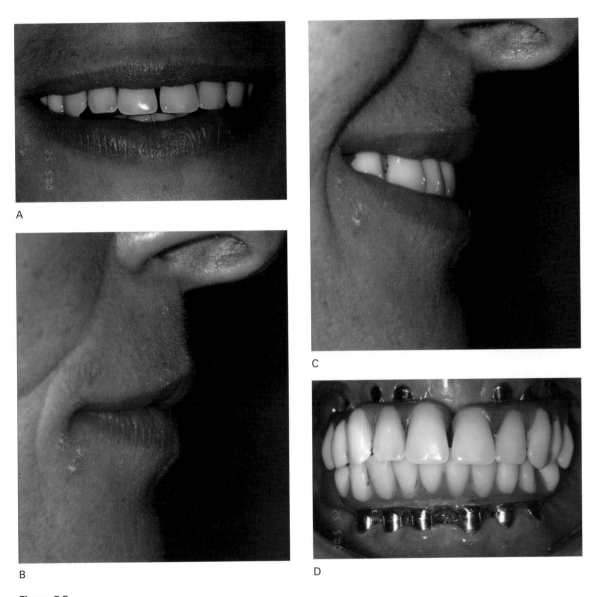

Figure 5.5

(A) An edentulous patient who had been treated with maxillary and mandibular fixed implant-supported bridges 6 years prior to these photographs. There is adequate lip support and good aesthetics during normal function. (B) The lip support in profile at rest. (C) The exposure of the maxillary bridge on smiling. (D) The intraoral appearance, showing the bridges that were constructed along the principles of Brånemark. The standard abutments protrude above the mucosa to allow good access for oral hygiene. The superstructure consists of a rigid gold casting and the prosthetic teeth and 'gumwork' are acrylic.

second molars in one jaw opposing the teeth in the other jaw that have a limited prognosis. Replacement of the opposing teeth may be straightforward with conventional dentistry or implants. In contrast, replacement may be impossible without implants involving major bone grafting, a treatment that the patient may not be willing to undergo.

2. The degree of ridge resorption. It is important to recognize not only the degree of resorption that would compromise implant placement but also that which would compromise aesthetics because of a high lip line or insufficient lip support (Figure 5.2). These factors should be assessed further using diagnostic wax-ups and diagnostic removable prostheses, as described previously.

3. Centric jaw relationship and protrusive and lateral excursions of the lower jaw. The vertical height within the existing and planned occlusal vertical dimension is another important factor. There may be insufficient height to accommodate the prosthesis from the implant head due to overeruption of the opposing teeth. The other extreme is where there is a large vertical space to be restored that would produce an unfavourable prosthesis/implant ratio (cf. crown/root ratio in natural dentition; Figures 5.3 and 5.4). The forces on the planned prosthesis are also increased where the prosthesis is likely to be cantilevered, either distally in a free end saddle (see Figure 5.14) or anteriorly where the jaw has resorbed relative to the required tooth position (see Figure 5.2). These factors assume greater importance in patients who exhibit parafunctional activities and who have limited bone volume and/or quality.

Additionally, in edentulous patients the degree of ridge and jaw resorption affecting soft-tissue support and maxillary/mandibular relationships should be evaluated (Figure 5.5). With progressive resorption, patients are more likely to acquire a pseudo class 3 jaw relationship and very poor lip support. The potential solutions to this problem are extensive bone grafting/osteotomy (Chapter 12) or provision of overdentures, which is dealt with in detail in Chapter 6.

Other points to remember in severely resorbed cases:

- A fixed bridge prosthesis will almost certainly require the addition of prosthetic gingivae (Figure 5.6).
- The restoration/implant height ratio is more likely to be unfavourable.
- Resorption of the ridge produces a smaller arc of bone to support the implants than the required arc to provide a functional and aesthetic prosthesis.

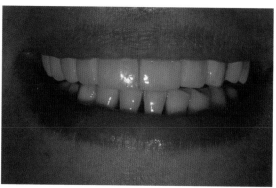

A

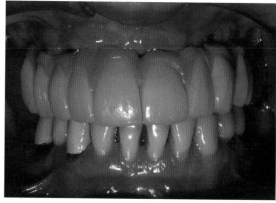

B

Figure 5.6

(A) A patient with a full-arch maxillary implant bridge. (B) The intraoral appearance of the maxillary bridge, showing that the residual ridge is very resorbed and the implant heads are palatally placed in a smaller arc. Adequate lip support and aesthetics are provided by the position of the teeth and the provision of prosthetic 'gumwork'.

Diagnostic set-ups

These should follow the principles described in the chapters on general planning (Chapter 2) and single tooth planning (Chapter 3). The larger the restoration, the more complex the evaluation. We would advocate the use of removable dentures with gum-fitted teeth (and labial flanges for comparison) to allow both the clinician and the patient to assess the potential end result (Figure 5.7).

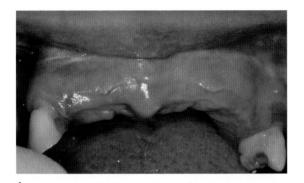

A

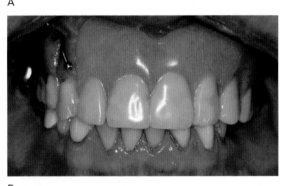

B

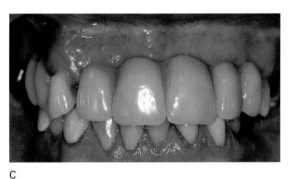

C

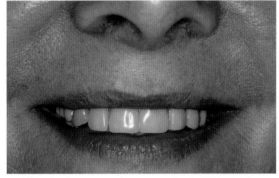

D

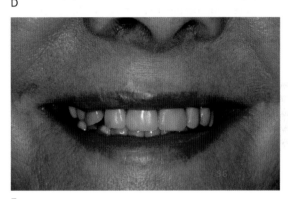

E

Figure 5.7

(A) A patient with extensive anterior tooth loss. (B) The removable partial denture that the patient had been wearing had a large labial flange to provide lip support (see Figure 5.7D). (C) A 'diagnostic denture' to determine the change in appearance with removal of the labial flange, and the position of the teeth in relation to ridge and potential implant placement. This denture can be duplicated to provide radiographic and surgical stents. (D) Lip support with the denture, including the labial flange. (E) Slight loss of lip support without the labial flange.

Radiographic examination

In some situations the simpler radiographic techniques of dental panoramic tomographs (DPTs) and conventional film tomography will be entirely adequate (see Chapter 4). However, complex cases often demand computed tomography (CT) scans, which can offer detailed multiformat images for detailed planning. They are particularly useful for cases involving:

1. Posterior mandible sites, particularly bilateral cases that are imaged by the same scan.
2. Large-span edentulous spaces in the maxillary arch. In the anterior region, thin ridges may be revealed where DPT images have suggested adequate bone height; in the posterior region, more detailed images of maxillary sinus extension are often required.

Computed tomography uses X-rays to produce sectional images, as in conventional tomography.

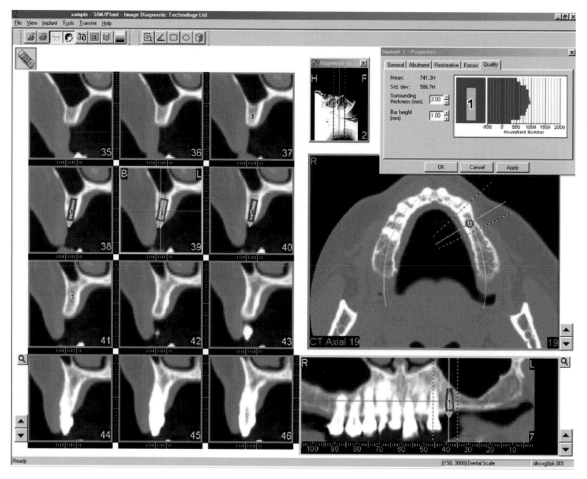

Figure 5.8

SIM/Plant™ (Columbia Scientific Inc, Maryland, USA) software view showing 'mock' implant placement in the maxilla. The images on the left numbered 35–46 are cross-sectional images. An implant has been placed and appears in sections 38–40. The mesiodistal position of the implant can be seen in the panoramic view (bottom right) and axial view above (CT Axial 19). The top right shows the alignment view (scout view), and a box which displays bone density values. (Courtesy of Image Diagnostic Technology, London, UK.)

High-resolution images are achieved by initially scanning in an axial plane, keeping the sections thin, and by making the scans contiguous or overlapping. The scans should be limited to the area of interest and avoid radiosensitive tissues such as the eyes. The patient's head is aligned in the scanner with light markers, and a scout view is obtained that gives an image similar to a lateral skull film. The radiation dose of this scout view is low and can be repeated if the alignment is incorrect. Generally, the mandible is scanned with slices parallel to the occlusal plane and the maxilla, using the same plane or one parallel to the floor of the nose. Deviation from this alignment will result in the cross-sectional slices not being in the same direction as the proposed implant placement (see pp. 38–42). In place of conventional film the radiation is detected by highly sensitive crystal or gas detectors and is then converted to digital data. These data can be stored and manipulated by computer software to produce the image. The software then allows multiplane sections to be reconstituted, the quality of which are dependent on the original

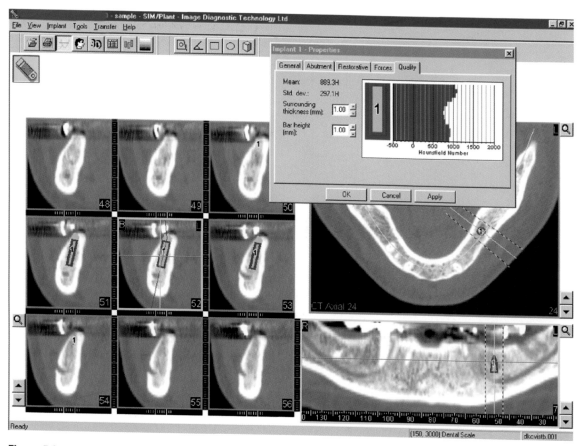

Figure 5.9

SIM/Plant™ (Columbia Scientific Inc, Maryland, USA) software view showing 'mock' implant placement in the mandible. The images on the left numbered 48–56 are cross-sectional images. An implant has been 'placed' and appears in sections 51–53 with its apex about 3 mm above the inferior dental canal and mental foramen (section 53). The mesiodistal position of the implant can be seen in the panoramic view (bottom right, which clearly shows the path of the inferior dental canal) and axial view above (CT Axial 24). The top right displays bone density values in relation to the implant. (Courtesy of Image Diagnostic Technology, London, UK.)

scan section thickness and integers between successive sections.

Images can be produced as:

1. Standard radiographic negative images on large sheets.
2. Images on photographic paper, often in book form.
3. Images for viewing on a computer monitor.

Heavy metals will produce a scatter-like interference pattern if they are present in the slice under examination and the interference will therefore appear in all the generated sectional images. Extensive artefacts may render a CT scan unreadable and can be produced by large posts in root canals or heavily restored teeth where the plane of examination passes through such a tooth as well as an area of critical interest.

In some instances, therefore, either a compromise has to be made in the direction of scanning or a different method of examination chosen (e. conventional tomography as described

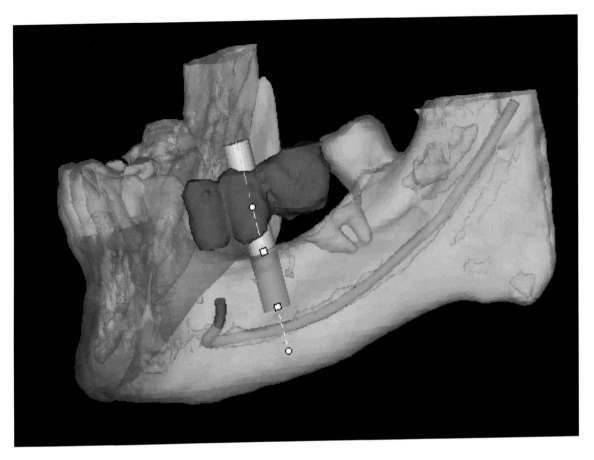

Figure 5.10

The new 'Surgicase' interactive software (Surgicase, Materialise NV, Leuven, Belgium) has additional three-dimensional capabilities. Implants can be placed and manipulated in this view and, as illustrated, the nerve can be highlighted within the jaw, using a transparency tool (courtesy of Image Diagnostic Technology, London, UK).

Chapter 3). Consideration should also be given to removing the offending metal prior to examination if appropriate in the overall treatment plan.

The various scan images can be measured for selection of implant length and diameter. Although the nominal magnification of the images is 1:1, some machines and cameras produce images where the magnification may vary. A scale is usually incorporated alongside the various groups of images and the real magnification can be determined from this. A correction factor then can be applied to measurements taken directly from the films.

In contrast to hard copies of the scans, one of the advantages of the computer-based image software programmes (e.g. SIM/Plant™) is that it is possible to produce images of implants (and their restorative components) that can be 'placed' within the CT scan (Figures 5.8–5.10). This enables the clinician to evaluate the relationships between the proposed implants and ridge morphology, anatomical features and adjacent teeth. When used in conjunction with a radiographic stent, the possibility of reproducing the orientation envisaged at the planning stage is greatly increased.

Table 5.1 Guide for implant numbers in various circumstances

Examples of types of replacement required	Suggested number of implants and prosthetic solution
Full-arch bridges in edentulous maxilla	At least five or six implants – preferably extending to second premolar region. Additional implants in molar regions recommended by many clinicians
Full-arch bridges in edentulous mandible	At least four or five implants in the region between the mental foramina. Additional implants in molar regions recommended by many clinicians
Missing molars	Two missing molars normally require three standard-diameter implants. Two wide-diameter implants could be used to support a bridge or two single tooth molar units.
Three missing maxillary anterior teeth	Two or three implants supporting a bridge. If there is sufficient space for three implants, consider three single tooth units
Four missing maxillary anterior teeth	Four upper incisors would normally require a minimum of three implants to support a bridge. If there is sufficient space for four implants, consider four single tooth units
Four missing mandibular incisors	Four lower incisors could be replaced using two implants and a fixed bridge. There is usually not enough room for more implants. The same solution may be adequate to replace mandibular canines and incisors (which is not usually the case in the maxilla)

Planning implant numbers and distribution

In planning fixed bridgework supported by implants there are recommendations regarding the minimum number of implants that would be required (Table 5.1). Increasing the number of implants allows for failure of an implant (or more than one) and may provide improved long-term predictability.

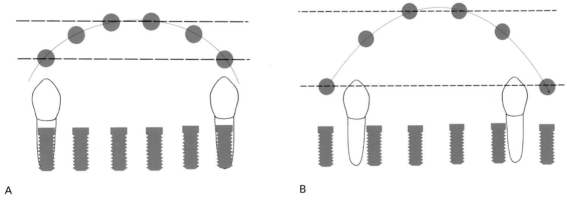

A   B

Figure 5.11

(A) An example of six implants arranged in the lower jaw in the region between the mental foramina, with the most distal implant in the first premolar site. In this case the anteroposterior distance between implants shown by the dashed lines is not very great because of the shape of the jaw. (B) In contrast, in this example the six implants have been arranged so that the most distal implants have been placed distal to the first premolars. The anteroposterior distance between implants has been increased greatly, providing an improved biomechanical arrangement. This arrangement could more adequately support distal cantilever extensions.

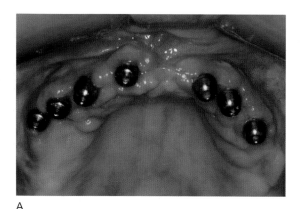

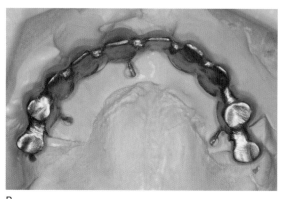

A

B

Figure 5.12

(A) Placement of seven implants in a maxilla that has been treated previously with buccal onlay grafts. The implants extend distally as far as the maxillary sinuses would allow. (B) The casting for the same patient, showing a single distal cantilever unit on each side.

Configuration and angulation of implants

The configuration of the implant sites, the angulation of the implant sites and the angulation of the implants have considerable impact on the structural/load-bearing capacity of the pros-

thesis. In edentulous full-arch cases it is important to distribute implants throughout the curve of the arch and to place implants distal to the canine sites (Figures 5.11–5.13). The possibility of extending the implant placement beyond the premolar zone into the molar zone depends upon the amount of available bone. Unfortunately,

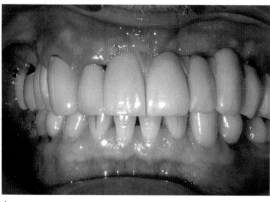

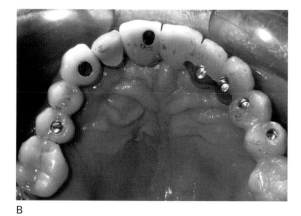

A

B

Figure 5.13

(A) A patient with a completed full-arch maxillary implant bridge. Where there was more resorption the teeth are more ridge lapped and there are small amounts of prosthetic gumwork (patient's left side). In other areas (patient's right side) the emergence profiles of the crowns are better. (B) An occlusal view of the full-arch bridge, which is screw-retained. It can be seen that the implant screw holes on the patient's left side are more palatally placed than on the right side, where they are close to the incisal edge.

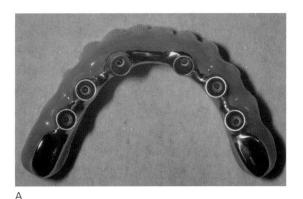 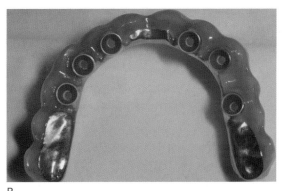

A   B

Figure 5.14

(A) A mandibular full-arch bridge (*ad modum* Brånemark) viewed from the undersurface, showing the distribution and arch form of the implant positions. One cantilever unit has been provided on each side. (B) Maxillary full-arch bridge (*ad modum* Brånemark) viewed from the undersurface, showing the distribution and arch form of the implant positions. Two cantilever units have been provided on each side, in this case, to improve aesthetics (see Figure 5.11).

adequate bone in these zones is not always present in completely edentulous jaws and presents the clinician with two choices:

1. Surgery to create sufficient bone (see Chapter 12).
2. Not utilizing the area for implant placement.

The latter situation may be overcome by distal cantilevering of a prosthesis but there are limits to this strategy (Figure 5.14).

In extensive edentulous zones in the partially dentate individual, the configuration of implants assumes the same degree of importance. It is generally recommended to avoid placement of

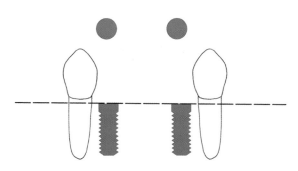

Figure 5.15

Two implants are always in a straight line! This arrangement may be entirely adequate for replacing the four lower incisors using two implants, and with favourable conditions could apply to the four upper incisors or the six lower anterior teeth (incisors and canines). However, it is generally considered an inadequate number for replacing two molar teeth with standard-diameter implants, where the advantage of a three-implant tripodization arrangement is recommended.

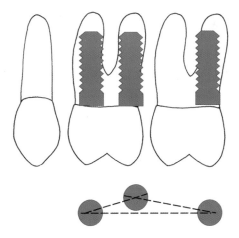

Figure 5.16

Three implants have been placed to support two molar units. The lower part of the figure represents a plan view with the middle implant offset slightly to produce a tripod arrangement (dashed lines) and improved biomechanical properties.

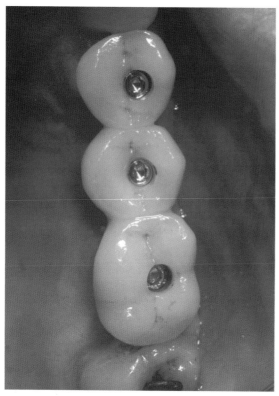

A

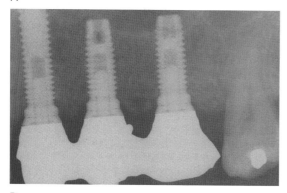

B

Figure 5.17

(A) A three-unit screw-retained maxillary bridge with the screw holes in the middle of the occlusal surfaces. The implants are not in a straight line. However, the degree of tripodization is small because of the width of available bone and the other prosthetic demands of implant placement. (B) Radiograph showing the three Nobel Biocare (Brånemark) implants supporting the bridge.

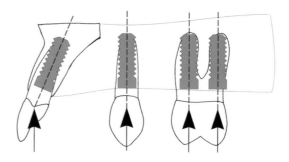

Figure 5.18

Forces directed through implants placed in the posterior jaw will usually be in the same long axis as the premolar and molar teeth. Labial angulation of the anterior implants means that normal forces are not directed down the long axis.

multiple implants in a straight line (Figures 5.15 and 5.16). In the situation where three implants are provided, offsetting one implant to produce a tripod arrangement is normally recommended (Figure 5.16). This will improve the situation even if the offset is minor, which is often the case in the posterior mandible and maxilla (Figure 5.17).

The angulation of the implant sites more or less mimics the angulation of the natural teeth, with modifications according to the design of the final prosthesis and the degree of ridge resorption. A surgical stent provides important guidance. If the final prosthesis is designed to be retrievable/screw-retained, the ideal angle of the implant passes through the cingulum area of the anterior teeth and the occlusal surfaces of the premolar/molar teeth (Figures 5.13 and 5.17). In a non-retrievable cemented prosthesis the angulation would be the same in the posterior teeth because this is also consistent with loading the implants through the long axis (Figure 5.18). However, in the anterior zone the angulation can be more labially inclined through the incisal tip or towards the labial surface, potentially improving the emergence aesthetics (see Chapter 9). However, force transmission through the anterior implants may be less favourable because it will be far removed from axial loading. Further consideration of the angulation and spacing of different implant designs is given in the surgical chapters (Chapters 9 and 10).

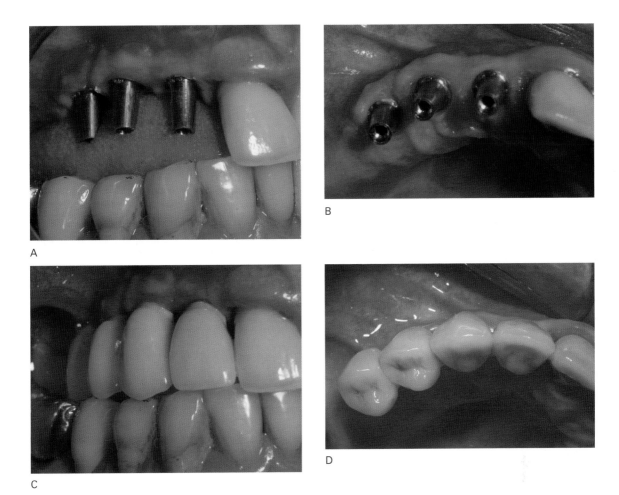

Figure 5.19

(A) The abutments show that there is labial angulation of the three implants in the right maxilla, which has undergone considerable resorption and lost some of its arch form. (B) A palatal view showing the same features. (C) The completed bridge has been cemented to the abutments (screw retention would have required angled abutments – see Chapter 14). The crowns are slightly cantilevered to the labial/buccal side. (D) An occlusal view of the completed bridge. No screw holes are visible because the bridge is cemented.

Fixed bridges or multiple single units

There is a trend to place an implant for each individual missing tooth, in which case it would be possible to restore each as a separate single tooth unit. This approach, although first appearing very logical, is difficult to achieve in practice and may not be as predictable in its outcome. There are a number of potential problems with this approach:

1. Some teeth, such as lower incisors, have a small mesiodistal dimension that is less than most implants.
2. Teeth can function perfectly well with very small amounts of intervening hard and soft tissue (less than 1 mm), unlike implants.
3. As teeth are lost and the jaws resorb, the perimeter of the arch decreases, thus reducing the space for implant placement. The implant spacing requirements are naturally affected by the system selected.

4. The angulation of natural roots in the healthy alveolus may be impossible to mimic in the resorbed jaw. Proclination of natural anterior teeth and anatomical variations such as crown/root angulations are difficult to mimic with implants.

5. Tapering of normal root forms may allow more teeth within a given area of jaw bone. Tapered implants may have an advantage in certain cases, although few designs mimic the pronounced tapering seen in some natural teeth.

6. Failure of a single implant in a multiple single-unit case requires replacement of that unit. The fixed bridge solution may still be workable with one implant less (Figure 5.20).

7. Provision of a fixed bridge with fewer implants than the teeth that are being replaced is more economical/cost effective.

8. The splinting afforded by the fixed bridge may improve the biomechanical properties.

The potential advantages of multiple single units are :

- More natural appearance
- No need for complex casting for precise fitting of multiple abutments
- Simpler prosthodontic procedures
- Patient can floss between units

But there are additional disadvantages:

- Multiple cementation of units
- Multiple paths of insertion and contact points

Provisional restorations

Removable dentures

The most simple provisional prosthesis is a complete or partial removable denture. When constructed in acrylic they provide an inexpensive and readily adjustable prosthesis that can be modified to produce a radiographic stent or duplicated and modified to produce a surgical stent. In cases where the implant surgery has been extensive, e.g. placement of four or more implants in an edentulous jaw, it is commonly recommended to avoid wearing the denture for

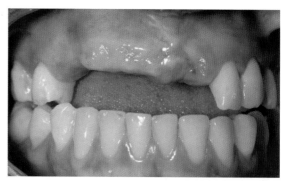

A

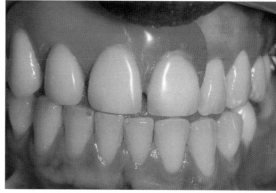

B

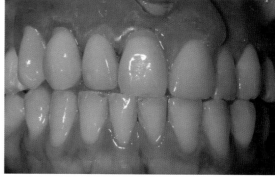

C

Figure 5.20

(A) A patient with loss of teeth 13,12,11 and 21. There is good ridge height and profile. (B) The patient's existing removable partial denture replaces the missing four teeth in a spaced arrangement. This implant solution would require four single tooth units. (C) The same patient with a diagnostic denture bearing five teeth to close the diastemas. This solution would require provision of a fixed bridge based on three implants. The siting of the implants under the teeth to be replaced would be quite different from the arrangement in (B).

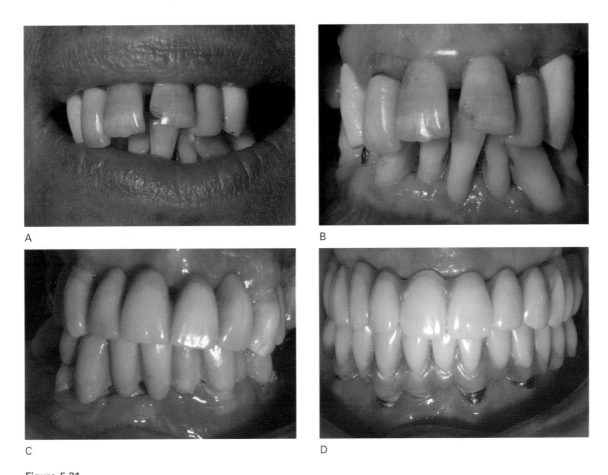

Figure 5.21

(A) This patient was very unhappy about the appearance of her natural teeth. (B) Intraoral examination revealed advanced periodontitis. The remaining teeth had a very poor prognosis. The patient did not wish to wear removable dentures at any time. (C) The majority of the teeth were extracted and periodontal treatment provided for the few remaining teeth. These teeth were used to support provisional/transitional bridges made of gold and composite. Implants were installed in the edentulous areas and, following a period of osseointegration, used to support new full-arch implant bridges. (D) The completed full-arch maxillary and mandibular implant bridges.

a period of at least 1 week. This avoids early transmucosal loading of the implants and allows adequate reduction of postsurgical oedema to take place, facilitating proper adaptation of the denture. A complete upper denture can usually be relined and refitted after 1 week, but the atrophic edentulous lower jaw often requires a period of 2 weeks of healing before a complete denture can be worn satisfactorily.

Fixed bridgework

Provisional fixed bridgework retained by full-coverage restorations may be the treatment of choice, particularly for patients having extensive treatment who are not prepared to undergo a period of time without a fixed restoration. This assumes the presence of a sufficient number of teeth to support the provisional or transitional bridge (Figure 5.21) or utilization of one of the transitional implant systems (these are very narrow-diameter implants that are placed between the definitive implants and are removed before the final prostheses is constructed). Fixed provisional bridgework enables ridge augmentation procedures to be carried out without the risk of transmucosal loading and the associated micro- movement affecting the healing, and should reduce complications. The bridgework may have to remain in place some considerable time, with frequent removal and replacement. Abutment teeth must be prepared adequately to allow for the casting of a metal framework of sufficient strength and rigidity and for the acrylic/composite. Allowance should be made for the fact that the bridge will have to be modified following abutment connection.

Treatment schedules

These are usually far more complex than those described for single teeth, but follow the same principles:

1. Initial consultation, clinical evaluation and radiographic examination, which often involves tomography.
2. Agreement of aesthetic/functional demands using existing prosthesis or diagnostic set-up/new provisional prosthesis. Decision on whether to provide a fixed bridge or an implant denture (see Chapter 6).
3. Treatment of related dental problems that could compromise implant treatment, including timing of further extractions and relationship to implant placement (see Chapter 11).
4. Planning number, type and location of implants in relation to planned prosthesis and available bone. Decision as to whether bone or soft-tissue augmentation is required prior to implant placement (see Chapter 12).
5. Arranging type of anaesthesia – local anaethesia, local anaesthesia plus sedation or general anaesthesia.
6. Surgical placement of the implants and provision of temporary prosthesis.
7. Healing phase to allow osseointegration according to established protocols and complexity of case.

8. Abutment connection and modification of prosthesis or construction of new implant-borne provisional prosthesis.
9. Number of appointments for prosthodontic treatment (see Chapter 14).

Conclusion

The treatment planning for extensive bridgework has a far greater number of variables to contend with and a number of alternative solutions. The patient needs to be made aware of these, but in any case will have to rely upon the treating clinician for guidance. Good recording, documentation and communication are required to maintain a good patient/clinician relationship. Patients should also realize that the maintenance requirements of extensive prostheses are likely to be much higher than those described for single tooth restorations.

Bibliography

Bahat O (1993). Treatment planning and placement of implants in the posterior maxillae: a report of 732 consecutive Nobelpharma implants. *Int J Oral Maxillofac Implants* **8**: 151–61.

Brånemark PI, Svensson B, van Steenberghe D (1995). Ten-year survival rates of fixed prostheses on four or six implants ad modum Brånemark in full edentulism. *Clin Oral Implants Res* **6**: 227–31.

Hebel K, Gajjar R (1997). Cement retained versus screw retained implant restorations: achieving optimal occlusion and aesthetics in implant dentistry. *J Prosth Dent* **77**: 28–35.

Naert I, Quirynen M, van Steenberghe D, Darius P (1992). A six-year prosthodontic study of 509 consecutively inserted implants for the treatment of partial edentulism. *J Prosth Dent* **67**: 236–45.

Rangert BR, Jemt T, Jorneus L (1989). Forces and moments on Brånemark implants. *Int J Oral Maxillofac Implants* **4**: 241–7.

Reddy S, Mayfield-Donahoo T, Vanderven FJJ, Jeffcoat MK (1994). A comparison of the diagnostic advantages of panoramic radiography and computed tomography scanning for placement of root form dental implants. *Clin Oral Implants Res* **5**: 229–38.

6
Diagnosis and treatment planning for implant dentures

Introduction

This chapter will describe the diagnosis and treatment planning of patients for implant dentures. These prostheses can be defined as complete or partial dentures, supported, retained or stabilized by one or more dental implants. In this book, the term 'denture' refers to a patient-removable prosthesis rather than, as in North America, a fixed or removable prosthesis.

The consequences of total tooth loss are well known and include bone resorption, changes in orofacial morphology and psychological effects. Treatment with conventional complete dentures has been shown to be reasonably successful when the residual alveolar ridges are favourable, when the dentures have been well made and when the patient is reasonably philosophical about wearing dentures (Fenlon et al., 2000). Such treatment has not been so successful, however, when:

1. The residual alveolar ridges are resorbed and even well-made dentures have poor support and stability.
2. Where movement of the dentures leads to discomfort, pain and poor function. This may be compounded by poor neuromuscular control in, for example, Parkinson's disease or following a stroke.
3. Where the dentures are not well tolerated because of emotional reasons or because of a strong gag reflex.
4. Where a single denture has poor stability because of opposing natural teeth. The worst combination is remaining maxillary teeth opposing a mandibular denture on a severely resorbed residual ridge.

These difficulties can be overcome by the use of osseointegrated implants to support, retain and stabilize dentures, and such treatment has been shown to be effective in longitudinal studies (Mericske-Stern, 1990; Mericske-Stern and Zarb, 1993; Jemt et al., 1996; Makkonen et al., 1997). Many of the principles of treatment with implant dentures are identical to those of treatment with conventional dentures.

Indications for implant dentures as definitive treatment

There are three main indications for implant dentures:

1. Where complete dentures have been worn successfully for many years but severe resorption (Figures 6.1 and 6.2) or loss of neuromuscular control now limits retention or stability, causing movement of one or both dentures; where the patient has accepted the tooth loss and does not really mind wearing dentures.

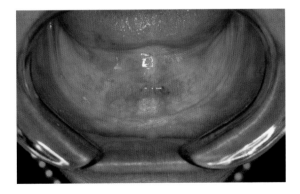

Figure 6.1

Resorbed mandibular residual ridge. The patient was experiencing discomfort and poor function owing to the poor support and poor stability of the mandibular denture.

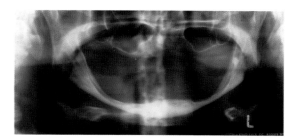

Figure 6.2

Dental panoramic tomograph (DPT) radiograph of same patient showing severe resorption of mandible.

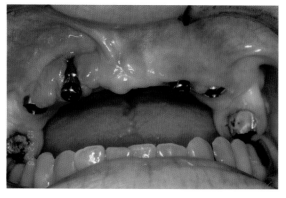

Figure 6.3

Partially dentate patient with posteriorly placed abutment teeth. Four AstraTech implants have been placed to support and retain the long span anterior base of a partial denture since a fixed restoration could not provide sufficient replacement of the resorbed tissues.

2. Where a fixed restoration cannot provide sufficient replacement of resorbed hard and soft-tissues to produce an acceptable appearance.
3. Where remaining natural teeth have an unfavourable distribution for retention and support of a removable partial denture (Figure 6.3).

Where conventional complete or partial dentures are not well tolerated because of emotional reasons, the patient may not accept implant dentures because these prostheses are still patient-removable and may still carry the 'stigma' of false teeth. In this situation, the patient may wish to settle for nothing less than a completely fixed implant bridge. Where conventional dentures are not well tolerated because of a strong gag reflex, it may be possible to provide a maxillary implant denture with reduced palatal coverage. If sufficient numbers of implants can be placed, with grafting if necessary, it may be preferable to plan for an implant bridge at the outset. In the mandible, as few as three implants in good quality bone have been used to retain implant bridges (Brånemark et al., 1999).

Where the complaint is of lack of confidence and fear of movement of the denture, implant stabilization of the denture may be indicated even though ridge resorption may not be severe. Where the residual ridges have undergone little resorption, however, there may be a shortage of vertical space for implant components.

Many alternative treatment plans in practice are developed because the patient finds the ideal treatment plan too expensive. This can lead to dissatisfaction in implant treatment because the apparently lower cost option may be denture-based whereas the ideal treatment is a fixed restoration. In reality, implant dentures require considerable maintenance (see Chapter 17). Not only do the dentures need repairing, relining or replacing but the various attachment mechanisms between the implants and the dentures are also subject to wear, fracture and loss and it is time consuming to replace them. The cost of this maintenance must be included in any comparison between the costs of fixed and removable implant restorations.

Indications for implant dentures as provisional prostheses

In those situations where a fixed implant bridge has been planned but some implants have failed, it may be necessary to provide a provisional implant denture until further implants can be placed. If the original clinical problem indicated a fixed solution, then that should be pursued. However, in such emergency situations, a failure rate of 72% for the remaining implants has been reported (Palmqvist *et al*, 1994).

Assessment of the patient

The commonest denture complaints are about looseness, pain or discomfort, inability to eat, poor appearance and poor speech. Fortunately, a strong gag reflex is not common and the majority of patients have come to terms with the loss of their teeth. A patient may still be embarrassed about the problem, however, and report an 'acceptable' concern. This may be one that is difficult to assess, such as vague discomfort, general looseness or difficulty in eating. For example, some patients may consider themselves rather vain if they complain about the appearance of the dentures and so tell you that they cannot eat. It should be possible to elicit the real problem, however, by a series of questions about the similarity of the present denture teeth to the original natural teeth.

The recommended method of history-taking is well covered in standard textbooks about conventional complete dentures and so will not be repeated here. What you are trying to find out is whether or not the patient's clinical situation comes under the indications mentioned above and whether or not the patient would benefit from implant treatment. Problems caused by faults in denture construction are generally resolved by better conventional dentures and these should certainly be attempted prior to implants unless it is evident that implant treatment is also indicated. Complaints about poor appearance cannot be resolved by implant treatment *per se* but by setting the denture teeth in a more natural position with reference to photographs of original teeth when available. Of course, if a patient has had teeth extracted because of unhappiness with their appearance, you will not be thanked if you suggest restoration of the original appearance!

The medical history should be discussed, although there are very few contraindications to conventional complete dentures because they, and the treatment stages required to make them,

are among the least invasive of any dental procedure. Some patients consider dentures as the *most* invasive dental procedure, being inextricably related to the extraction of the natural teeth. Psychological problems caused by the latter may be helped by implant treatment but the outcome may be uncertain: unresolved conflict over the loss of the teeth may lead to an irrational response to treatment.

Putting implants into bone is a surgical procedure and contraindications to surgery have been discussed in Chapter 1. Prosthodontic contraindications would include lack of space in which to place components and parafunctional forces greater than those that the components can bear. However, if the implants themselves can withstand these forces, then you and the patient must accept that there will be more maintenance and repairs of the dentures than normal. The alternative is greater potential for pain and bone resorption with conventional complete dentures. The patient must be informed prior to treatment so that any subsequent explanation as to why bits keep breaking off the dentures is not perceived to be a lame excuse.

Severe mental illness has generally been included in lists of contraindications for implant treatment because of the difficulties of reasonable informed consent. However, the mental problems that lead to severe denture intolerance and failure to come to terms with the loss of the teeth are the same as those that would pose difficulties were implant treatment to fail. For patients in this group, it is crucial to know the likely response to failure of treatment. It is a difficult area to judge and referral to a clinical psychologist or psychiatrist may be necessary.

Examination of the patient and the existing dentures

The face and mouth should be examined in a systematic manner for pathological conditions. Extraorally, the amount of lip and cheek support provided by the existing dentures should be noted, as well as the occluding vertical relationship with the dentures in place. Intraorally, the resorption of the residual alveolar ridges should be recorded as mild, moderate or severe. The sulci should be examined for displaceability, width and depth. A ball-ended burnisher is useful for examination of displaceable tissue and fibrous replacement of ridges. The vibrating line of the palate should be graded as being a broad area or sharply demarcated, and the depth of the hamular notches should be noted. The position of the coronoid process should be noted because it sometimes occludes the pterygomaxillary fossa in lateral movements of the mandible. The mucosa should be examined carefully and any inflammation, ulceration, sinuses, retained roots, etc. noted. The quantity and quality of saliva should be assessed.

The existing dentures should be examined for basic details such as:

1. Extension
2. Occluding vertical relationship
3. Occlusal plane
4. Anterior and posterior tooth position
5. How the teeth meet and slide over each other
6. Shape and colour of the denture teeth
7. Contour and colour of the denture base material

It is generally accepted that the occluding vertical relationship of conventional complete dentures must allow for sufficient freeway space and that the denture teeth should meet evenly when the patient closes in the retruded position.

Examination of the dentures out of the mouth will reveal whether or not there may be sufficient space for components should implant treatment be considered and give an approximate idea of where the implants should be placed. This is obviously easier the better the technical quality of the dentures. If they have been made at the correct vertical relationship with a correct occlusal plane, then the thickness of the denture can be measured with a calliper. This is the maximum space available from which something must be subtracted to allow for denture teeth.

Where existing dentures have too many technical errors to be useful in assessing the proposed implant position, a trial set-up (Figure 6.4) will be needed as part of the special investigations. When grafting is planned, such a trial set-up will indicate how much space is available for the graft when the space for the components and teeth is subtracted (Figures 6.5, 6.6).

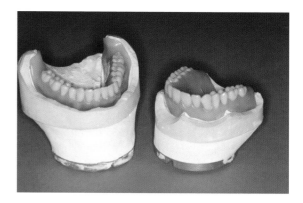

Figure 6.4

Completed trial set-up of denture teeth on casts which had been mounted on articulator using facebow record and interocclusal record.

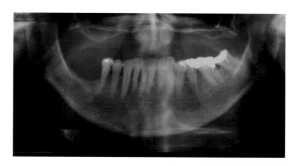

Figure 6.5

DPT radiograph of patient with severe resorption of maxilla necessitating grafting in order to place implants.

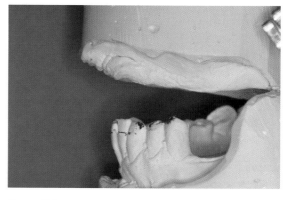

Figure 6.6

Articulated diagnostic casts showing space available for graft, prosthodontic components, and teeth.

By this stage you have listened to your patient and examined the mouth and existing dentures, and it should be possible for you to arrive at a provisional diagnosis. This may include:

1. Moderate or severe alveolar ridge resorption
2. Unstable dentures
3. Incorrectly constructed dentures with one or more errors of base extension, tooth position, occlusion, etc.
4. Poor adaptation to dentures after loss of teeth
5. Pathological conditions such as retained roots, denture ulcers, hyperplasia, etc.

Other special investigations may include radiographs to complete the diagnosis and referrals to specialists for suspicious ulcers, etc. If the clinical situation comes under the indications mentioned earlier, you will certainly be thinking of implant treatment and a radiographic examination will be needed.

Radiographic assessment

The standard view is the dental pantomogram with some way of working out the magnification. This can be done by taping a trident device with known tine lengths to the skin in the area to be assessed (Figure 6.7). The bone height on the film then can be calculated by reference to the known enlargement of the image of the trident. Many dental panoramic tomograph (DPT) machines now produce films to a known magnification and the bone dimension can be measured directly using a ruler supplied by the manufacturer. Alternatively, transparent overlays with printed images of different length implants to known magnifications can be used to select proposed implant size directly. There is some horizontal distortion with all DPT machines.

A lateral skull view can be useful for the anterior maxilla and mandible (Figure 6.8). But to assess accurately the amount of bone in other areas a sectional tomogram will be required. For example, a Scanora machine (Soredex Orion, Helsinki, Finland) will provide sections or a full computed tomography (CT) scan can be used. A stent with radiographic markers is required to match the films with the clinical sites.

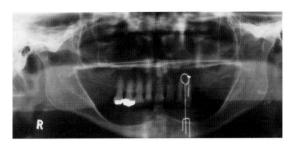

Figure 6.7

DPT radiograph showing image of trident with tines of known length.

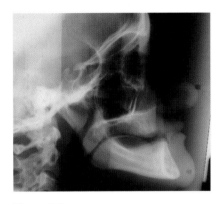

Figure 6.8

Lateral skull radiograph showing midline of mandible. The thickness and density of the cortical bone and the cancellous bone can be clearly seen.

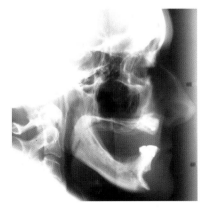

Figure 6.9

Lateral skull radiograph of patient who has had onlay grafts to anterior maxilla to increase width of available bone. The grafts were taken from the anterior mandible and are secured by titanium screws to the existing maxillary bone.

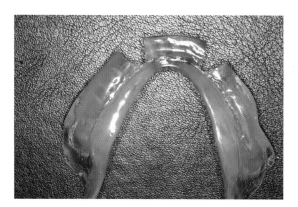

Figure 6.10

The mandibular trial denture shown in Figure 6.4 has been duplicated in clear acrylic resin. Guide holes have been cut in the canine region of the stent and opened out buccally.

For mandibular implant dentures, a DPT film will probably suffice because the implants need only be placed in the canine region. This film will also indicate whether or not grafting will be required for lack of ridge height but it is less useful for assessing ridge thickness. Palpation of the ridge thickness is useful in the anterior mandible but can be very misleading in the maxilla where the palatal mucosa is thick.

The sections, either from a lateral skull view or from tomograms, will indicate the quality and quantity of bone available for implant placement. In our experience, grafting is rarely needed in the mandible but is needed in the maxilla when either the vertical height or width is insufficient. It is beyond the scope of this section to go into detail about grafting (see Chapter 12) but, in outline, bone grafts for implant dentures may be onlay or interpositional. For maxillary implant dentures for patients with severe bone resorption, onlay grafts (Figure 6.9) are generally sufficient: there is no need to reposition the alveolar ridge to improve appearance because the denture flange can be used to restore the soft-tissue contour.

Diagnosis and treatment planning

By this stage, sufficient information should be known to confirm the diagnosis and to decide

what treatment is appropriate. If the patient's clinical situation comes under the indication categories mentioned above, you can decide whether or not implant treatment is indicated, whether or not there is sufficient bone of good quality and whether or not there are any contraindications to the treatment. The outcome may be that new conventional dentures are indicated and that there is no real indication for implant treatment. Having said that, it could be argued that all edentulous patients would benefit from two implants in the mandible to support the denture and to prevent further bone resorption. Certainly, if there were evidence of fairly rapid bone resorption even though the patient was not suffering any problem, it would be good clinical practice to inform the patient of the fact and suggest treatment. The effect of implant treatment in the mandible on a conventional maxillary complete denture must also be considered and it may be necessary to consider implants in both jaws. Fixed implant bridges may be indicated with or without grafting; these restorations are covered in Chapter 5.

Once treatment has been decided, the next step is to plan the sequence of the stages. Unless the existing dentures are technically correct, a trial set-up is essential to decide proposed tooth position (Figure 6.4) and to confirm the amount of space for the components. Once tooth position is confirmed, a stent can be made from the trial denture (Figure 6.10) or duplicate of the existing denture (Figure 6.11). Guide holes are then cut in the stent to indicate the proposed implant position and opened out buccally or lingually so that the guide pins used during implant placement can be directly observed (Figure 6.12). In general, the proposed implant position should be that which allows the components to be sited in the thickest part of the denture resin and within the normal contour.

Prosthodontic components available

Nobel Biocare

This manufacturer offers various bars and ball attachments for implant dentures. The original 2-mm diameter round bar and small clip system

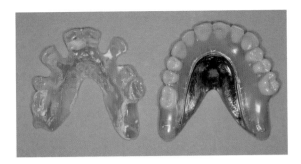

Figure 6.11

A stent has been made from a duplicate of an existing denture.

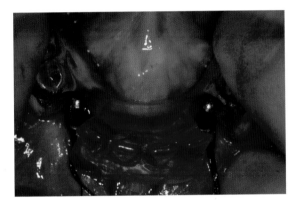

Figure 6.12

Mandibular stent in place during implant placement. The guide pins placed into the implants can be seen emerging in the intended position.

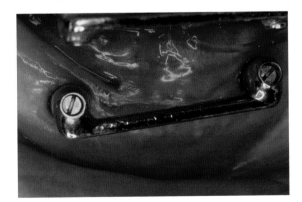

Figure 6.13

NobelBiocare 2-mm diameter round bar soldered buccally to gold cylinders on two mandibular implants to avoid encroachment on lingual sulcus.

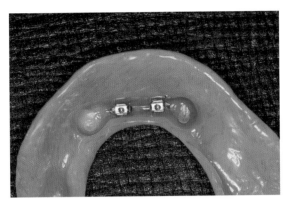

Figure 6.14

Fitting surface of denture showing two clips for NobelBiocare round bar.

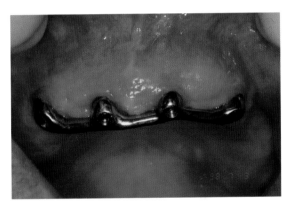

Figure 6.15

NobelBiocare Macro-Ovoid bar on four maxillary implants.

has been expanded to now include macro and micro ovoid bars and macro and micro U-shaped bars, all with clips that can be cut to the required length (Figures 6.13–6.16).

These preformed gold bars can be soldered to gold cylinders, 3 and 4 mm in height, that are screwed to standard abutments ranging in length from 3 to 10 mm. Fixture head gold alloy cylinders (Figures 6.17 and 6.18) and titanium alloy cylinders also are now available. These were introduced with single-stage implants, where the external hex is placed supramucosally to reduce

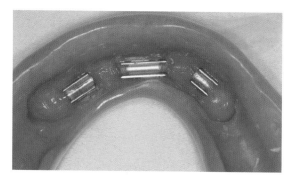

Figure 6.16

Fitting surface of mandibular denture showing custom length clips for NobelBiocare Macro-Ovoid bar.

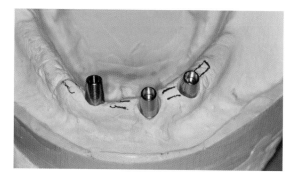

Figure 6.17

Mandibular cast with three NobelBiocare fixture head gold alloy cylinders. These cylinders can be adjusted to obtain lowest profile for bar.

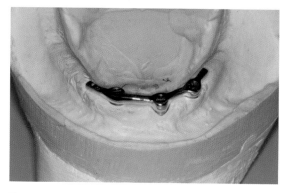

Figure 6.18

Mandibular cast with low profile bar constructed on NobelBiocare fixture head gold alloy cylinders.

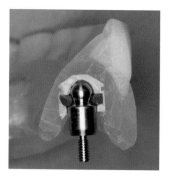

Figure 6.19

NobelBiocare standard ball attachment. A mandibular implant denture has been sectioned through a retention cap in the canine region and a ball attachment with sleeve placed in position. The ball attachment is screwed into the implant and the sleeve fits around the external hex. The driver engages an internal hexagon on the top of the ball attachment.

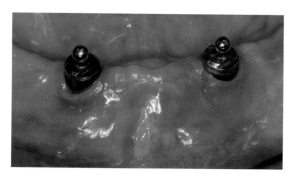

Figure 6.20

NobelBiocare 2.25-mm ball attachments in place on two mandibular implants. The ball attachment is screwed into the implant retaining the sleeve around the external hex. The driver engages the flat surfaces on the collar of the ball attachment.

the overall height of the supramucosal components. They are very useful, however, for rather superficially placed implants to obtain a low bar profile.

The original standard ball attachment consisted of a ball-headed titanium screw and a 3–5.5-mm sleeve similar to the standard abutment sleeve (Figure 6.19). The matrix consisted of a plastic cap (with rubber O-ring), 5.5 mm high and 7.2 mm in diameter, that was processed into the denture. The ball-headed titanium screw has now

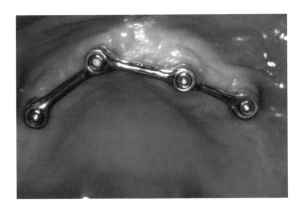

Figure 6.21

AstraTech 1.9-mm diameter round gold alloy bar soldered to gold alloy cylinders on four maxillary implants (photograph courtesy of Mrs C Morgan).

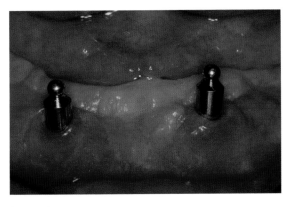

Figure 6.22

AstraTech ball attachments on two mandibular implants. These attachments are solid and are screwed into the internal cone of the AstraTech implants via the flat surfaces just below the ball.

been replaced with a gold alloy screw but the ball attachment is only available for regular platform implants. Some years later, Nobel Biocare introduced a 2.25-mm ball attachment (Figure 6.20) with a six-tined adjustable gold alloy matrix or a titanium alloy matrix with replaceable stainless-steel circlip. The circlip can be replaced by unscrewing the cover. The gold matrix is 2.3 mm high and 3.7 mm in diameter. The titanium alloy matrix is 3.1 mm high and 3.7 mm in diameter. The gold matrix is processed into the acrylic resin of the denture base. Only the retention portion of

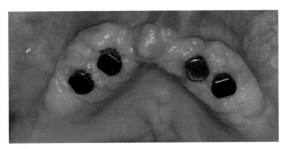

Figure 6.23

AstraTech magnet system. The TiN coated keepers have been screwed into 45° uni-abutments in four maxillary implants. A driver engages the flat surfaces of the keepers.

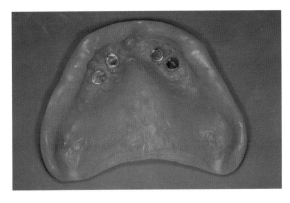

Figure 6.24

AstraTech magnet system. The fitting surface of the maxillary denture showing four titanium encapsulated steel alloy magnets.

the titanium alloy matrix is processed into the acrylic resin, positioned by a mounting sleeve. The circlip and cover are attached after the denture is finished. The 2.25-mm ball attachments are available for narrow and regular platform implants.

AstraTech

This manufacturer supplies a 1.9-mm diameter round gold alloy bar, 50 mm in length, with small riders (clips) manufactured by Cendres and

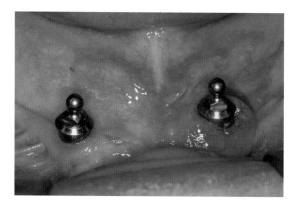

Figure 6.25

ITI/Straumann retentive anchor. The ball attachment screws into the implant with the driver engaging the flat surfaces.

Metaux. The bar is soldered to gold alloy cylinders that are screwed to 20° or 45° uni-abutments ranging in length from 0 to 6.0 mm. There is a small ball abutment (Figure 6.22), in lengths of 0–6.0 mm, with an adjustable four-tine gold alloy matrix that is processed into the acrylic resin of the denture. There is also a magnet system that has a TiN-coated keeper that screws into a 45° uni-abutment with a titanium-encapsulated steel alloy magnet in the denture (Figures 6.23 and 6.24).

ITI/Straumann

This manufacturer supplies mini and regular egg-shaped gold alloy bars and clips (Dolder bars: manufactured by Cendres and Metaux, Biel-Bienne, Switzerland). The bar is soldered to a gold alloy coping that is screwed to the Octa (now SynOcta, Institut Straumann, Waldenburg, Switzerland) abutment. ITI/Straumann also supply mini and regular titanium bars and clips for laser welding to titanium copings as well as plastic burn-out patterns for casting titanium bars and copings. There is a small ball attachment (Figure 6.25: listed as a retentive anchor) that screws directly into the ITI/Straumann implant (there is no abutment as such) with an adjustable four-tine gold alloy matrix and a titanium alloy matrix with replaceable stainless-steel circlip that appears identical to the Nobel Biocare matrix.

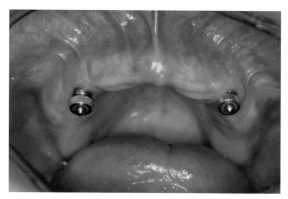

Figure 6.26

3i ball attachments have been screwed into NobelBiocare implants. The matrices are in place on the ball attachments and are attached to the denture with autopolymerizing resin via an intraoral procedure. The red O-rings are fitted to the matrices for this procedure and are removed and replaced with the white O-rings.

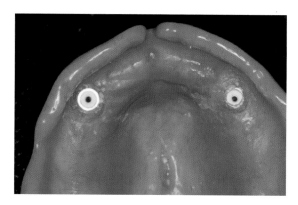

Figure 6.27

Fitting surface of maxillary denture. The red O-rings have been replaced with the white O-rings. The rubber O-rings are easily removed and replaced with a flat plastic instrument.

3i

This manufacturer provides a range of components that fit other manufacturers' implants. Their small ball attachment was available a year before the Nobel Biocare 2.25-mm ball attachment and has a very low profile matrix with rubber ring requiring as little as 3 mm of vertical space (Figures 6.26 and 6.27). The matrix is attached to the denture by autopolymerizing resin as an intraoral procedure. There is also a castable ball attachment for use on non-parallel implants in conjunction with a UCLA (University of California at Los Angeles) abutment. A preformed round gold alloy bar and clips is supplied as well as the Hader bar and plastic clip system.

Other manufacturers

There are several other manufacturers who offer bar/clip systems and ball attachments, e.g. Friatec and IMZ.

Choosing the implant system and retentive device

Mandibular dentures

In general, two to four implants placed between the mental foramina have been suggested, with the denture being retained by clips onto a bar joining the implants, by ball attachments onto the individual implants or by magnets. Bars have been round or ovoid to allow some rotation of the denture but it has been shown that the bar configuration does not appear to be significant (Wright and Watson, 1998).

The results from medium- and long-term studies, however, have shown that two implants placed in the canine region are sufficient to stabilize a mandibular denture (Mericske-Stern, 1990; Chan et al., 1995). Moreover, two ball attachments have been shown to be as effective as a bar and clip system (Naert et al., 1998). The implants for ball attachments should be parallel for best results, although manufacturers state that divergences of up to 10° are acceptable. The 3i's system has a castable ball so that divergent implants can still be used for ball attachments.

The major systems that we have used (Nobel Biocare, AstraTech, ITI/Straumann) have all been shown to be effective in stabilizing mandibular dentures, whether by bar and clip systems, by ball attachments, or by magnets (Mericske-Stern, 1990; Jemt et al., 1996; Makkonen et al., 1997; Davis and Packer, 1999). Ball attachments have been shown to be as effective as bar and clip systems, so they should be the first choice because they are simple to use, require less laboratory work and produce no dead space space for overgrowth of soft tissue.

We have no particular recommendations as to which implant system should be used in the mandible: all three major systems appear equally effective. The ITI/Straumann implant has a slight disadvantage in that no compensation is possible if the implant is placed too superficial. The other systems have varying lengths of abutments. The Nobel Biocare system has implant head gold or titanium cylinders that enable a very low profile for their bar/clip system.

If there is sufficient space, the standard Nobel Biocare ball attachments appear to be the simplest and the most durable. The implant should be placed so that the retention cap will be sited within the thickest part of the acrylic resin and within the normal contour of the denture (Figure 6.19).

Where the implants are divergent, a bar and clip system can be used or the 3i castable ball. The amount of space available must be sufficient for both the bar and the clip to lie within the contour of the denture. The final decision as to the exact position of the bar should be made after the final set-up of the implant denture teeth. It may be necessary to solder the bar lingual or buccal to the gold cylinders to enable the clip to be positioned within the contour of the denture or to avoid encroaching on the lingual sulcus (Figure 6.13). The original Nobel Biocare round bar worked well but the small clips sometimes fractured. The later ovoid bars, both micro and macro, come supplied with long clips that can be cut to size. Occasionally, these clips come out of the acrylic resin entirely. The ITI/Straumann bar and clip (the Cendres and Metaux Dolder bar) appears to be the most durable bar/clip combination and we have occasionally used this bar on other manufacturers' gold cylinders.

A disadvantage of any bar and clip system is that there will be a dead space in the denture into which soft tissue can proliferate. Various suggestions have been made to reduce the dead space, including the lowest possible profile of bar or the use of silicone rubber inserts to fit around the bar. The amount of space available will be shown by the trial set-up and the appropriate system can be selected.

Maxillary dentures

The consensus appears to be that the minimum number of implants in the maxilla for an overdenture is four and that they should be splinted by a bar. The retention device can be a clip or clips directly onto the bar, or studs or other attachments can be soldered to the bar with matrices in the denture. Most studies show higher failure rates for implants in the maxilla but they had too many variables to enable comparisons to be made between various retention systems. One study followed 49 patients for up to 10 years, comparing the Nobel Biocare round bar and clip system with the Nobel Biocare standard ball attachments, and found no difference between the two retention systems (Bergendal and Engquist, 1998). What appeared to be more significant was the quality of the bone, because the bulk of failures occurred in poor quality bone. It would seem sensible to place four or more implants in poor quality bone and join them together. For the maxilla, it may be more important to select an implant system with the best success rate in poor quality bone, such as one with implants that have a roughened surface.

For bar and clip systems, the implants need to be spaced so that there is room for clips between the implants. Most manufacturers have clips that can be adjusted for length. Clips can be placed on cantilevered bars but the added strain will lead to occasional solder joint failure and a higher rate of clip fracture or dislodgement.

Owing to the greater difficulties experienced in providing maxillary overdentures on single attachment systems, some clinicians advocate placement of as many implants as possible, with the provision of a milled or spark-eroded bar to support a removable bridge with a flange. This is one of the most technically demanding and expensive prosthetic options and is not covered in this book.

Single-stage or two-stage implants

There are no real advantages or disadvantages of either approach from a prosthodontic point of view. Certainly, the patient will get the finished implant denture in a slightly shorter time but the existing denture may have to be highly modified in order for it to be worn safely while the implants are deemed to be integrating. If the denture can be modified with an appropriate soft material, it will probably be more stable over healing abutments after a single-stage procedure than over the edentulous ridge following the implant placement in a two-stage procedure. Single-stage implant placement has been shown to be effective for mandibular implant dentures (Cooper et al., 1999).

Bibliography

Bergendal T, Engquist B (1998). Implant-supported overdentures: a longitudinal prospective study. *Int J Oral Maxillofac Implants* **13**: 253–62.

Brånemark PI, Engstrand P, Ohrnell LO, Grondahl K, Nilsson P, Hagberg K, Darle C, Lekholm U (1999). Brånemark Novum: a new treatment concept for rehabilitation of the edentulous mandible. Preliminary results from a prospective clinical follow up study. *Clin Implant Dent and Related Research* **1**: 2–16.

Chan MFW-Y, Johnston C, Howell RA, Cawood JI (1995). Prosthetic management of the atrophic mandible using endosseous implants and overdentures: a six year review. *Br Dent J* **179**: 329–37.

Cooper LF, Scurria MS, Lang LA, Guckes AD, Moriarty JD, Felton DA (1999). Treatment of edentulism using AstraTech implants and ball abutments to retain mandibular overdentures. *Int J Oral Maxillofac Implants* **14**: 646–53.

Davis D, Packer M (1999). Mandibular overdentures stabilised by AstraTech implants with either ball attachments or magnets. *Int J Prosthod* **12**: 222–9.

Fenlon MR, Sherriff M, Walter JD (2000). An investigation of factors influencing patients' use of new complete dentures using structural equation modelling techniques. *Comm Dent Oral Epidemiol* **28**: 133–40.

Jemt T, Chai J, Harnett J, Heath MR, Hutton JE, Johns RB, McKenna S, McNamara DC, van Steenberghe D, Taylor R, Watson RM, Herrman I (1996). A 5-year prospective multicentre follow-up report on overdentures supported by osseointegrated implants. *Int J Oral Maxillofac Implants* **11**: 291–8.

Makkonen TA, Homberg S, Niemi L, Olsson C, Tammisalo T, Peltola J (1997). A 5-year prospective clinical study of AstraTech dental implants supporting fixed bridges or overdentures in the edentulous mandible. *Clin Oral Implants Res* **8**: 469–75.

Mericske-Stern R (1990). Clinical evaluation of overdenture restorations supported by osseointegrated titanium implants: a retrospective study. *Int J Oral Maxillofac Implants* **5**: 375–83.

Mericske-Stern R, Zarb GA (1993). Overdentures: an alternative implant methodology for edentulous patients. *Int J Prosthod* **6**: 203–8.

Naert I, Gizani S, Vuylsteke M, van Steenberghe D (1998). A 5-year randomised clinical trial on the influence of splinted and unsplinted oral implants in mandibular overdenture therapy. Part 1: Peri-implant outcome. *Clin Oral Implants Res* **9**: 170–7.

Palmqvist S, Sondell K, Swartz B (1994). Implant-supported maxillary overdentures: outcome in planned and emergency cases. *Int J Oral Maxillofac Implants* **9**: 184–90.

Wright PS, Watson RM (1998) Effect of prefabricated bar design with implant-stabilized prostheses on ridge resorption: a clinical report. *Int J Oral Maxillofac Implants* **13**: 77–81.

PART III

Surgery

7
Basic factors in implant surgery

Introduction

After planning, the surgical execution of implant placement is the next critical procedure in the attainment of successful osseointegrated implants. The most important factors to control in implant surgery are:

1. A sterile technique avoiding contamination of the implant surface.
2. Avoiding damage to the bone by thermal injury during the drilling process.
3. Careful preparation of the bone site so that the implant is stable at placement.
4. Placement of the implant in an aesthetically and functionally acceptable position.
5. Avoidance of excessive loading in the healing period. Some protocols advocate no loading for 3–6 months. Newer protocols that allow immediate loading depend upon very careful control of the magnitude of loading (see Chapter 1).

Poor control of these factors can lead to failure of osseointegration, which may be manifested subsequently as:

1. Infection at the implant site.
2. Implant mobility or the implant may be rotated when attempting to detach or attach a component.
3. Pain from inflammation in the bone surrounding the implant. This may be manifested as pain on pressure on the implant.
4. A radiolucent space surrounding the implant that is consistent with fibrous encapsulation. However, a failed implant may have a normal radiographic appearance.

Under these circumstances the failed implant would have to be removed and treatment recommenced or an alternative sought.

Avoidance of thermal injury to the bone

Bone cells will be damaged irreversibly if the temperature is raised in the bone to 47°C for more than 1 min. Bone cell death will result in more extensive resorption and failure of osseointegration. This is avoided by:

- careful cooling of the bone and drills with copious sterile saline
- use of sharp drills
- control of the cutting speed

Coolant is applied to the external surface of the drills or via the internal aspect in specially designed internal irrigation drills. The harder and more dense the bone, the more difficult it is to maintain adequate cooling. In situations where the bone is dense, the surgeon runs the risk of overheating the bone as the depth of the drilling increases. This can be minimized by accepting shorter implant preparations as advocated in the Straumann system or by improving the cooling efficiency of the bone preparation. The Frialit 2 system (Friatec AG, Mannheim, Germany), unlike the other systems described in this text, uses internally irrigated drills in addition to external irrigation (Figure 7.1). The drills are extremely efficient at cutting bone and the likelihood of burning the bone must be low, provided that the drills are replaced regularly (20 preparations) and care is taken to ensure that the irrigant solution is not blocked in its passage to the working tip.

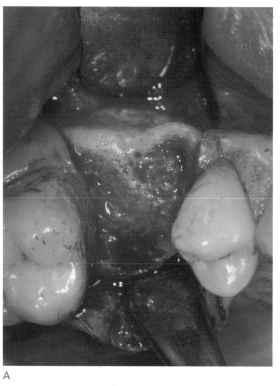

A

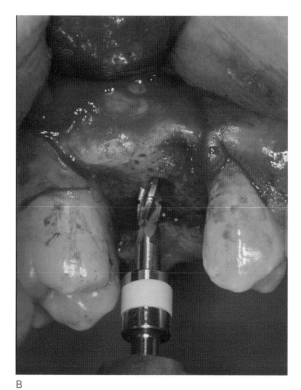

B

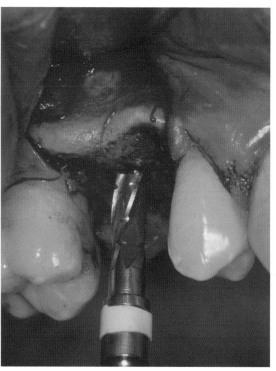

C

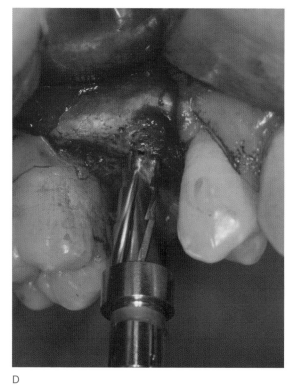

D

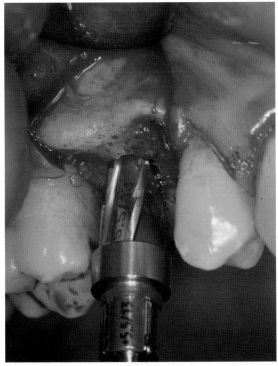

E

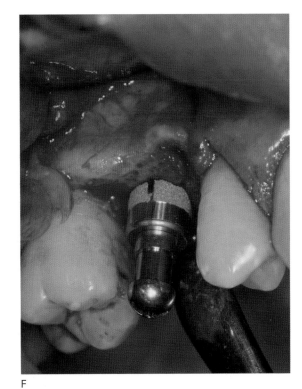

F

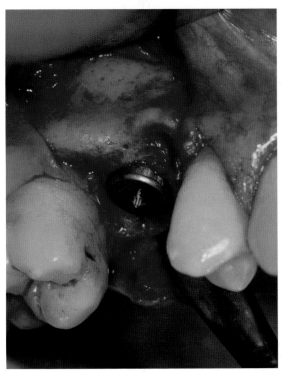

G

Figure 7.1

A series of photographs illustrating surgical preparation and placement of an implant with the Frialit 2 system. At all stages the drilling procedure is cooled by internal and external irrigation with sterile saline. (A) Buccal and palatal flaps have been raised to expose the bone at the upper second premolar site. (B) A 2-mm diameter twist drill is used to establish the initial angulation and depth of the site. The drill has cross-cut grooves showing the length of preparation. In most cases the site is started with a round bur that readily penetrates the outer cortex of bone. (C) A 3-mm diameter twist drill enlarges the site and confirms the depth to accept a 13-mm long Frialit 2 implant. (D) The first of the stepped Frialit drills enlarges the site to accept a 4.5-mm diameter implant. (E) The second of the Frialit stepped drills is used to enlarge the site to accept a 5.5-mm diameter implant. (F) A 13-mm long, 5.5-mm diameter Frialit 2 implant has been pushed into the site with the placement head (ball-shaped device on top of the implant). It is then gently but firmly tapped into place until all the plasma-sprayed surface is within bone. (G) The placement head is simply removed to reveal the sealing screw, which protects the inner part of the implant during the healing process.

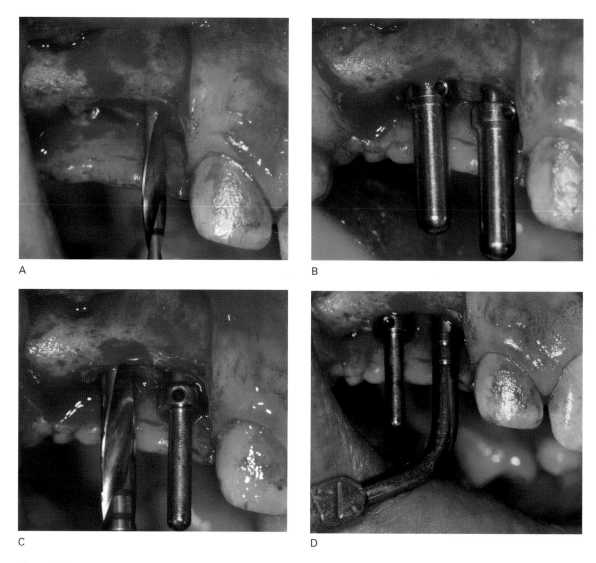

Figure 7.2

A series of photographs illustrating surgical preparation and placement of two implants with the Brånemark system (Nobel Biocare AB, Göteborg, Sweden). At all stages the drilling procedure is cooled by external irrigation with sterile saline. (A) Flaps have been raised to reveal the bone ridge. The initial entry point of the site has been achieved with a round bur. A 2-mm twist drill is used to establish the angulation and depth of the site. The drill is marked with black bands at the implant lengths. (B) The position and angulation of the two implant sites is verified with direction indicators. These should be viewed from various angles and checked against the surgical stent and the opposing teeth (by asking the patient to close and gently touch the indicators – they should be directed to the buccal cusps of the lower teeth). The angles can be adjusted slightly at this stage. (C) Provided that the position and angulation are satisfactory, the sites can be enlarged with a 3-mm twist drill following the same line. The surgeon is helped by reference to an indicator retained in the adjacent site and by using a pilot drill that enlarges the top part of the site from 2 mm to 3 mm. (D) Both sites have been drilled to 3 mm in diameter. A direction indicator is in the distal site and a measuring probe is being used to verify the depth of the anterior site. (E) The bone cortex is countersunk to accept the implant level with the bone crest. The level of countersinking is varied according to many factors, including available bone height, bone quality, interocclusal space, aesthetic demands and emergence profile of the planned restoration. It is helpful to judge this against the surgical stent. (F) The threaded implant is inserted using slow revolutions of the handpiece and is cooled with sterile saline irrigation. The implant is either a 'self-tapper' or the site is pre-tapped according to bone hardness and operator preference. (G) The

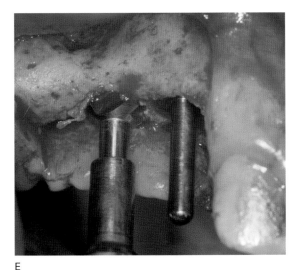

E

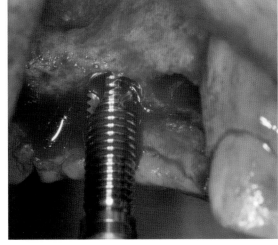

F

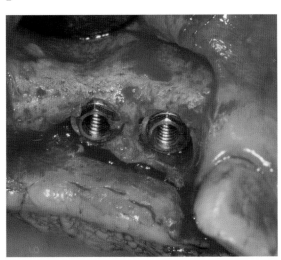

G

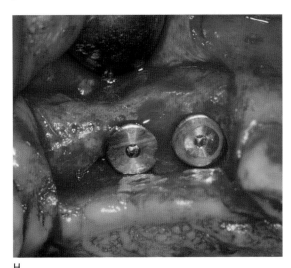

H

implants in place. They have at least 2 mm of intervening bone and about the same between the anterior implant and the adjacent tooth. (H) Cover screws have been placed on the implant heads to protect the inner aspect of the implant during healing. They are level with the surrounding bone. (I) The flaps are closed and the implants left buried for 3–6 months in the classical Brånemark two-stage submerged protocol.

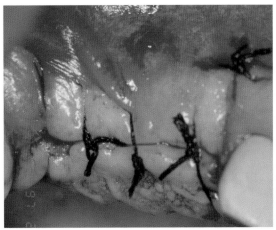

I

In all systems the implant site is prepared with small-diameter drills in the first place and then the site is gradually made larger with increasing-diameter drills (Figures 7.1 and 7.2). In addition to minimizing heat production, the initial use of small-diameter drills also allows modifications to the initial angle or site of preparation when required. The drills should be sharp. This is easier to ensure using new disposable drills for each case, as in the Nobel Biocare/Brånemark protocol, compared with the other systems considered in this book. However, the sophisticated design of the step-shaped internally irrigated drills in the Frialit system (see Figure 7.1) would be expensive to fabricate in a disposable form, therefore a record of the number of sites prepared (and the hardness of the bone) is useful in determining when drills should be replaced. This also applies to the Straumann and Astra systems.

The cutting speed of the drills during the main preparation of the sites is approximately 1500–2000 rpm. The flutes of twist drills may be clogged up with bone debris, and therefore it is important to withdraw them from the preparation site at regular intervals during the preparation process to wash away the debris and cool the drill. If the site needs to be tapped, as in the original Brånemark protocol, this is done at speeds comparable with those used to insert screw-threaded implants (approximately 20 rpm).

Ensuring good initial stability of the implant

The surgical preparation aims to provide an implant that feels stable following insertion. This can be judged by:

- simple clinical evaluation (dependent upon operator experience)
- torque insertion forces – these can be set on the drilling unit and are usually between 10 and 45 Ncm. Some units record the torque and provide a printout
- periotest values – the mobility can be measured with an electronic instrument that was originally designed to measure tooth mobility

- resonance frequency analysis – this latest device measures the stiffness of the implant within the bone through electronic vibration and recording

The last two methods have been used mainly in experimental studies but could find a clinical application. An implant that is loose within the prepared site will not osseointegrate. In the early phases of healing the implant must not be subjected to forces that will cause movement of the implant, even if the movement is small. It has been suggested that micromovement up to 100 µm may be compatible with healing by osseointegration, but beyond this fibrous encapsulation is more likely to occur. It is not possible to offer comparative data between implants in this respect. However, various approaches can be adopted to ensure a stable implant with the different implant systems. Initial stability of the implant depends upon:

1. Length of the implant
2. Diameter of the implant
3. Design of the implant
4. Surface configuration of the implant
5. Thickness of the bone cortex and how many cortices the implant engages
6. Density of the medullary bone trabeculation
7. Dimensions of the preparation site compared with that of the implant

The philosophy of what constitutes adequate implant length varies between systems. The original Brånemark concept was that of bicortical stabilization. This required that an implant extended from the superficial cortex of the edentulous ridge to the inferior cortex of the anterior mandible or the nasal floor or floor of the antrum in the maxilla. This is clearly not possible in the posterior mandible because of the presence of the inferior dental canal and in this situation shorter implants with unicortical fixation are used. Bicortical fixation is probably only advantageous in areas of poor bone quality in the medullary space. The Straumann system routinely uses shorter implants of 8–12 mm in length, and fixation and surface area are improved by using solid screws (hollow screw now only available for single tooth replacement) with surface treatments of either plasma-sprayed titanium or sand blasting and acid etching (see

Chapter 1). This type of implant may be a good choice for bridgework in the posterior mandible and posterior maxilla, where there may be little height of available bone.

There is one other important proviso about implant length, and that is to ensure that there is adequate vertical space when the patient opens his/her mouth to permit insertion of the planned length of implant together with its insertion device. The latter could include the handpiece head, handpiece connector and implant mount. Although many systems offer low-profile versions of these components, the length of the implant may be the most critical feature. This is not usually a problem for the anterior region of the mouth but is very important in the molar regions. Some systems such as Straumann have a gauge that can be used to assess this factor (Figure 7.3).

Most systems produce implants in wider diameters to improve stability and strength (see Chapter 4). The increased diameter provides an overall greater surface area and theoretically may provide the equivalent of bicortical stabilization by engaging both buccal and lingual cortices.

The Brånemark system implant has also been modified as an alternative approach to improve stabilization in areas of limited bone height and limited bone quality. The modification to the implant for poor quality bone has been to produce a slightly tapered implant with a double helical thread. This means that it requires half the number of rotations to seat it and it will cut more efficiently in softer bone. The surface of the implant is like the rest of the Brånemark system – machined – and therefore the response of the bone to the surface will presumably be the same, the only difference being a higher degree of initial stability.

The Frialit 2 system provides a different approach to this problem. The surface area of the implants is increased considerably by having a stepped cylinder design, a range of different diameters and a surface that is treated. The Frialit 2 push-fit implant can be used in practically all situations and may have advantages over a screw design in soft bone. The Frialit 2 is also available in a screw design. Each of the stepped cylinders has an individual thread and it only requires three rotations to ensure full seating of the implant. The threaded implant may have better initial stability in bone that is more dense and is partic-

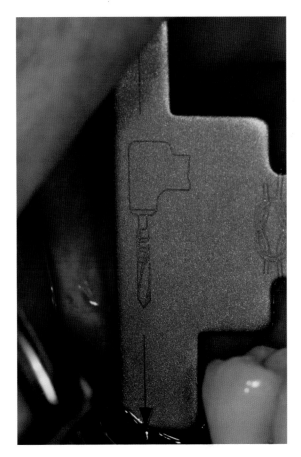

Figure 7.3

The Straumann measuring device is used to check that there is adequate inter-arch space to accommodate the handpiece and drill.

ularly recommended in immediate replacement protocols (see Chapter 11).

The initial stability of an implant can be improved easily by inserting an implant into a site that is prepared smaller than the implant. This approach is used in the AstraTech system to good effect (see Chapter 10, Figure 10.1). Therefore, when using a 3.5-mm diameter implant the site is routinely prepared to a diameter of 3.2 mm and the implant is self-tapped into position. If, however, the bone at the site is very dense, the surgeon is advised to prepare the site to a diameter of 3.35 mm. Similar recommendations are given with the 4-mm. diameter AstraTech implant, with twist drills of 3.7 and

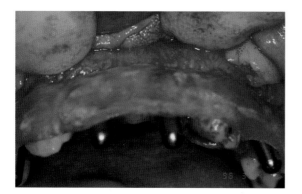

Figure 7.4

A rigid cold-cure acrylic stent reproducing the labial faces of the missing central incisors. Direction indicators have been placed in the initial preparation sites to assess against the stent.

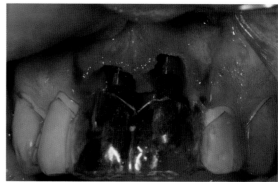

A

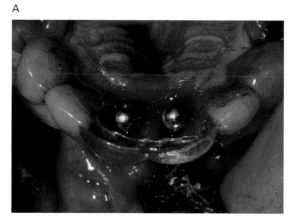

B

Figure 7.5

(A) A clear plastic 'blow down' stent constructed on a cast from the diagnostic set-up. It has been trimmed to follow the cervical margins of the teeth. With short edentulous spans these stents are rigid and stable enough, but the plastic is generally too flexible for longer spans. Direction indicators show the initial preparation sites. (B) An occlusal view of the stent, with direction indicators showing that the angle of the sites is through the cingulum region of the crowns, allowing screw retention of the restorations.

3.85 mm according to the available bone density. The AstraTech implant surface is blasted (with titanium oxide giving a 5-μm rough surface), which may do little to improve initial stability but has been shown to achieve higher bone-to-implant contact in the healing period compared with a machine surface. This is also true of the plasma-sprayed surfaces (Frialit and Straumann) and the SLA (Sand blasted–Large grit–Acid etched) surface of the Straumann.

Placement of the implant in an acceptable position

This is dealt with in considerable detail in the chapters on single teeth (Chapter 9) and fixed bridges (Chapter 10). Problems should be avoided by:

1. Careful planning
2. Use of surgical stents
3. Reviewing each stage of the preparation process

Surgical stents should be constructed using the diagnostic set-ups or provisional prosthesis. They should be rigid enough to prevent distortion and stable to minimize movement (Figure 7.4). Stents constructed in cold-cure acrylic using adjacent teeth for stability are ideal. The stent helps the surgeon with the mesiodistal positioning of the implant (avoiding placement in the embrasure spaces) and the buccolingual positioning and angulation. In replacing anterior teeth it is particularly important to provide the profile of the buccal aspect of the prosthesis, including the cervical margin, to give the planned emergence profile (Figure 7.5) in order to optimize aesthetics.

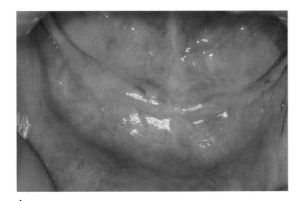

A

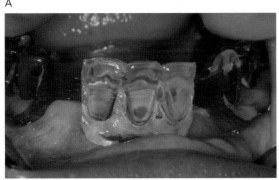

B

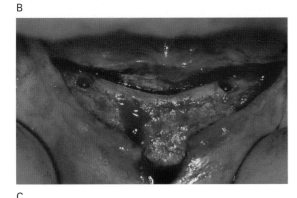

C

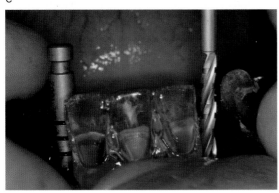

D

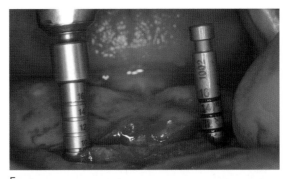

E

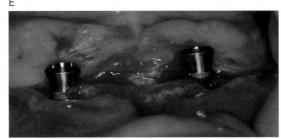

F

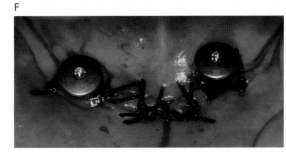

G

Figure 7.6

A series of photographs illustrating surgical preparation and placement of Straumann implants in a mandibular denture case. (A) The atrophic mandibular ridge with little keratinized mucosa. (B) A cold-cure acrylic stent has been constructed and tried in the mouth. The stent is a duplicate of the patient's denture, with slots cut in the regions of planned implant placement (right and left canine). At this stage it helps to plan the location and extent of the incisions. (C) Flaps have been raised and the sites started using a round bur to penetrate the hard cortex. The incision preserves keratinized tissue on the labial and lingual aspects. A midline labial incison helps initial reflection and reduces tension. (D) The stent in position with a depth gauge/indicator post in the patient's right side and a twist drill on the left side. The stent is removed to allow complete preparation of the site but is inserted at different stages to check on position and alignment. (E) The right site is being tapped and there is a depth indicator on the left side. Both show a depth of 10 mm, which is the planned insertion length of the solid-screw 4.1-mm diameter implants. (F) The implants have been placed with the polished collars above the bone crest. (G) Closure screws have been attached to the implants and the flaps have been sutured.

It is more difficult to provide a stable stent in an edentulous jaw. Under these circumstances the stent needs to be extended onto stable mucosa (which is more readily accomplished using the palate) but still allow access and retain stability once the mucoperiosteal flaps are raised. In completely edentulous jaws and long-span edentulous spaces it is important to construct stents in a material that is sufficiently rigid to retain its shape; if it was flexible it would compromise implant positioning (Figure 7.6).

The stages of placement can be reviewed using indicator posts in the prepared sites. These can be evaluated against the surgical stent (Figures 7.5 and 7.6). It is recommended that the surgeon reviews the angles of the indicator posts from various aspects. Failure to do so can lead to surprising errors.

The position of the indicator posts should also be reviewed in relation to the opposing dentition. In the buccal segments in a patient with a normal buccopalatal relationship, the maxillary indicator should be directed towards the buccal cusps of the lower teeth and the mandibular indicators towards the palatal cusps of the maxillary teeth. This ensures that the implant is placed in the central fossa area of the tooth and forces are directed down the long axis.

The level of the head of the implant should be placed to allow adequate vertical space from the opposing dentition and to produce good aesthetics. These important issues are dealt with in detail in the following chapters.

Preoperative care, anaesthesia and analgesia

Basic preoperative care should include:

1. Antiseptic rinsing of the oral cavity and perioral skin. Chlorhexidine gluconate (2% or 1.2% proprietary rinses for 1 min) is recommended.
2. Administration of analgesics. Oral analgesics (such as 200 or 400 mg of ibuprofen or a comparable alternative) are usually sufficient in most outpatient cases. Control of pain is more effective if analgesics are given prior to surgery and the levels maintained to prevent development of severe pain.
3. Administration of antibiotics. This used to be a routine procedure. Placement of one or a few implants under ideal circumstances probably does not warrant antibiotics. Where antibiotics are indicated (e.g. multiple implants where bone is exposed for long periods of time or grafting is carried out), the clinician could use a standard protocol (e.g. 3 g of amoxicillin preoperatively, followed by a 5-day course).

Antibiotic and analgesic regimes will differ according to the status of the patient, the viewpoint of the clinician and the country where the treatment is being carried out. It is therefore beyond the remit of this book.

Anaesthesia

Many cases can be managed satisfactorily with local anaesthesia, depending upon the skill and experience of the surgeon and the attitude of the patient. The magnitude and duration of implant surgery are considerably increased with multiple implant placement, especially where more than one quadrant is involved. As a general indication, it is worthwhile considering sedation techniques in procedures likely to exceed 1 h (e.g. the equivalent of the placement of three implants or more for the experienced operator). Prolonged difficult procedures and those requiring extensive grafting may require general anaesthesia.

Local anaesthesia has advantages over general anaesthesia. In particular the conscious patient is able to cooperate by performing normal jaw movements in centric and lateral excursions to help verify the appropriate implant positioning. The vasoconstrictor in the local anaesthetic is useful in providing improved haemostasis and prolonged analgesia. Longer acting local anaesthetics may be particularly useful in this type of surgery.

Basic flap design and soft-tissue handling

Some surgical texts describe implant placement without flap elevation but this can readily lead to lateral perforation of the bone in inexperienced hands. It is more suited to single implant placement directly into extraction sockets, and this is considered in Chapter 11. Flap design (see Chapter 8) and elevation should achieve complete exposure of the edentulous ridge, including any bone concavities and identification of important anatomical structures. The flap also should be closed easily with sutures under minimum tension, with incision lines based upon sound bone as in any good surgical practice.

Elevation of flaps is best accomplished using periosteal elevators with a fairly sharp edge, especially where the bone ridge is uneven. Fibrous and muscle attachments that tether the flap margins may need to be released by sharp dissection. Flaps should be elevated to allow good visualization of the ridge form but not excessive in opening tissue spaces unnecessarily. However, good reflection of the soft tissues on the lingual aspect of the lower premolars is advised because implant preparations in this area may inadvertently perforate the lingual plate in a natural concavity and damage a branch of the sublingual artery. This can result in extensive bleeding in the unreflected tissue that is not noticed by the surgeon and results in a deep-seated sublingual haematoma. This may present some time within 24 h postoperatively and has been reported to threaten the patient's airway.

Before closure of the flaps it is important to check that there is no residual bone debris or clot beneath the flaps by careful irrigation with sterile saline and inspection with suction. The flaps are carefully closed with sutures of the surgeon's choice, either non-resorbable or resorbable. In most cases, simple interrupted no. 4/0 black silk sutures are satisfactory. Vertical mattress sutures are recommended by some operators where a more secure seal is required, e.g. over a grafted site. Finer no. 7/0 polypropylene sutures (as used in plastic surgery) are recommended by others, in which case a larger number are required and fine suturing instruments are mandatory. However, the most important factor is to ensure that the wound closure is free of tension. In difficult cases requiring flap advancement, periosteal releasing incisions, vertical relieving incisions and stabilizing sutures remote from the wound edges can be helpful. Firm pressure with moist packs should be applied to re-adapt the flaps and control bleeding.

Basic postoperative care

Patients should be prescribed appropriate analgesics, antibiotics if indicated and a chlorhexidine mouthrinse. They should be advised to use ice packs to reduce swelling and bruising, which does not usually occur with simple cases. Postoperative pain should not be severe. Pain should not arise from the bone because this would indicate poor technique and damage, possibly leading to failure. Surgery close to the inferior dental nerve may result in transient altered sensation and the patient should be made aware of this possibility.

In many cases patients are advised not to wear their removable dentures for 1–2 weeks in order to avoid pressure on the wound and implants. This requirement is probably still valid with implant surgery in the edentulous mandible. It is acceptable for the patient to wear a removable denture after surgery with placement of a small number of implants, where swelling is less likely and there is good wound and denture stability. However, the denture normally needs to be relieved and a soft lining added. The patient should be seen 1 week later for suture removal and further adjustment to their denture if required. Patients who are provided with a fixed provisional prosthesis have an advantage in this respect, but may need adjustment to the undersurface of the pontics to accommodate soft-tissue changes.

Bibliography

Brånemark PI, Zarb GA, Albrektsson T, eds (1985). *Osseointegration in Clinical Dentistry*. Chicago: Quintessence Publishing.

ten Bruggenkate CM, Krekeler G, Kraaijenhagen HA, Foitzik C, Osterbeek HS (1993). Haemorrhage of the floor of the mouth resulting from lingual perforation during implant placement: a clinical report. *Int J Oral Maxillofac Implants* **8**: 329–34.

Eriksson RA, Albrektsson T (1984). The effect of heat on bone regeneration: an experimental study in the rabbit using the bone growth chamber. *J Oral Maxillofac Surg* **42**: 705–11.

Eriksson RA, Adell R (1986). Temperatures during drilling for the placement of implants using the osseointegration technique. *J Oral Maxillofac Surg* **44**: 4–7.

Ivanoff CJ, Sennerby L, Lekholm U (1996). Influence of initial implant mobility on the integration of titanium implants: an experimental study in rabbits. *Clin Oral Implants Res* **7**: 120–7.

Jaffin R, Berman C (1991). The excessive loss of Brånemark fixtures in type IV bone. *J Periodontol* **62**: 2–4.

Lekholm U (1998). Surgical considerations and possible shortcomings of the host sites. *J Prosth Dent* **79**: 43–8.

Meredith N (1998). Assessment of implant stability as a prognostic determinant. *Int J Prosthod* **11**: 491–501.

8
Flap design for implant surgery

Introduction

This chapter deals primarily with flap design for partially dentate cases, describing most examples in the aesthetic zone for single implant placement. The same principles are applicable to larger edentulous spaces. The last section briefly describes some aspects of flap design in the edentulous jaw.

Flap design in the aesthetic zone

Some surgical texts describe implant placement without flap elevation but this can readily lead to lateral perforation of the bone in inexperienced hands. It is more suited to single implant placement directly into extraction sockets, which is considered in Chapter 11. Flap design and elevation should achieve adequate exposure of the ridge, including any bone concavities, and identify important anatomical structures. The flap also should be closed easily with sutures under minimum tension, with incision lines based upon sound bone as in any good surgical practice.

A midcrestal incision can be employed in most cases. The incision can be extended within the gingival crevices of adjacent teeth (Figure 8.1A) and the mucoperiosteum can be elevated quite extensively in an apical direction to allow adequate visualization of the bone contour.

However, in most cases we advocate the use of relieving incisions to aid flap reflection and exposure (Figure 8.2). The relieving incisions next to teeth require particular attention. The incisions can be kept vertical and parallel overlying sound bone so that, on closure, the flap's

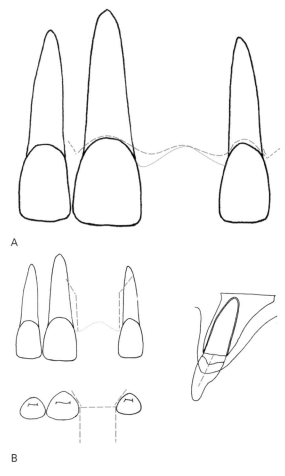

A

B

Figure 8.1

(A) An incision on the crest of the edentulous ridge is extended in the gingival crevices of the adjacent teeth to allow adequate exposure of the ridge. (B) A normal incisor space with a midcrestal incision. The vertical relieving incisions on sound bone are flared at their apical extent. The relieving incisions extend a short distance into the palatal mucosa to allow adequate elevation.

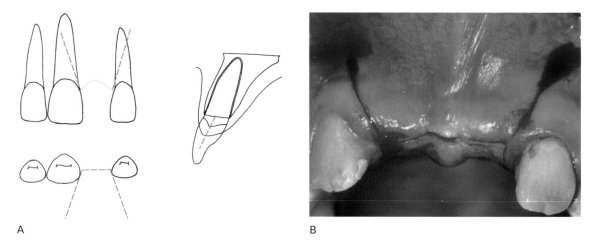

A

B

Figure 8.2

(A) It is advised to avoid placing oblique relieving incisions over prominent root surfaces because recession may result if there is an underlying bony dehiscence. A broad base to the flap is not necessary for survival because the blood supply and nutrient bed for mucosal flaps are excellent. (B) A midcrestal incision leaving papillae *in situ*. The oblique relieving incisions do not pass over the adjacent root surfaces.

nutrition is not compromised. The apical extent can be flared if improved in visualization of the apical bone contour is needed. It is important to avoid placing obliquely inclined relieving incisions over prominent root surfaces, because the wound can break down if there are underlying bone dehiscences and gingival recession can result (Figure 8.1B).

On placing relieving incisions or reflecting the flaps, care should be taken to protect important anatomical structures such as the mental nerve. Elevation of flaps over the incisive canal region has minimal consequences in terms of resulting paraesthesia, and bleeding is seldom a problem. Short relieving incisions into the palate are also helpful and do not need to be extended so far as to cut any major vessels.

Where there is little keratinized tissue it is sometimes useful to locate the crestal incision towards the palatal aspect in the maxillary arch, which has considerably more keratinized tissue as it extends onto the palate (Figure 8.3). This design is also a useful strategy in cases where bone augmentation procedures may be required on the labial aspect, to ensure adequate wound closure remote from any implant surfaces, graft materials or GBR membranes. However, in these latter cases it is probably prudent to place reliev-

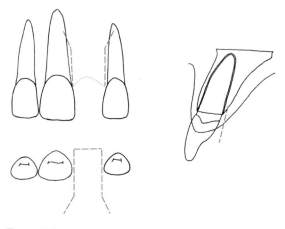

Figure 8.3

The crestal incision has been made on the palatal aspect of the ridge. Reflection of the flap may be slightly more difficult and the wound margins are more remote from the implant head. This was once considered to be important in submerged implant surgery.

ing incisions at least one tooth, lateral to the area of augmentation treatment (Figure 8.4).

The main controversy in flap design for single tooth implants is whether to involve and reflect

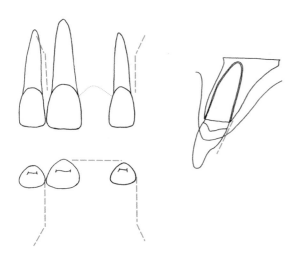

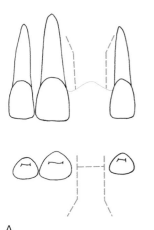

Figure 8.4

If augmentation procedures are thought to be required, it is prudent to base incision lines more remotely to avoid exposure of grafted materials. The relieving incisions have therefore been made one tooth wide, laterally on each side, and the crestal incision has been made towards the palatal side.

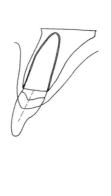

Figure 8.5

(A) The wide central incisor space allows an adequate width flap to be developed in the middle of the space, while allowing preservation of the papillae. (B) A clinical example showing preservation of the papillae on the adjacent teeth in this wide central incisor space. The flap design and reflection have provided good visualization of the bone during implant insertion. (C) The same case with the flap nicely approximated with just two crestal sutures. Relieving incisions may require suturing if they tend to gape.

A

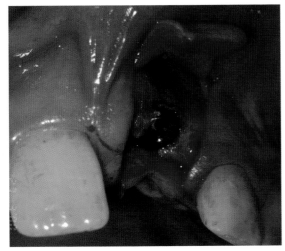

B

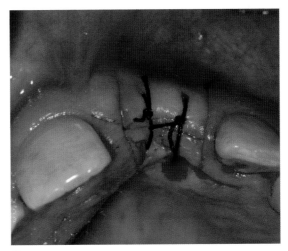

C

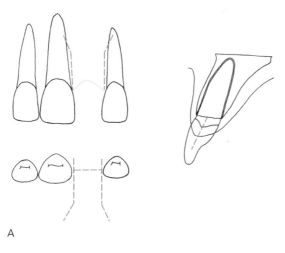

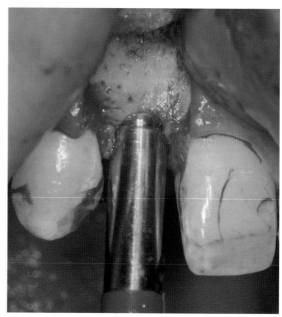

Figure 8.6

(A) The narrower incisor space (as is often the case with lateral incisors) does not allow an adequate width of flap and avoidance of disturbing the proximal papillae, which are routinely raised in this flap design. (B) A narrow maxillary lateral incisor is being replaced with a narrow-platform 3.3-mm diameter Nobel Biocare implant. The flap design has elevated all the soft tissue in the space and the parallel labial relieving incisions are at the line angles of the adjacent teeth.

the adjacent papillae or not. Avoidance of papilla reflection aims to preserve the aesthetics of these structures which are difficult or impossible to reconstruct if lost (Figure 8.5).

However, in many cases the single tooth space is narrow mesiodistally and elevation of the papillae may be unavoidable (Figure 8.6). If one can only preserve a narrow strip of soft tissue on the proximal surfaces of the adjacent teeth, it may have its blood supply compromised to such an extent that full reflection of the tissue would be no more damaging. The present authors have routinely elevated papillae as in the flap design shown in Figures 8.1 and 8.5, with no detriment to the soft-tissue profile subsequently. We would therefore recommend:

1. In sites that are less than or equal to 7 mm mesiodistally, to reflect the papillae.
2. In sites that are 8 mm or greater, a mesiodistal crestal incision of 5–6 mm will allow non-reflection of an adequate width of papillary tissue to recommend the technique.

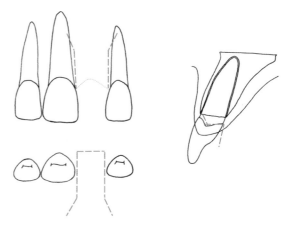

Figure 8.7

Where the soft tissue of the ridge is thick, a split-thickness incision can be employed that produces a 'halving joint'. This is designed to minimize the chance of breakdown of the incision but can only be made in thick tissue where this problem is less likely to occur anyway.

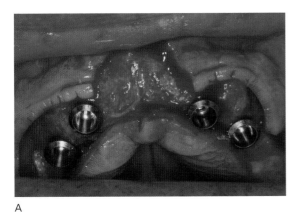

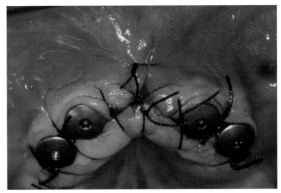

A   B

Figure 8.8

(A) Flap design in the edentulous maxilla being treated with non-submerged Straumann implants. The crestal incision has been made towards the palatal aspect of the planned placement site. This allows retention of more keratinized tissue on the buccal aspects of the implants. A midline labial relieving incision helps flap reflection and lengthens the flap margin to improve adaptation around the implant collars. (B) The flaps are sutured with simple re-adaptation and no resection of tissue.

3. If doubt exists as to the need to expose anatomical structures such as the incisive nerve or if augmentation techniques may be indicated, then the wider flap design incorporating papillae is again recommended.

The incisions described above are simple incisions through epithelium, connective tissue and periosteum down to bone. More sophisticated incision lines can be used where the tissue is thick in order to produce overlapping flap margins rather than a simple butt joint (Figure 8.7). This requires incision through the epithelium at one point, horizontal extension of the incision in the midzone of the connective tissue and a vertical incision down through the periosteum. The resulting 'halving joint' may provide more secure coverage in areas where bone augmentation is planned.

Additional considerations in edentulous jaws

As described in the previous section, a midcrestal incision can be employed in most cases. Where there is little keratinized tissue, e.g. in the case of the resorbed edentulous mandible, it is recommended that the incision is made in the middle of this tissue to retain some keratinized mucosa on each side of the wound. The maxillary arch has considerably more keratinized tissue as it extends onto the palate, and it is sometimes useful to locate the crestal incision towards the palatal aspect. This strategy can be used to relocate more keratinized tissue on the buccal surface of the non-submerged implant (or the same at abutment connection surgery).

In the edentulous maxilla or mandible, a midline labial relieving incision extending into the sulcus enables the surgeon to elevate under the periosteum more easily, especially where the crest of the ridge is knife-edged or uneven. The relieving incision also reduces tension on the buccal flap, making retraction much easier (Figure 8.8).

Flap design in abutment connection surgery

Flap design for abutment connection surgery is important because it gives the surgeon a chance to modify the soft-tissue profiles. Many of the points raised also apply to handling of the flaps in single-stage non-submerged implant surgery.

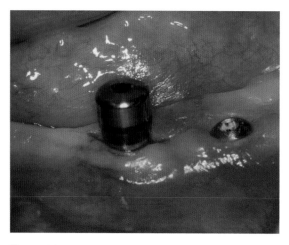

Figure 8.9

Small incisions over an AstraTech implant allow connection of a healing abutment. The implant to the right has
the cover screw exposed.

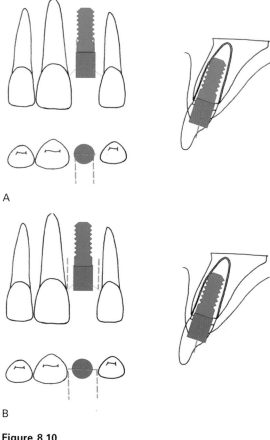

A

B

Figure 8.10

(A) The relieving incisions are made at the line angles of
the abutments and may subsequently break down. (B) The
more remote relieving incisions are more likely to heal
uneventfully and do not generally compromise the papillary form.

In general, incisions are made directly over the
implant heads unless the surgeon wishes to
relocate some of the available keratinized tissue
more on one aspect than the other. In severely
resorbed jaws with minimal keratinized tissue it
is important to preserve it all, and in some cases
soft-tissue grafting may be required. Small crestal
incisions over the implant head and minimal soft-
tissue reflection to allow abutment connection
are easier with systems that have an internal
abutment/implant connection such as AstraTech
(Figure 8.9). In the Brånemark system, we would
generally advocate more extensive exposure of
the implant head to facilitate abutment connection, and to allow visual checking of the fit prior
to radiographic verification. In some cases bone
grows over the implant head and this has to be
removed with small hand chisels (our preference), burs or purpose-designed mills, taking
care not to damage the implant. More flap reflection is required if bone removal is needed, including the use of relieving incisions. It is important
to have relieving incisions remote from the edges
of the transmucosal abutment (or collar of a non-
submerged implant) where the wound may break
down at these points because the flap margins
are not based upon sound tissue (Figure 8.10).

In some circumstances the initial straight-line
incision can be closed around the abutments
without resecting/reshaping tissue, provided that
a good soft-tissue profile is achieved. This is
easier where the mucosa is relatively thin or
elastic. In other circumstances the flaps need to
be reshaped by making curved incisions to
match the shape of the abutments. Instead of
simply excising this tissue, it is often worthwhile
adopting the strategy described by Palacci, of
retaining the attachment of this tissue at one end
and rotating it around the abutment to ensure

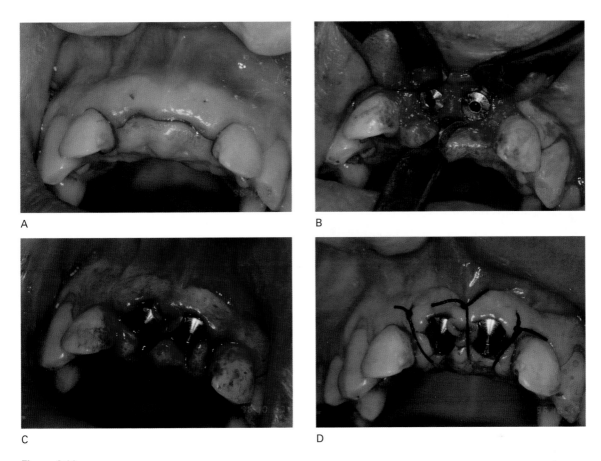

Figure 8.11

A series of clinical illustrations of abutment connection surgery. (A) A crestal incision over the heads of the implants extends just into the crevice of the adjacent teeth. (B) Good flap reflection has allowed removal of bone, which has grown over the cover screws, with a hand chisel. (C) The flaps are re-adapted around healing abutments. The flaps are reshaped and the tissue that would normally be excised is preserved and rotated between the healing abutments. (D) The flaps are closed with simple interrupted sutures.

good coverage of the bone (Figure 8.11). This will aid the soft-tissue profile but will not necessarily produce papillary height between adjacent abutments as originally described. Papillary form is more dependent on the presence of natural adjacent teeth with good gingival attachment on the proximal surface and careful development of adjacent emerging crown profiles.

The healing abutment length should be chosen so that it just emerges through the soft tissue and does not require too much modification of the provisional prosthesis. There has been a vogue for advocating different width healing abutments to match the size of the tooth being replaced, thereby developing a more appropriate soft-tissue form at an early stage. However, the width of the healing abutment can be extreme and can compromise the soft-tissue profile. We would advocate using healing abutments that are slightly narrower than the tooth being replaced and then 'stretching' the tissue with the final or provisional prosthesis.

Conclusion

This chapter has simply dealt with the issue of flap design. Suturing and postoperative care were dealt with in Chapter 7. The following chapters deal with the finer points of implant placement.

Bibliography

Palacci P, Ericsson I (2000). *Esthetic implant dentistry: soft and hard tissue management.* Chicago: Quintessence Publishing.

9

Surgical placement of the single tooth implant in the anterior maxilla

Introduction

This chapter deals with some of the most important issues of implant placement that are directly applicable to Chapter 10 on fixed bridgework. Single tooth restorations may be the most aesthetically demanding of all implant restorations because they are most frequently used to replace maxillary anterior teeth where they can be judged against adjacent natural teeth. In order to produce the optimum aesthetics the restoration should emerge from the soft tissue at the same level and contour as the natural teeth. This is facilitated by good pre-existing soft tissue and bone contours, meticulous planning, precise positioning of the implant at surgery and a high standard of prosthodontics. The ideal situation is where there has been no or minimal bone loss and the soft tissues are perfectly contoured around the adjacent natural teeth.

Controlling variables in implant placement

All implant placement relies upon a good three-dimensional perspective by the operator. There are relatively few variables that affect this:

1. Mesiodistal positioning
2. Buccolingual positioning
3. Angulation of the long axis of the implant
4. Vertical positioning of the implant head

All of these variables are easier to consider when judged against a surgical stent that provides information on the position and shape of the labial face of the restoration. A typical sequence of single tooth implant surgery is illustrated in Figure 9.1.

Mesiodistal and buccolingual positioning

These are decided upon with the initial penetration of the drill into the bone site (Figure 9.1D). The mesiodistal positioning is relatively straightforward and in most instances will be in the middle of the single tooth gap (Figure 9.2), unless there is planned spacing to accommodate a wider diastema on one side of the restoration.

However, in many instances bone resorption will affect the buccolingual position of the ridge and the angulation, factors that are more difficult to cope with, especially for the inexperienced clinician (Figure 9.3). The site also may be affected by localized ridge defects or the presence of anatomical structures such as the incisive canal (Figure 9.4).

Buccolingual angulation of the implant

The implant can be placed in the same long axis as the crown. This is shown in the clinical series (Figure 9.5) and diagrammatically in Figure 9.6A, where the implant/crown has been placed at the average angle from the Frankfurt plane of 110°. The long axis of the implant and abutment passes through the incisal tip of the crown. This is a common situation and dictates that the

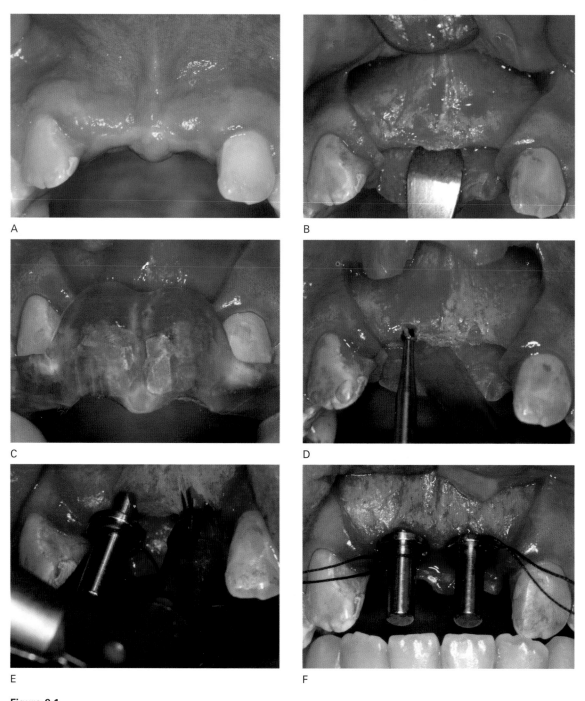

Figure 9.1

A series of photographs showing the placement of two AstraTech single tooth (ST) implants to replace both maxillary central incisors. (A) The preoperative situation showing good ridge form. (B) Buccal and palatal flaps have been elevated. (C) A cold-cure acrylic stent has been tried to assess the position of the labial faces of the central incisors to the underlying ridge. (D) The outer cortex of the ridge is penetrated with a round bur in the appropriate mesiodistal and buccolingual positions. (E) The angulation of the sites is developed with twist drills of increasing dimensions. This is the first twist drill of 2.5 mm in

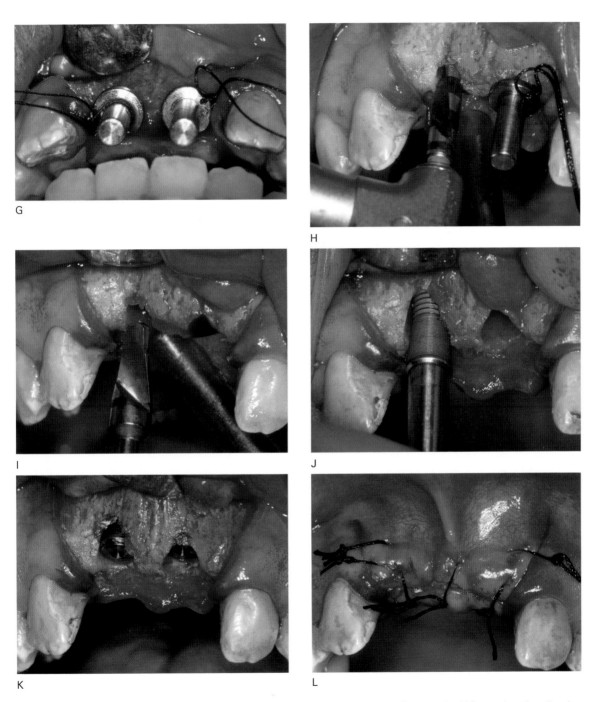

diameter. Changes to the angulation can be made at the early stages of drilling. Reference should be made using direction indicators (in patient's right site) and the stent. (F) and (G) Direction indicators (with safety sutures attached) placed in both sites. (H) After establishing that the site positions and angulations are satisfactory, the sites are enlarged with a 3.2-mm twist drill. (I) The sites are prepared with a conical drill to accept the conical head of the ST implant. (J) The ST implant is inserted, initially by hand on the implant inserter and then using a handpiece at slow revolutions. (K) The implants have been placed with their heads just below the crest of the bone. This is to allow a good emergence profile of the central incisors, which are quite wide compared with the implant head (4.5 mm). (L) Closure of the flaps in this submerged two-stage protocol.

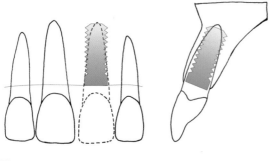

Figure 9.2

The implant is placed in the middle of the gap of the tooth it is replacing, in the same position as the root would have been. This is also indicated in the lateral view in this ideal-istic situation where minimal or no bone loss has occurred.

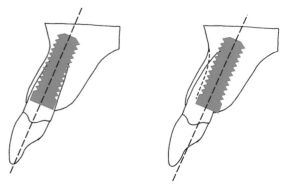

Figure 9.3

The diagram on the left shows an implant in the long axis of the root in an ideal situation. The more common situa-tion is illustrated in the diagram on the right, where the implant has been positioned palatally as the ridge has resorbed in this direction. The angulation of the implant has been maintained and now passes through the cingu-lum of the incisor such that a screw-retained retrievable restoration would be possible. There is, however, suffi-cient bone volume to allow proclination of the implant so that the angle passes through the incisal tip.

crown is cemented to the abutment. In some cases the profile of the bone ridge dictates a more labial inclination of the implant.

In Figure 9.6B the implant has been angled a further 10° labially, with the crown maintaining its previous position/angulation. The long axis now passes labial to the incisal edge and produces a slight crown/implant angulation that mimics the crown/root angulation seen in many natural incisor teeth. This angulation may produce very good aesthetics, giving a natural form and prominence to the labial cervical margin similar to the adjacent teeth, i.e. an optimum emergence profile (Figures 9.7 and 9.8). Increased labial angulation (Figure 9.6C) by a further 10° will still produce a restorable aesthetic solution, but beyond this the restora-tive problems will increase to a point where it may be impossible to provide an acceptable restoration (Figure 9.6D).

In contrast, resorption of the bone ridge towards the palate may promote more palatal angulation of the implant. Figure 9.9 shows progressive 10° angulations of the implant towards the palate. Up to 10° palatal angulation

there is little compromise, although there will be a tendency towards a less favourable buccal cervical contour/emergence profile. As the palatal angulation increases there will be a need to make up the loss of cervical contour by progressive ridge lapping of the restoration. This results in a restoration that does not emerge from the soft tissues but a ridge lap that 'sits' on the tissues in a similar way to a conventional pontic in fixed prosthodontics (Figure 9.10). The only advantage of the palatally angled implant is the possibility of access to the abutment screw through the cingulum of the restoration permit-ting a screw-retained restoration rather than a cemented one. The screw-retained design of single tooth restoration is less important than it used to be because of lower incidences of abutment screw loosening (through better design and adequate tightening of abutment screws using controlled torque devices).

Figures 9.6 and 9.9 would suggest that an acceptable angle would be between 20° proclined and 10° retroclined to the 'ideal/ normal' long axis. Angulations outside these parameters will compromise the aesthetics and

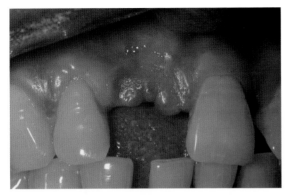

A

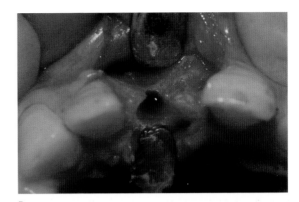

B

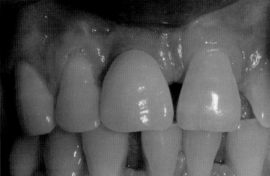

C

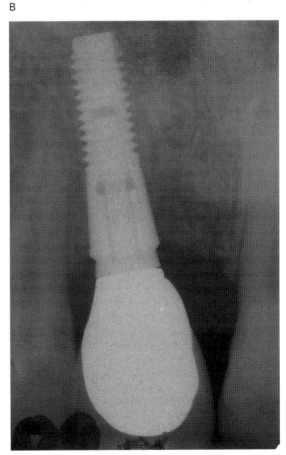

D

Figure 9.4

A series of photographs illustrating the effects of palatal placement of the implant. (A) A patient with a missing maxillary central incisor. (B) Flaps have been raised and the implant site prepared in the available bone. It is slightly palatal because of loss of labial bone, and slightly distal because of the presence of a prominent incisive nerve canal. (C) The completed result showing satisfactory aesthetics, but with the implant crown slightly ridge lapped to compensate for the palatal placement. (D) A radiograph of the completed case showing bone levels at the top of this AstraTech single tooth (ST) implant.

test the skills of the prosthodontist to the limit where the implant is unrestorable or aesthetically unacceptable. The following points should help to avoid this situation:

1. Good preoperative assessment and planning
2. Grafting of sites where these difficulties are predicted
3. Utilization of surgical stents and guide pins at

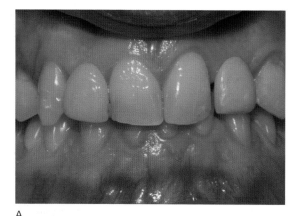

A

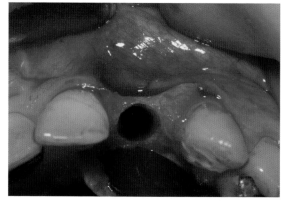

B

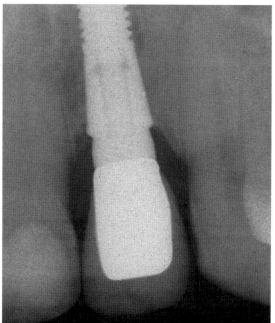

C

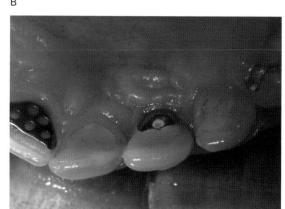

D

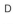

E

Figure 9.5

A series showing replacement of a maxillary lateral incisor with an AstraTech single tooth (ST) implant where the implant angle is through the incisal tip. (A) Initial presentation showing that left and right maxillary lateral incisors had been replaced previously with resin-retained bridges. The left bridge had failed and is being replaced with an implant restoration. (B) Preparation of the site is complete. There has been little labial resorption, allowing very good placement and an angulation that passes close to the incisal tip. (C) The completed case showing good aesthetics and emergence profile of the implant crown. (D) Palatal view of the cemented implant crown, showing normal contour and a small vent hole to allow escape of excess cement. (E) Radiograph of completed case, showing bone at the top of the implant and the good emergence profile of the restoration.

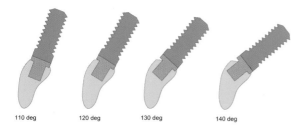

Figure 9.6

Implants drawn at various angles from the Frankfurt plane, with 110° considered to be the average root angulation in a class I incisor relationship. The crown of the restoration has not had its angulation changed, and in each case the implant and abutment have been progressively labially inclined by 10° increments.

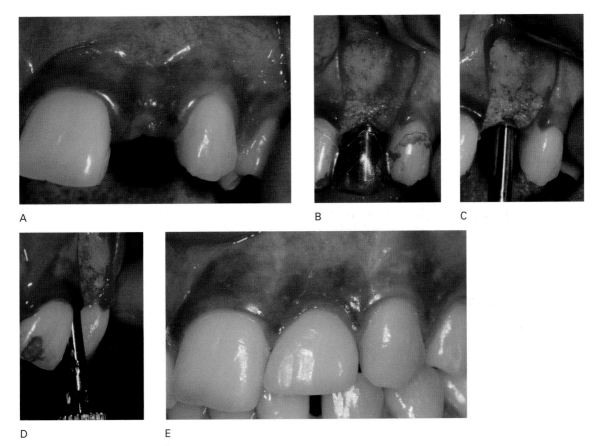

Figure 9.7

A series showing replacement of a maxillary lateral incisor with labial angulation of the implant. (A) The wide missing lateral incisor space. (B) The stent in place, with a direction indicator in the initially prepared site. (C) The implant has been inserted and the inserting device is still connected. The midlabial part of the implant shows a very small (1-mm) dehiscence and the proximal sides are just below the crest of the interdental bone. (D) A side view of the implant inserter showing quite marked labial angulation of the implant, corresponding to a line through the midlabial point of the crown. It is also apparent that the natural teeth have a pronounced crown/root angulation. (E) The completed result showing good aesthetics of this cemented implant crown.

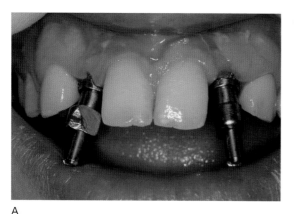

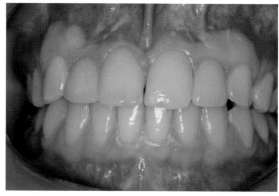

A   B

Figure 9.8

Replacement of both maxillary lateral incisors in a young patient. (A) This photograph shows the impression copings on the implants during the prosthodontic phase. There is a labial angulation of both implants compared with the adjacent natural teeth. (B) The completed result showing good emergence profiles.

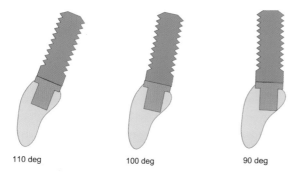

110 deg   100 deg   90 deg

Figure 9.9

Implants are drawn at various angles from the Frankfurt plane, with 110° considered to be the average root angulation in a class I incisor relationship. The crown of the restoration has not had its angulation changed, and in each case the implant and abutment have been progressively palatally inclined by 10° increments.

each stage of the preparation to check on angulation and vertical positioning of the implant head

The above guidelines are approximate (and relatively crude 10° increments) and each case should be judged on its own merits, particularly with regard to patients who have pronounced natural crown root angulations and/or class 2 or 3 incisal relationships.

A difficult angulation problem encountered at the time of surgery may be reduced by preparing the initial entry site of the implant towards the palatal, which would allow a change in angulation and keep the implant preparation within the bone contour.

An alternative strategy is available with the Straumann system, which produces an implant with an angle at the head of the implant of 15° that mimics a natural crown/root angulation (see Chapter 1). This implant is a push-fit design so that the angled aspect can be positioned at the exact required plane.

Vertical positioning of the implant head

Figure 9.2 shows a frontal view of the ideal arrangement of the implant in the middle of the space in the long axis of the tooth with the head

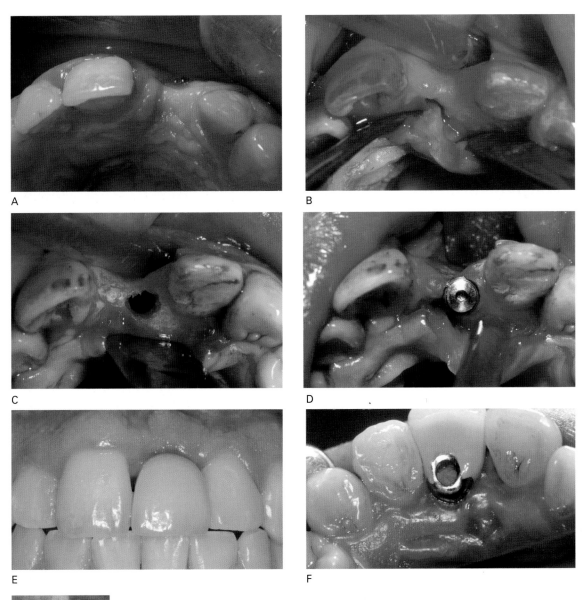

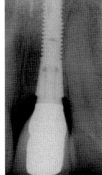

Figure 9.10

A series showing marked palatal positioning of an implant replacing a maxillary central incisor. (A) Occlusal view of the ridge form showing labial concavity. (B) Elevation of the flaps reveals a large incisive canal, further compromising the site. (C) The site has been prepared in the available bone volume without compromising adjacent structures. (D) An AstraTech single tooth (ST) implant has been placed. (E) The completed result showing compromised aesthetics because of the palatal positioning of the implant. The crown is ridge lapped. The area would have required a moderate-sized graft to overcome this. The patient was prepared to accept the compromise, particularly as the cervical area did not show during normal function. (F) Palatal view of the completed case, showing the access hole to the abutment screw. The crown is cemented to a standard abutment, but the crown/abutment assembly could be removed or the abutment screw tightened through this access hole. (G) Radiograph of completed case showing good contour/mergence in this plane, concealing the ridge lap profile in the buccopalatal plane.

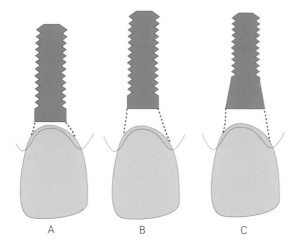

Figure 9.11

Labial view of emergence profile contours from implants placed at different vertical levels apical to the desired restoration. (A) Very abrupt profile. (B) The more ideal profile. (C) The profile has been altered by maintaining the vertical level but increasing the diameter of the head of the implant.

of the implant 3 mm apical to the cervical/gingival margin of the restoration. There should be little variation in the angle of the implant in this plane and most of the variation relates to the vertical level of the head of the implant. The distance of 3 mm between implant head and adjacent tooth cement/enamel junction is quoted because it usually allows a smooth transition of restoration profile from an implant of average diameter (4 mm) to the natural crown contour/dimensions of maxillary central incisors or canines (Figure 9.5E). An implant head that is too close to the crown (Figure 9.11A) will necessitate an abrupt, highly angulated profile and the possibility of unaesthetic exposure of the abutment or implant head. An implant head that is located further apically will allow a very

smooth transition profile (Figures 9.11B and 9.1K), but if this is too extreme it will produce less favourable restoration/implant height ratios. The deeply placed implant head may be more difficult for the prosthodontist to deal with and failure to maintain soft-tissue height will compromise the aesthetics.

The emergence profile therefore depends upon:

1. The size of the crown to be replaced
2. The diameter of the implant/abutment
3. The vertical distance between implant and crown cervical margin

In systems such as the Frialit 2, an implant diameter can be selected to match more closely the size of the tooth it is replacing. The vertical level of the implant is still very important to maintain soft-tissue aesthetics.

Conclusions

It should be clear from the preceding discussions and diagrams that the angulation, buccolingual position and the vertical level of the implant head have a marked effect on the contour and aesthetics of the single tooth restoration. It is very important that the clinician who is surgically placing the implant has a thorough appreciation of these factors. The utilization of a stent indicating the labial aspect of the planned restoration will help to avoid many of the potential problems, particularly for the inexperienced operator. The placement of an implant in an unrestorable or unaesthetic position must be avoided and in situations where the bone profile, position or quantity is compromised, grafting should be carried out to correct this, ideally as a separate procedure prior to implant placement (see Chapter 12).

10
Implant placement for fixed bridgework

Introduction

The planning and placement of implants for fixed bridgework follows the basic rules set out for those described in the chapter on single teeth (Chapter 9) but with more complications of site selection, the relationship between adjacent implants and their relationship to the planned prosthesis. Ideally all of these factors will have been resolved in the planning phase, with careful matching of the radiographic data, diagnostic set-ups and clinical verification. However, despite the most careful planning there are occasions when modifications have to be made at surgery and it is under these circumstances that it is advantageous if the surgeon has knowledge of the prosthodontic implications, either through his/her own experience or through that of an attending prosthodontic specialist.

The requirements for surgical stents, anaesthesia, flap design and soft-tissue handling are dealt within the chapter on basic surgery (Chapter 7).

Implant positioning and installation

When placing multiple implants it is especially helpful to be able to refer to a written plan of site location, estimated implant length and implant diameter and relevant radiographs and study casts. Following elevation of the flaps the surgical stent is tried in and referred to at various stages during the site development. The proposed sites of the implants are marked in the cortical bone with a round bur. The initial positioning is checked against adjacent teeth and anatomical structures, tooth positions on the stent, bone contour at the site and implant spacing. Spacing is required between adjacent implants (and implants and teeth) for an adequate width of bone (at least 1 mm and preferably 2 mm) and an adequate zone of soft tissue (2–3 mm). The angulation of the site is then developed with a twist drill. Remember that modifications to the position and angle can be made only at the early stages of the preparation process (e.g. the 2-mm twist drill stage). The length of the site is then established and the system protocol is followed with increasing diameters of drills until the preparation is complete and the implant can be placed (Figure 10.1).

Implant spacing in multiple implant placement

This was dealt with in some detail in the planning chapters (Chapters 4 and 5) but it is helpful to remind the surgeon with appropriate illustrations. The spacing requirements will vary with the system being used. In cases treated with the Brånemark system (Figure 10.2), the standard implants used are 3.75 or 4 mm in diameter in the threaded portion and 4 mm in diameter at the implant head. The routine recommendation is to place implants at a 7-mm centre-to-centre spacing, which would allow a 3-mm bone width between the outer surfaces of the implants. As described above, this can be reduced to as little as 1 mm at the bone level. However, this may not give sufficient soft-tissue width in many

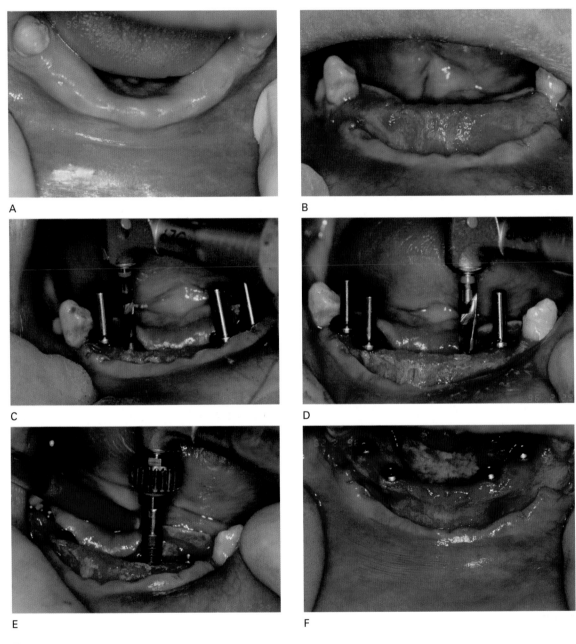

Figure 10.1

A series of photographs illustrating placement of AstraTech implants in the anterior mandible in a patient with severe hypodontia. (A) The preoperative view of the anterior mandible. (B) Flaps have been raised buccally and lingually to reveal the ridge form. The location of the mental nerve is checked radiographically and clinically. (C) The four implant sites are prepared with a 2.5-mm twist drill, following perforation of the cortex with a round bur. Direction indicators are placed sequentially in the prepared sites to help the surgeon maintain an acceptable degree of parallelism. The direction indicator posts should be checked against the stent and the opposing dentition. The widths of the indicator posts also give information about the diameter of the implants and the spacing between them. (D) Once the surgeon is satisfied with the location and angulation of the initial preparation, the sites can be enlarged with the next diameter of twist drill, in this case 3.2 mm. The direction indicator posts still give important guidance to maintain the angulation at the individual sites. (E) A 3.5-mm diameter implant is inserted into the prepared site. (F) All implants have been placed and cover screws inserted. The flaps are then closed with sutures.

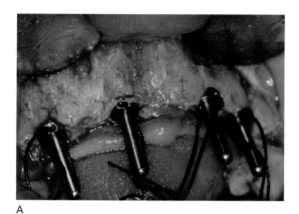

A

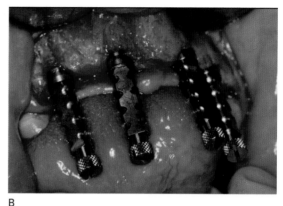

B

Figure 10.2

Placement of Brånemark implants in the anterior maxilla. (A) The sites have been prepared to a 3-mm diameter and the direction indicators have been placed to review the angulation and spacing. There is ample space in this case, with centre-to-centre spacing between implants of about 8 mm. (B) The implants have been placed and transfer copings attached to them. An impression recording the position of the implants was then taken to allow construction of a provisional bridge that could be fitted at the abutment connection surgery 6 months later.

cases, especially as the manufactured abutments have a wider diameter than the implant head (Figure 10.3). The standard Estheticone (Nobel Biocare, Göteborg, Sweden) abutment is the most commonly used manufactured component and has a width of 4.5 mm. Therefore, with a 1-mm spacing at the bone level two adjacent abutments will touch, leaving no space for a soft-tissue cuff. In most instances, therefore, the standard 7-mm spacing recommendation is much safer.

The spacing problem may be eased by utilization of a system where the abutment is narrower than the implant head. This the case with the AstraTech system illustrated in Figure 10.1. Standard implants are either 3.5 or 4 mm in diameter at the implant head but the conical abutment fits within the head of the implant. The reduced width of the abutment at the implant head expands to a maximum diameter that matches the implant diameter at a distance of 2 mm above the head of the implant. This conical profile allows a good soft-tissue cuff to be formed and therefore permits slightly closer positioning of the implants than is the case for the Brånemark system when using standard manufactured abutments.

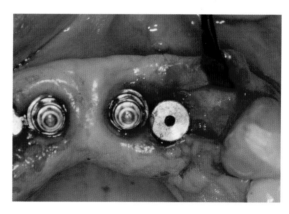

Figure 10.3

An example of Brånemark implants that were placed too close together. The implants in the central incisor sites (those with abutments connected) have good spacing between them, in contrast to the minimal space between the implants in the lateral incisor sites (cover screws in place).

The Straumann system (Figure 10.4) requires different considerations. A standard 4.1-mm diameter implant (measured in the endosseous part) has a transmucosal collar that enlarges to

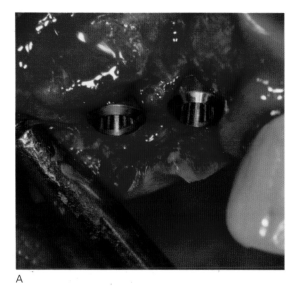

A

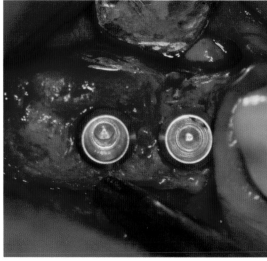

B

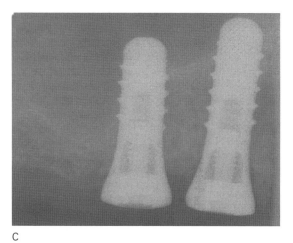

C

Figure 10.4

A series of photographs showing the installation of Straumann implants. (A) Two Straumann implants have been inserted in the maxilla distal to the canine. (B) An occlusal view of the implants showing a gap of about 2 mm between the outer aspect of the polished collars and the same gap between the anterior implant and the tooth. (C) A radiograph of the implants with closure screws in place. The shape of the implants means that there is more space between them at the bone level than at the soft-tissue level.

4.8 mm in diameter at the top. The implants should be placed so that there is at least a 1-mm gap between adjacent collars at their maximum width, which gives an additional soft-tissue space apical to this (and in turn an adequate dimension of bone). As with the AstraTech system, the abutments have a narrower diameter than the implant head and therefore do not encroach upon the space further.

The Frialit system requires a different approach. In this system the implant sites are first prepared to an acceptable final depth (Figure 10.5). The sites are then widened with successive stepped conical drills that exactly match the range of implants of diameters 3.8, 4.5, 5.5 and 6.5 mm, therefore the initial siting of the implant centres is very dependent upon the planned diameter of the final implant. If there is a miscalculation and it appears that the implants of the planned diameter will be too close, then a narrower preparation and implant would have to be utilized. Unlike the previously described systems, the Frialit implants are tapered apically and therefore it is easier to provide adequate bone between implants in the apical zone. However, this is not so much of a problem as the coronal aspect where the breach in the epithelium occurs, where complications are far more likely in terms of inflammation or aesthetics.

The other factor to remember is to allow adequate space between the implant and an adjacent tooth (Figures 10.4B and 10.5C–F). The initial selection of the site has to take into account:

- the planned diameter of the implant
- the proximal contour of the tooth
- allowance of a minimum of 1 mm of bone between implant and root
- allowance of adequate space for the proximal soft-tissue papilla
- a path of insertion of the implant that is not affected by the tooth contour.

Implant angulation

Guide pins placed in the developing implant sites should be checked against the surgical stent and the opposing dentition, and modifications made as necessary. The angulation of the implant sites more or less mimics the angulation of the natural teeth, with modifications according to the design of the final prosthesis and the degree of ridge resorption. If the final prosthesis is designed to be retrievable/screw-retained, the ideal angle of the implant passes through the cingulum area of the anterior teeth and the occlusal surfaces of the premolar/molar teeth. In a non-retrievable cemented prosthesis the angulation would be the same in the posterior teeth because this is also consistent with loading the implants through the long axis. However, in the anterior zone the angulation can be inclined more labially through the incisal tip or towards the labial surface, potentially improving the emergence aesthetics (see Chapter 9 on single tooth implants). However, the force transmission through the implants may be less favourable because it will be far removed from axial loading (Figure 10.6). Therefore, within a given zone of the jaw the implants are placed more or less parallel to one another. Placement of multiple guide pins is very helpful and should prevent unacceptable angulation of the implants (Figures

10.1C, D and 10.2A). Manufactured abutments allow quite large angular variations between implants, and customizable abutments can be used if these values are exceeded (Chapter 14). For example, implants may be angled more than usual to engage more bone length at sites next to the maxillary sinus (see Chapter 12).

Level of the implant head

The last factor to consider in implant placement is the level of the implant head. This level will dictate:

1. available vertical space to the occlusal plane or incisal plane for abutments and restoration
2. vertical space for the emergence profile of the restoration

Submerging the implant head may provide much needed space to accommodate abutments and restoration in individuals with little vertical space, for instance patients with minimal ridge resorption. More often, ridge resorption is to such an extent that submergence of the implant head is not required other than to optimize the emergence profile and aesthetics. The deeper the implant head, the easier it is to make a gradual smooth transition to the emerging crown. In contrast, it will have an adverse effect on the ratio of the height of the restoration to the implant length (equivalent of the crown/root ratio). This can therefore produce unfavourable force distribution and leverage.

It is perhaps easiest to contrast the effects of implant head level between submerged systems such as the Brånemark or AstraTech with that of a non-submerged system such as the Straumann. In the prescribed use of the Brånemark implants, the implant head is countersunk to a point that allows the cover screw (which protects the external hexagon) to be level with the crest of the bone ridge. This facilitates soft-tissue coverage and minimizes the chance of subsequent wound dehiscence and implant loading. However, in order to achieve this the implant site is countersunk and this places the implant head either within the superficial cortex or below this if the cortex is thin. This may therefore negate one of the prime aims

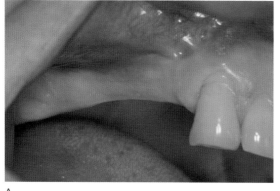

A

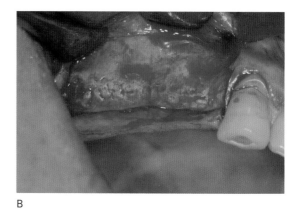

B

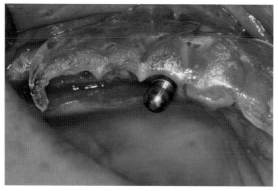

C

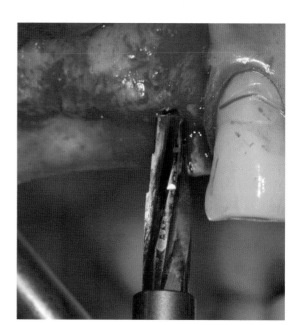

D

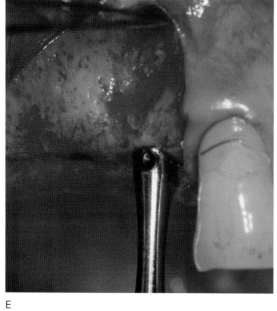

E

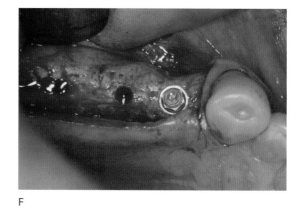

F

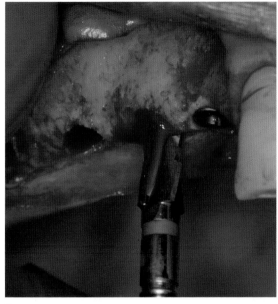

G

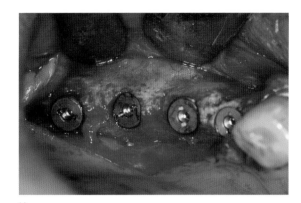

H

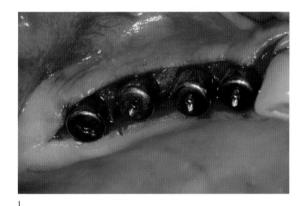

I

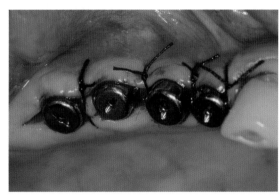

J

Figure 10.5

A series of photographs showing the installation of four Frialit 2 implants in the posterior maxilla. (A) The edentulous posterior maxilla prior to surgery. (B) Buccal and palatal flaps have been raised to expose the ridge adequately. (C) An acrylic stent in place to evaluate the position and direction of the mesial site that has been prepared with the 2-mm diameter drill. (D) The mesial site preparation is completed with a 3.8-mm diameter stepped drill. (E) The 3.8-mm diameter stepped screw implant has been inserted level with the crest of the ridge. The 'dot' on the inserting device should be on the buccal aspect to facilitate the prosthodontic procedure. (F) An occlusal view of the mesial implant in place—note the space between it and the tooth. Initial preparation of the distal sites has been started. (G) The distal site is completed with a 4.5-mm stepped drill (colour code blue). (H) All four implants have been inserted. The three distal implants are 4.5 mm in diameter (blue) and the mesial implant is 3.8 mm in diameter (yellow). (I) Abutment connection surgery with healing abutments. (J) Suturing of the flaps around the healing abutments.

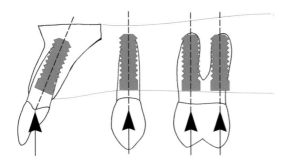

Figure 10.6

Forces directed through implants placed in the posterior jaw will usually be in the same long axis as the premolar and molar teeth. Labial angulation of the anterior implants means that normal forces are not directed down the long axis.

of bicortical stabilization with this system. Countersinking could therefore be viewed as being destructive for the cortical anchorage, which could be critical in areas of poor bone quality, such as the posterior maxilla. It is even more pertinent when one considers that in the first year of loading the implant there is bone resorption to the level of the first thread, further accentuating loss of previous cortical bone. However, the advantage of countersinking is that the abutment implant junction is placed sufficiently far apically to allow a good emergence profile of the restoration and an aesthetic subgingival placement of the restoration margin. The design of the AstraTech system allows placement of the implant head at the level of the crestal bone without countersinking and thereby preserves cortical bone. This is because the

standard implant head has nearly the same diameter as the main threaded portion of the implant and the cover screw fits within the implant head. This system is therefore very useful in the resorbed maxilla, which may have little crestal cortex, because it can be used to utilize fully the limited bone height and maintain cortical anchorage.

The standard design of the Straumann implant has a smooth transmucosal collar that is 2.8 mm in length. In areas of thin mucosa the implant head will be above the mucosa and the aesthetics may be compromised. However, the Straumann aesthetic line has a reduced height of transmucosal collar because the plasma-sprayed/ SLA surface coating extends further onto the collar area. The interface is placed at the level of the cortical bone (or countersunk further) to produce a submucosal implant/ abutment junction.

Conclusion

The surgeon must be very familiar with the system that he/she is using in multiple implant placement because of the large number of variables. The dimensional comparisons of the various implant systems used in this book are described in Chapter 1 and an appreciation of their differences and respective dimensions is vital to the clinician planning the treatment and those providing the surgical and prosthodontic phases of treatment. The surgeon may have to modify the plan during surgery and can only do this if he/she has an extensive range of implants at his/her disposal and knowledge of the prosthodontic requirements.

11

Immediate and early replacement implants

Introduction

In many cases implants are placed at sites where teeth have been lost many months or years previously. Traditional implant surgical protocols such as that described by Brånemark advocated leaving extraction sites for 12 months to allow complete healing and maturation of bone. However, the resorption of bone over extended time periods often led to a situation where there was insufficient bone for routine implant placement. Protocols have therefore developed in which implants are placed at the time of extraction of the tooth, or soon after, before significant bone resorption occurs.

Timing of implant placement

There are various recommendations regarding timing of implant placement following tooth extraction. Basically the implant can be placed immediately following extraction during the same surgical procedure ('immediate implant placement') or following a delay of a few weeks, in which case it has often been referred to as 'delayed-immediate'. This latter term is rather clumsy and this protocol will be referred to as 'early placement' in this text. The differences between 'immediate' and 'early' placement are summarized in Table 11.1.

The 'early' protocol errs on the side of caution and is therefore possibly more predictable, although there are no comparative studies to support this statement. It may offer an advantage when it is used with submerged implant protocols because the soft-tissue healing that occurs between extraction and implant placement facilitates flap coverage. The choice of protocol also depends upon the difficulty of the case.

The 'immediate' protocol is more applicable if an anterior tooth is being replaced. The extraction should be relatively straightforward, the socket not too large to compromise implant stability (Figures 11.1 and 11.2) and the provision of a temporary restoration should be simple. In contrast, a case requiring multiple and/or difficult extractions and temporization may be best handled in a separate dedicated surgical operation to that of implant placement. Most of the following considerations apply to anterior tooth replacement, because the situation with multi-rooted teeth is usually far more compromised

Table 11.1 Summary of immediate and early implant placement

	Immediate placement	Early placement
Timing	Implant placement at the same surgical procedure as tooth extraction	Implant placement 2–6 weeks following tooth extraction
Advantages	• Reduced number of surgical procedures • Optimizes visualization of extraction socket • Flap elevation may be unnecessary	• Allows resolution of any infection • Allows soft-tissue healing to cover socket • May allow early healing of bone (woven bone)
Disadvantages	• Contraindicated if overt infection is present • Caution required if extraction sufficiently traumatic to complicate healing process	• Additional surgical procedure required • May be insufficient bone to achieve primary stability of the implant

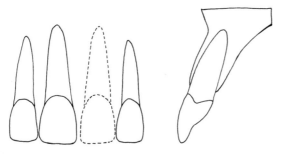

Figure 11.1

The central incisor root is longer and wider than the lateral incisor. The distance between the apex of the root and the floor of the nose varies considerably. The bone apical to the root may be important to secure initial stability of the implant.

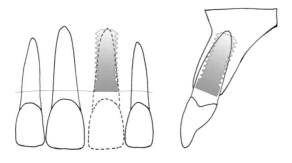

Figure 11.2

A standard 4-mm diameter implant of the same length as the central incisor root may only just attain stability in the apical portion. A longer implant could be used.

owing to the larger extraction sockets and less bone apical to the socket.

Assessment

The assessment for immediate/early placement follows the same guidelines as discussed in previous sections but with additional features related to the effect of the extraction socket on the implant placement. It has been stated already that the area should be free of overt infection and if any doubt exists the implant surgery should be delayed and, if necessary, appropriate antibiotics given.

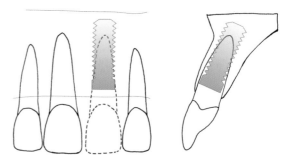

Figure 11.3

A longer 4-mm diameter implant has been placed more apically in a site prepared apical to the apex of the socket close to the floor of the nose. The apical bone provides good stability for the implant. There is a reduction in the space between the implant and the socket walls., The alternative strategies are illustrated in Figures 11.6 and 11.7.

The main factors to assess are obtained from good-quality radiographs of known magnification and include:

1. Size and shape of roots (Figure 11.1)
   - length
   - width
   - taper
   - number of roots in the case of molars
2. Bone support (Figures 11.2 and 11.3)
   - height of marginal bone supporting the tooth root
   - distance between apex of root and anatomical limit of bone (e.g. floor of nose, maxillary sinus, inferior dental neurovascular bundle)
3. Difficulty of extraction procedure
   - simple elevation/forceps
   - surgical procedure involving bone removal

Tooth/root extraction

It is essential to carry out the tooth/root extraction as atraumatically as possible in order to prevent:

1. Fracture of the socket walls
2. Loss of the labial plate of bone

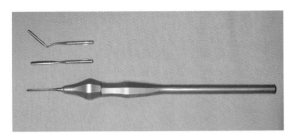

Figure 11.4

Periotomes with different-designed ends to allow dilatation of the socket and atraumatic extraction.

3. Excessive trauma to the socket wall that could lead to necrosis of bone or a localized osteitis.

In most cases it is recommended to use gradual and careful loosening and elevation of the roots with specifically designed periotomes (Figure 11.4). These allow gradual dilatation of the coronal part of the socket and severance/rupture of the periodontal ligament fibres. The periotome should be worked circumferentially around the root, working gradually deeper until the tooth is elevated with little force. Careful forceps extraction is also permissible, particularly if small rotational movements are effective and leverage against the labial plate of bone can be avoided. In some cases exposure of the alveolus through flap elevation is necessary, which allows inspection of the bone and effect of the transmitted forces upon it. Surgical bone removal should be kept to a minimum and performed with copious irrigation if burs are used.

Following successful removal of the root, any granulation tissue should be curetted from the socket and any inflamed periodontal pocket tissue should be excised. Some clinicians recommend routine curettage of the socket wall to remove residual periodontal ligament fibres, although there is little evidence to support this protocol (and it is not performed by the present authors). Implant placement should be postponed if any doubts exist regarding the likelihood of persistent infection or the possibility of osteitis due to traumatic removal of the tooth root. Under these circumstances and in planned early-placement protocols the soft tissue should be closed as much as possible with sutures. Soft-tissue closure can be facilitated by flap advancement following releasing incisions and incision of the periosteal surface of the flap. Antibiotics should be given where appropriate.

Implant placement

Preparation of implant sites within extraction sockets may not be as easy as it first appears. In immediate placement the socket will have been curetted as necessary. With the early-placement protocol the soft tissue is elevated to allow re-inspection of the socket and removal of any ingrowth of soft tissue. Any woven bone should be left undisturbed. The surgical preparation (with drills matched to the system being utilized) more or less follows the angulation of the socket, provided that the tooth was in a satisfactory position and that an implant angle through the incisal tip or labial to it is acceptable (Figures 11.2 and 11.3). However, in some cases involving the maxillary anterior teeth the bone on the palatal aspect of the socket is the best to provide a good site preparation to secure implant stability (Figure 11.5). It may also provide more palatal angulation of the implant to facilitate screw retention of the prosthesis if this is desirable. It is helpful if the initial preparation of the site is started with a round bur, which readily penetrates the socket wall. Drilling into an angled surface within a

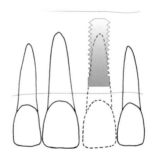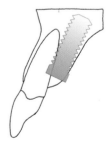

Figure 11.5

At times, the most suitable bone to secure stability of the implant is on the palatal aspect of the socket, especially where the labial plate is very thin or has been lost. However, the implant will be palatally placed and aesthetics may be compromised. A thin labial plate may be compressed to reduce the volume of the residual socket.

socket is more difficult than into a relatively flat crestal platform of bone. A standard sequence of drills follows the round bur and the angulation of the site is checked against the stent and opposing teeth. It is usually more difficult to check the angulation with the standard indicators present in most surgical kits because they are too short and unstable within the socket. The angulation can always be checked with a twist drill removed from the handpiece.

In most cases it is essential to prepare the site apical to the natural socket to ensure implant stability and predictable osseointegration into mature bone (Figure 11.3). In situations where there is little or no bone available apical to the socket, then a wider diameter implant has to be selected or the procedure delayed to allow adequate bone healing of the socket. The level of the implant head is usually placed just within the socket or slightly apical, according to the aesthetic requirements as discussed in Chapters 3 and 9. A more apically placed implant head often reduces the size of gap between implant surface and socket wall (Figure 11.3), but there is a limit to this compensatory strategy.

Implant selection

It is very helpful to overlay the radiograph with transparent outlines of the implant design to be considered in the various lengths and diameters available. Ideally the implant should be slightly bigger than the root it is replacing, to ensure a good fit in the prepared site within the socket and hence a high degree of initial stability. This is one of the claimed advantages of a system specifically designed for this purpose, such as Frialit. The Frialit 2 has a stepped cylinder design of various diameters to make it easier to achieve these objectives (Figure 11.6). The other implant system that is good in these situations is the AstraTech single tooth (ST) implant (Figure 11.7). This has a wider conical collar (available in 4.5- and 5-mm diameters at the top) that gives a good fit in most anterior tooth sockets, and the apical threaded portion gives good initial stability, especially if it can be extended into bone apical to the socket. This latter feature is the main way of achieving good stability with parallel screw-threaded design implants. Ideally there

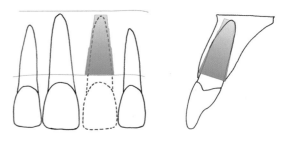

Figure 11.6

A stepped cylinder implant (Frialit 2) developed for immediate replacement has a wide enough diameter and length to almost obliterate the socket. This implant also has a series of threads to help stability in the immediate replacement situation.

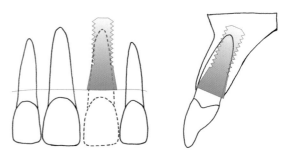

Figure 11.7

An AstraTech ST implant has an apical threaded portion that can be used to engage bone apical to the socket and provide good stability. The conical microthreaded collar is wider at the top (4.5 or 5 mm) and reduces the dead space.

should be 4-5 mm of sound bone apical to the socket to prepare and engage with an implant of sufficient length. With implants of a parallel-sided design there is often a gap between the coronal part of the socket and the implant surface (Figure 11.2 and 11.3). The size of the gap is critical. A gap of 1–2 mm should fill with bone and osseointegration should occur. Where the gap is larger, this may be grafted, preferably using autogenous bone collected from the site preparation or an adjacent area of suitable donor bone. In addition, it is often possible to reduce the size of the gap by compressing the walls of the socket using finger pressure or by gentle fracturing of the thin coronal walls of the socket

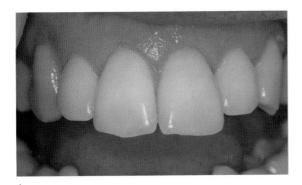

A

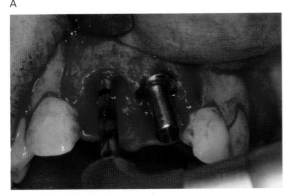

C

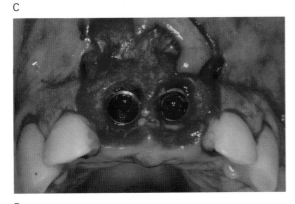

D

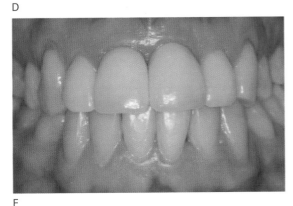

F

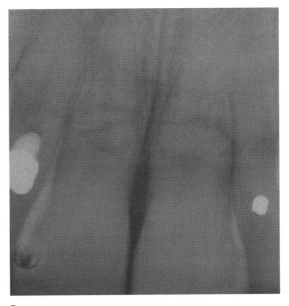

B

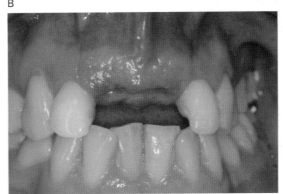

E

Figure 11.8

A series of photographs showing immediate implant place-ment for replacement of maxillary central incisors with AstraTech ST implants. (A) Preoperative photograph showing aesthetic natural teeth. (B) Radiograph showing fractures of roots in the cervical third. (C) Flaps have been raised and the roots carefully elevated. The sites are being prepared within the sockets. A stent (not shown) has been used to check the position of the guide pin in the partially prepared site. (D) The AstraTech ST implants have been placed. Stability is achieved by extending the implant length apical to the natural socket. There is only a small void on the labial aspect of the implants that will fill in with bone without recourse to grafting. (E) The area has healed very well 2 weeks after surgery. There is complete soft-tissue coverage. The implants were left buried for 6 months. The abutment connection surgery for this case is illustrated in Chapter 8 (Figure 8.11). (F) The completed result 2 years after crown cementation on prep-able abutments.

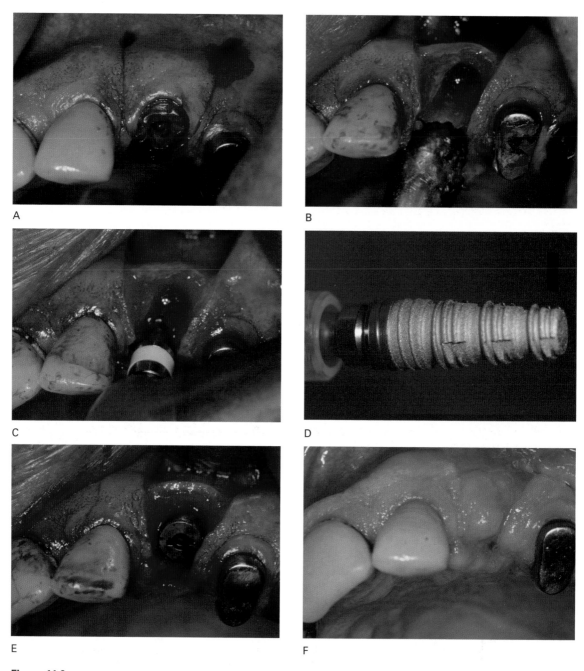

A

B

C

D

E

F

Figure 11.9

A series of photographs showing immediate replacement of a maxillary canine in a patient with dentinogenesis imperfecta, using the Frialit 2 system. (A) The crown of the maxillary canine has fractured and worn after many years with a conventional restoration. The flap design is evident. (B) The root has been carefully elevated. (C) The initial preparation of the socket with the twist drill. The length of the preparation is established and then increasing widths of stepped drills are used according to the final diameter of the implant that can be accommodated at this site. (D) The chosen implant: a 4.5-mm diameter threaded stepped cylinder (Frialit 2). This design achieves very good stability by preparing the lateral walls of the socket and is aided by the threads. (E) The implant completely fills the prepared site without any voids. (F) The healed soft tissue showing complete closure at 2 weeks post-surgery.

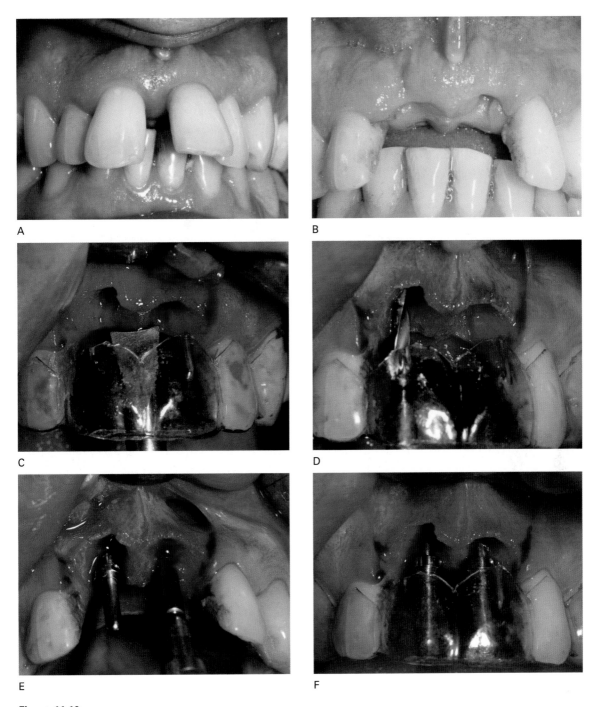

Figure 11.10

A series of photographs showing early placement of two Brånemark implants to replace the maxillary central incisors. (A) The maxillary central incisors have drifted and are very mobile due to extensive root resorption. (B) Four weeks following extraction of the incisors, soft-tissue healing of the sockets is good. The patient has been wearing a Rochette provisional bridge, which has been removed to allow installation of the implants. (C) Buccal and palatal flaps have been raised

continued overleaf

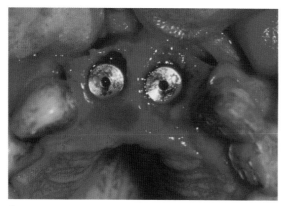

G

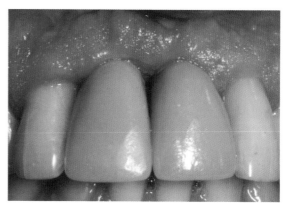

H

and residual soft tissue has been removed from the sockets. A plastic stent, based upon a diagnostic set-up and provisional Rochette, is stabilized on the adjacent teeth. The measuring indicator, held palatally, has a width of 7 mm (corresponding to the recommended centre-to-centre distance between two Brånemark 3.75-mm implants). (D) A 2-mm twist drill is used to prepare the initial implant angulation. (E) A guide pin is placed in the right central incisor socket and the left site is being enlarged from 2 to 3 mm in diameter. (F) The guide pins show the position and angle of the prepared sites within the sockets in relation to the stent. (G) The implants have been placed and the cover screws connected. The implants are towards the palatal aspect of the sockets. The small voids labially were grafted with osseous coagulum collected from the drilling process. (H) The completed result showing the two single tooth implants in an acceptable aesthetic position.

with a suitable instrument. Most of the foregoing discussion is mainly applicable to placement into an anterior single root socket and it is not usually possible with molar sites.

The sequence of implant placement in extraction sockets is shown in Figures 11.8–11.10, which illustrates some of the points mentioned above and how the different systems cope with this situation.

Conclusion

Immediate and early implant placement protocols can offer highly predictable results, which in clinical trials have been shown to be as good or even better than traditional protocols. However, there are many potential factors that have to be appreciated and accounted for if one is to emulate these success rates.

Bibliography

Becker W, Becker B (1990). Guided tissue regeneration for implants placed into extraction sockets and for implant dehiscences. Surgical techniques and case reports. *Int J Period and Rest Dent* **10**: 376–91.

Gomez-Roman G, Schulte W, d'Hoedt B, Axman-Krcmar D (1997). The Frialit-2 implant system: five-year clinical experience in single tooth and immediately postextraction applications. *Int J Oral Maxillofac Implants* **12**: 299–309.

Rosenquist B, Grenthe B (1996). Immediate placement of implants into extraction sockets: implant survival. *Int J Oral Maxillofac Implants* **11**: 205–9.

Salama H, Salama M (1993). The role of orthodontic extrusive remodelling in the enhancement of soft and hard tissue profiles prior to implant placement: a systematic approach to the management of extraction site defects. *Int J Period and Rest Dent* **13**: 312–33.

12
Grafting procedures for implant placement

Introduction

The overriding requirement for successful implant placement is to have enough bone volume of sufficient density to enable an implant of the appropriate size to be placed in a desirable position and orientation. Many of the grafting procedures described in this chapter have been developed as localized procedures to overcome small anatomical limitations. There is also a need occasionally to employ more complex techniques to change the entire alveolar ridge form that may additionally involve an associated change in skeletal base.

As well as the obvious osseous component to this problem there are also many situations where the soft tissue in the area of proposed implant placement is deficient. The soft tissues play a vital role in maintaining the peri-implant environment, long-term health and also contribute greatly to the resulting aesthetics, particularly in the anterior region. The peri-implant soft tissues must be able to maintain their structural integrity during normal function and oral hygiene procedures.

Grafts therefore may be employed to:

* enable implant placement
* enhance aesthetics and improve soft tissues
* change the pre-existing jaw relationship

The initial planning stages as described in previous chapters take on even greater levels of importance in potential graft cases. By their very nature they are more difficult to plan and execute and the end result may fall short of both the clinician's and patient's expectations. It is important that all the alternatives are considered and presented to the patient so that they can make an informed decision with regard to their treatment. In particular, it is important to consider whether a compromise solution using prosthetic techniques may be more desirable and achievable as well as more predictable in the long term. Another alternative is to consider whether the utilization of the various implant designs may overcome the problem.

Bone graft materials

The degree of bone grafting required for implant placement varies from localized deficiencies to cases where there is a need to change the entire arch form and/or jaw relationship. There exist, therefore, a great many techniques and materials to facilitate such grafting procedures, many of which may be used in combination. The interaction between the graft and the surrounding host bone is very important and is the subject of much research. Although some grafts will act merely as space fillers, the ideal graft will be osseoconductive and osseoinductive. Osseoconduction is the property of promoting bone growth from the surrounding host bone onto the surface of the graft material, using the graft as a framework. The graft material in such cases may be resorbed or remain virtually intact, depending on the material used. Osseoinduction is the ability to promote *de novo* bone formation remote from the host bone even within noncalcified tissues. Bone morphogenetic proteins and other bone-promoting factors have this latter property.

Autogenous bone grafts

The ready availability of autogenous bone has always meant that it is the first choice of bone grafting material for many clinicians. However, patient acceptance of autogenous bone harvesting may be low, given the potential morbidity associated with such techniques. Although a great amount of research and clinical time has been spent over many years to develop substitutes for autogenous bone, it remains the gold standard by which all other materials are judged and is the material of choice for the present authors. Its main advantages are:

• Availability
• Sterility
• Biocompatibility
• Osseoinductive potential
• Osseoconductive potential
• Ease of use

The graft acts as a scaffold for the ingrowth of blood vessels and as a source of osteoprogenitor cells and bone-inducing molecules. The graft is eventually resorbed as part of the normal turnover of bone.

Other graft materials

Although the gold standard for bone grafting remains the patient's own bone, the limitations on the amounts available (particularly from sites other than the iliac crest) mean that there remains a great demand for alternative graft materials. Xenografts are derived from another species, allogenic grafts (allografts) from a member of the same species and alloplasts are synthetic materials.

The macro- and microstructure of these grafts have an enormous influence on their efficacy. The pore diameter and volume are therefore of great importance. The ideal characteristics of a substitute bone graft material have been described (Hammerle, 1999) as:

• Sterile
• Non-toxic
• Non-immunogenic
• Osteoconductive or osteoinductive
• Favorable clinical handling

• Resorption and replacement by host bone
• Synthetic
• Available in sufficient quantities
• Low in cost

Allogenic grafts

Bone derived from cadavers has been used widely in orthopaedics and implant dentistry as well as periodontics. The graft may be freeze-dried or decalcified freeze-dried bone allograft (DFDBA), both of which are thought to be a good source of bone morphogenetic protein. It is harvested from donors with well-documented medical histories and tested for the common infective antigens. It is therefore considered to be a reasonably safe source of grafting material. The grafts are produced as particulates with a reasonably uniform grain size or as sheets and large blocks. They are osteoconductive, providing a framework for new bone growth, and should be resorbed as part of the normal turnover of bone but some particles appear to remain intact for some time after the graft has been placed. The ability of DFDBA to induce new bone (osteoinductive) formation has been the subject of a great amount of research with conflicting results. This is thought to be due partly to the differences in the way humans react to graft materials as opposed to animal models, and partly to the differences in the source and processing of DFDBA grafts.

Demineralized laminar bone sheets are available in varying thicknesses of 20–700 µm, and those of 100–300 µm have similar physical properties to Gore-Tex™ (WL Gore and Associates, Flagstaff, AZ, USA), allowing them to be used as membranes for guided bone regeneration (GBR) procedures.

Despite the rigorous testing of the donors there remains the possibility of some cross-infection from the graft and the development of other sources of graft materials is likely to reduce the demand for allografts in the future.

Deproteinized bovine bone mineral

Deproteinized bovine bone mineral (Bio-Oss®, Geistlich Pharma, Wolhusen, Switzerland) has similar properties to human cancellous bone, both in its macrostructure and its crystalline content. The physical properties are also close to those of the bone that it is used to replace. As a purely mineral graft it is osseoconductive and is thought to undergo resorption, although this has been found to be variable. When used in a particulate form it is mixed with the patient's blood and packed into the defect. Some authors have described improved results when combining this with a membrane to protect the clot. Because it is available in large quantities it has been used in sinus lift procedures instead of autografting (Yildirim, 2000). The particles also may be used as a filler to increase the volume of autogenous graft material. In addition, the graft material is available as thin sheets of bone to cover and protect defects while retaining their shape as described above for allografts. The use of bovine material, albeit in a purely mineral and non-antigenic form, may not be completely acceptable to some clinicians or indeed some patients.

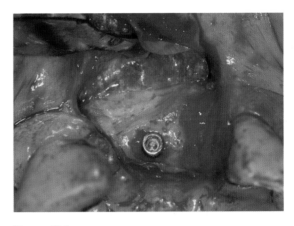

Figure 12.1

The use of screws or pins may be advocated in the absence of autogenous bone to retain the shape of the defect and stabilize the membrane, thus optimizing healing. Here, a Memfix™ (Institut Straumann, Waldenburg, Switzerland) tenting screw has been placed in the middle of the defect to prevent the soft tissues from collapsing, thereby reducing the volume of bone created.

Alloplastic graft materials

Synthetically produced materials have the advantage of having no risk of cross-infection but may still give rise to an antigenic response. Their physical properties can be manipulated to a great degree and they may be used also in combination with bone-promoting molecules to enhance their effectiveness. They act as a framework for bone formation on their surface and are therefore osseoconductive. They include:

- Hydroxyapatite
- Calcium Phosphate
- Tricalcium Phosphate (TCP)
- Bioactive Glasses
- Calcium Carbonate

Guided bone regeneration

Guided bone regeneration (GBR) membranes were originally developed to promote new tissue growth within a protected volumetric defect for periodontal regeneration. The desire to promote new bone growth without resorting to grafting procedures led to widespread use of this technique in implant surgery. The main aim is to

allow ingress of bone cells to promote bone formation within the defect. The original membranes were expanded polytetrafluoroethylene (PTFE, Gore-Tex™). It is a non-resorbable material that requires removal at second-stage surgery. The need for removal led to the development of resorbable membranes made of synthetic polymers such as polylactate and polyglycolic acid, as well as collagen membranes. Resorbable materials should be functional for between 3 and 6 months after insertion. However, they may be resorbed or lose their shape too quickly and limit the amount of bone regeneration achieved.

The creation and maintenance of a volumetric defect is critical and this may be improved by reinforcing PTFE membranes with titanium strips. Further enhancement of the space-maintaining properties is achieved by the use of fixation pins and screws that serve to 'tent' the membrane (Figure 12.1). This can be achieved also by placing small bone chips within the defect, which will also act as osseoconductive/osseoinductive grafts (Figure 12.2). Cortical bone within the defect is perforated with surgical burs to promote osteogenic cells to occupy the space created (Figure 12.3).

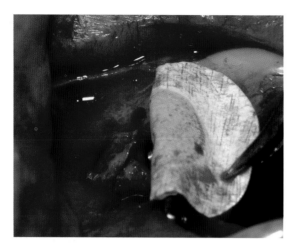

Figure 12.2

Small bone chips have been placed under a PTFE membrane to maintain the volume of the graft site; the underlying cortical bone also has been perforated with a small round surgical bur.

Guided bone regeneration is also commonly used at the time of implant placement to repair small fenestrations and dehiscences around implants (see Figure 12.18A). It should be remembered that any such bone created will not function to stabilize the implant at the time of placement and that initial implant stability remains the overriding priority. The amount of new bone created can be quite substantial but the degree to which it becomes osseointegrated is variable. The amount of bone to implant contact of the newly generated bone is thought to change with time and loading. Guided bone regeneration is most predictable when attempting to increase the buccolingual dimension, but increasing the vertical dimension using this technique is very difficult and unpredictable.

Although membranes are designed to allow the passage of nutrients, they nonetheless tend to compromise the blood supply to the overlying soft tissues. This can result in breakdown of the soft tissues, exposure of the membrane and infection. This may result in a net loss of bone in the surgical area or failure of implants to osseointegrate. It is important that all incisions are kept as remote from the grafted area as possible and that the wound is sutured hermetically and without undue tension. Supporting the tissues

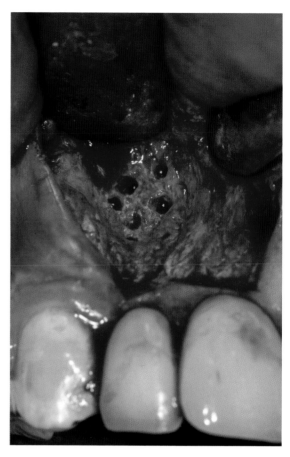

Figure 12.3

Perforation of the host bed with surgical drills allows proliferation of bone cells and vascular tissue underneath membranes and between the donor site and grafted bone material.

with sutures that take large bites and 'sling' the flaps can reduce tension at the wound edges.

Intraoral harvesting and grafting of autogenous bone

Autogenous bone grafts may be taken as trephine or block specimens both from intra- and extraoral sites. Fairly large grafts may be taken from the interforaminal region of the mandible. This procedure can be performed under local

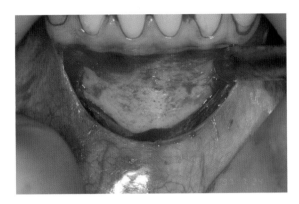

Figure 12.4

By using a wide-based flap close to the mucogingival junction, a large portion of the anterior mandible may be exposed. Owing to a thick labial plate, the roots of the lower teeth are not visible and care must be taken to avoid traumatizing the teeth.

anaesthesia. Great care is required in order to avoid compromising the nerve/blood supply to the anterior teeth. Careful radiographic assessment of the region is important preoperatively in order to ascertain the amount of bone available. Once the mucoperiosteal flap has been raised via a sulcular incision to give wide exposure of the mandible, the graft can be outlined leaving at least 3 mm of clear bone below the apices of the incisor teeth (Figure 12.4).

The root contours often can be visualized directly once the alveolus is exposed. For harvesting blocks of bone the surgeon has a number of choices:

* Fissure burs
* Oscillating saws
* Rotating discs
* Trephines

The authors prefer the use of high-speed diamond discs in either straight or contra-angled handpieces when obtaining large bone blocks (Figure 12.5). These have the advantage of limiting the depth of cut to 2–3 mm, as well as having excellent guards to prevent soft-tissue trauma. Copious saline irrigation is required throughout this procedure. It is vital to cut completely through the outer cortex so that the graft can be cleaved from the underlying cancellous bone (Figure 12.6).

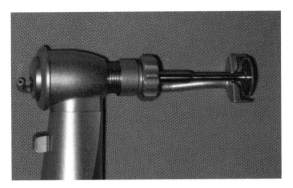

A

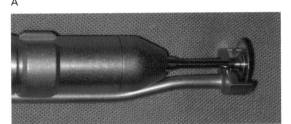

B

Figure 12.5

Contra-angled and straight handpieces for the use of diamond discs for bone grafting (FRIOS MicroSaws, Friatec, Mannheim, Germany). Owing to the guards, these may be used in fairly confined spaces without traumatizing the adjacent soft tissues.

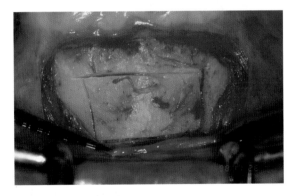

Figure 12.6

The diamond discs cut very fine lines at a controlled depth, minimizing the chance of causing damage to adjacent structures. It is important to ensure that the cuts meet at each corner to allow elevation of the block. Bleeding from the depths of each cut indicates that the cuts are completely through the cortex and into the cancellous bone. Attempting to elevate the block while the cortical layer is intact will cause fracture of the graft.

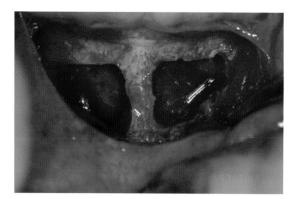

Figure 12.7

In order to harvest a large graft from the anterior mandible, the blocks are taken in two pieces, enabling outfracture without using too much force and reducing the risk of breaking the blocks. Note the depth of the graft sites, which have been deepened by harvesting of the underlying cancellous bone.

In some areas the initial cuts may have to be deepened using standard fissure pattern burs to the desired depth. Care is required to limit the cuts to within the body of the mandible because lingual perforation may lead to haemorrhage of the lingual soft tissues, which can be difficult to arrest. Once the outline cuts have been completed the graft can be elevated using osteotomes or curved chisels specifically designed for that purpose. Large blocks that extend across the midline can prove difficult to elevate and may need to be divided and delivered in two pieces (Figure 12.7).

Trephine specimens also may be harvested from the chin and there are many different sizes of trephine available for this purpose (Figure 12.8D).

Figure 12.8

(A,B) Trephine donor sites from the lower retromolar area. This region can yield good-quality bone grafts but the size of the grafts can be limited. By increasing the size of the access flap, the ascending ramus may be used as a donor site—in such cases the use of diamond discs may be easier and the size of the graft is increased. (C) The amount of bone available from trephine specimens is variable; in dense bone the graft may be largely cortical as shown. In areas of low density, such as the maxillary tuberosity, there may be little bone recovered. (D) Trephines of various sizes are available to allow for different graft sizes as well as limitations of access in certain regions. It is useful to have depth indication lines on the outer aspect to allow the surgeon to judge the depth of the cut being made.

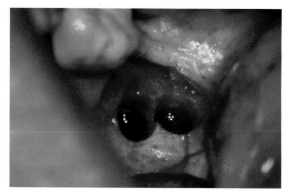

A

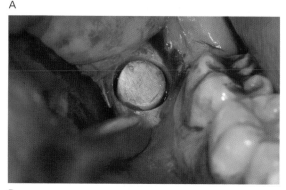

B

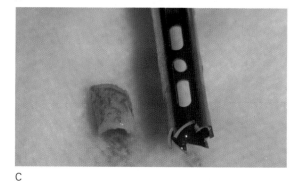

C

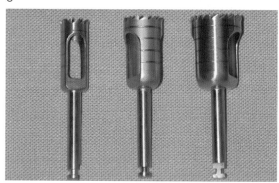

D

Access to this region with fairly unwieldy handpieces and large trephines can make this a more difficult procedure than taking blocks, unless extensive soft-tissue reflection has been achieved. Once the corticocancellous block has been removed, further harvesting of cancellous chips can be undertaken from the graft bed as well as cortical chips from the wound edge. Control of any bony haemorrhage is important before soft-tissue closure, and for this the authors prefer carboxymethylcellulose mesh packed into the graft bed, although bone wax may be preferred by some operators. Others advocate packing the defect with bone substitutes held in place with barrier membranes in order to minimize any potential change in the bony profile. Good closure of the soft tissue at the donor site is critical because the tendency for wound breakdown is quite high and a hermetic-type wound closure should be aimed for.

Other intraoral harvesting sites are available but may be more limited in the amount of bone available. Trephine specimens taken from the mandibular retromolar area can provide good-sized grafts of high-density bone (Figures 12.8A,B); the maxillary tuberosities also may be used but the bone density in this region may be poor. Larger blocks may be gained from the ascending ramus and external oblique ridge/coronoid process, as well as the buccal aspect of the body of the mandible, using the diamond discs described.

The amount of bone harvested from any site while using cutting instruments can be increased by employing harvesting sieves within the suction apparatus (Figure 12.9). These collect the osseous coagulum produced during drilling, which is considered to have good osseoinductive potential. Owing to aeration and hydration during cutting, the volume of coagulum produced can be significant, particularly if fairly coarse rotary instruments have been used. The coagulum forms a paste-like substance that is readily manipulated and can be placed in any residual voids between graft and recipient bed. Where a change in alveolar profile is sought, the graft needs protection with a space-creating membrane or mesh.

Intraoral bone harvesting has become more popular with the introduction of some of the techniques above and is particularly attractive in that the dental surgeon is working in a familiar

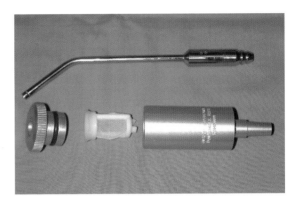

Figure 12.9

A bone trap used for harvesting bone chips and osseous coagulum during bone preparation with rotary instruments. The white plastic filter collects the bone, which then can be used to pack small voids; this part is disposable. Fairly large quantities of material may be collected using this method, particularly when using fairly coarse cutting instruments such as twist drills.

environment. The fact that these procedures can be performed under local anaesthesia with a relatively low morbidity also makes them the treatment of choice for small grafts. However, if there is a need for larger blocks of bone, extra-oral donor sites are required. Historically the site of choice has been the iliac crest because bone is readily available in large volumes (Figure 12.10). However, this requires an appropriately trained surgeon, a general anaesthetic (unless trephine specimens are considered adequate) and the procedure is associated with a significant morbidity.

Once the graft material has been harvested, it can be shaped to fill the defect with irrigated burs or hand instruments such as rongeurs and chisels. Ideally the graft should be adapted to give a close fit to the recipient bed, with any small residual deficiencies made good with bone chips and osseous coagulum. The recipient bed should be perforated with round surgical burs to promote bleeding from the underlying cancellous bone, to encourage vascularization and union of the graft.

The success of the graft, like that of the implants, is dependent on the stability of the graft and the associated blood clot. The graft should, therefore, be held firmly in position

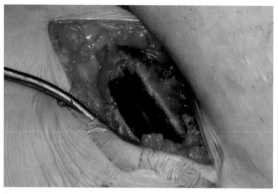

A

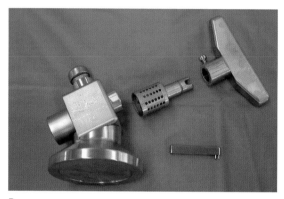

B

Figure 12.10

(A) The favoured extraoral site for bone harvesting remains the iliac crest, from where substantial blocks of bone and significant amounts of cancellous chips may be harvested. (B) A bone mill can be used to fragment large bone grafts to produce a particulate graft that is more readily packed into voids and awkward or confined spaces. Such grafts may be useful in sinus lift procedures using a delayed implant insertion protocol (see section on sinus lift procedures).

using wires or titanium screws (Figure 12.11B). Further stability and protection of the graft may be achieved by using titanium mesh or barrier membranes to cover the graft. These may be stabilized using small screws or tacks. The use of barrier membranes in particular has been advocated to reduce the amount of resorption of the graft that occurs in the healing phase, which may be as much as 50% over 6 months (Hammerle, 1998). However, the use of membranes also poses an increased risk of infection, particularly if this becomes exposed. The

present authors do not advocate the use of membranes with block grafts but accept that they may be necessary with particulate/milled grafts.

Wound closure at the grafted site must be complete, with great emphasis on achieving a hermetic seal with as little tension on the soft-tissue flaps as possible. This can be difficult to achieve with large changes in bone profile and may require further soft-tissue reflection and periosteal relief to advance the soft tissues. Due consideration should be given to the potential problems of closure and in particular placing relieving incisions remote from the grafted site when gaining surgical access. The potential for wound breakdown over grafted areas is higher and carries with it a high morbidity. Patients should receive appropriate pre- and postoperative antibiotics to minimize the risk of infection.

Figure 12.11 (right)

(A) View of the upper jaw showing the left canine region requiring grafting prior to implant placement. The crestal ridge profile appears to be of adequate dimensions on the right but there is a significant buccal concavity present on the left. (B) Two cortico-cancellous blocks have been trimmed to shape and secured using 2.0-mm diameter titanium screws which engage the residual ridge. Prior to this the host site cortical plate is perforated with a small surgical drill (See Figure 12.3.) The grafts are larger than the required ridge profile to allow for some resorption during healing. Any spaces between the grafts and the host bed are packed with cancellous bone chips and osseous coagulum. Further osseous coagulum is packed between and over the grafts to produce a smoother profile to the grafted site. (C) Three months later there has been little resorption of the grafts but this underlines the importance of placing larger grafts than are ultimately required. Protection of the grafts with membranes or titanium mesh may reduce the amount of resorption but can increase the risk of infection and total loss of graft material. (D) A direction indicator in place after drilling with a 2.5-mm twist drill to show the planned implant orientation and adequate available bone on the buccal aspect. (E) Placement of an implant in an ideal orientation without any dehiscences or fenestrations has been facilitated by the use of the grafts.

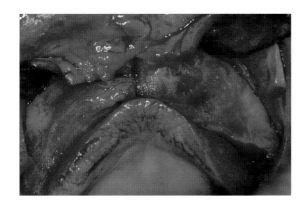

A

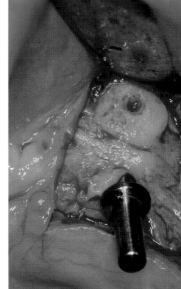

D

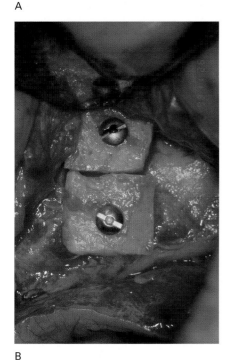

B

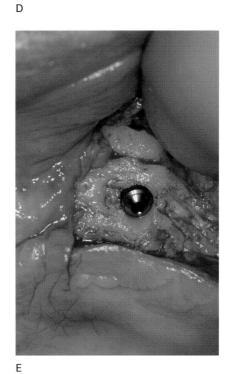

E

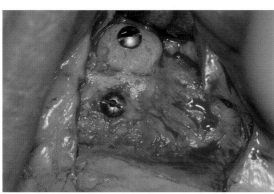

C

The length of time between grafting and implant placement has been the subject of much controversy. When using onlay grafts the authors prefer a time interval of 3 months, whereas in GBR techniques it may be better to delay implant placement for up to 6 months. Screws and membrane tacks are readily removed at the time of implant placement but the complete removal of PTFE membranes can be difficult to achieve. When placing implants in areas that have recently undergone an onlay graft, great care is required not to cleave the graft off the underlying alveolus. Incremental drilling procedures and low forces at placement are therefore mandatory.

Surgical management of large alveolar defects

More demanding ridge defects arise from long-standing tooth loss and denture wearing, as well as trauma and as a result of some pathological conditions. Grafting in such cases may be undertaken to allow implant placement but also to change the profile of the alveolus to enable placement of implants in a more ideal orientation. Long-standing tooth loss can lead to a considerable change in skeletal relationships (pseudo-class III jaw relation) that may need correction. Treatment of cases with gross loss of vertical height of the alveolar ridge without grafting would necessitate the use of short implants, which may be considered undesirable because it results in a poor crown/prosthesis to implant ratio that may cause biomechanical failure in the long term (Figure 12.12). Bone grafting techniques should not only increase the volume of bone but also create an implant bed of good-quality bone to ensure long-term implant success.

Large grafts taken from the iliac crest can be fashioned to produce an entire new alveolar form. This technique is favoured in cases where there is a skeletal base discrepancy or where a large change in the vertical component of the ridge is required, particularly where there is a desire to reduce the height of the prosthesis. Onlay grafting can be performed as a one- or two-stage procedure, with the implants used to secure the graft in the one-stage approach (Figure 12.13). This requires that there is enough

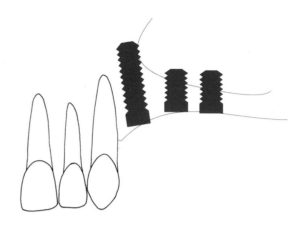

Figure 12.12

Placing implants into the residual ridge will require the use of short implants and a poor implant/crown ratio. An onlay graft would increase the bone volume, allowing the use of longer implants as well as reducing the height of the prosthesis (see Figure 12.13).

residual basal bone to secure the implants and graft. In full-arch cases at least six implants are required to achieve this. In the two-stage approach, implant placement should take place around 3 months after the graft procedure.

In cases where the vertical height of the maxillary ridge is inadequate, inlay grafts may be the treatment of choice. Large inlay grafts spanning the entire maxillary complex in combination with a Le Fort 1 down-fracture have been used successfully, particularly in cases where a change in skeletal relationship is desirable. This technique preserves the intraoral ridge profile but allows substantial gains in available vertical height for implant placement (Figure 12.14).

Sinus lift procedures

Loss of alveolar ridge height, particularly in combination with pneumatization of the edentulous posterior maxilla, means that there is frequently a lack of bone height for implant placement. It is also often the case that any residual bone in this area is of poor quality. Sinus floor grafting procedures were developed by Tatum in the late 1970s to overcome these

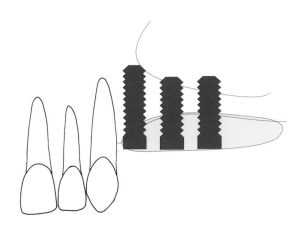

Figure 12.13

Onlay grafts may be secured to the residual alveolus provided that there is enough bone to stabilize the implants. Soft-tissue closure may be difficult in these situations.

problems and have been used with great success worldwide following the principles described by him. There is little evidence of disturbances to sinus drainage following this procedure.

In the classic approach, a bony window or trapdoor is created in the buccal sinus wall to gain access to the sinus. It is vital that clear radiographs are available preoperatively to show the topography of the sinus, particularly the presence of any bony butresses or septa that prevent elevation of the window (Figure 12.15A). In addition, it is useful to ascertain the buccopalatal dimension of the sinus to ensure that the trapdoor created will have space to rotate upwards within the sinus cavity (Figure 12.15B). The presence of any sinus disease or a history of recurrent sinus infections are contraindications to this procedure.

The procedure can be carried out under local anaesthesia, and the use of infraorbital blocks is advocated. Good access is obtained through a wide-based soft-tissue incision with its boundaries remote from the proposed point of entry to the sinus. Commonly, the sinus wall is thin and the sinus cavity can be seen as a bluish grey area on the bone surface. This is helpful in delineating the trapdoor, which must be cut over the sinus cavity or it will be impossible to elevate.

Where the sinus wall is thick the surgeon has to rely on the preoperative radiographs or computed tomography (CT) scans to mark out the shape of the window. The window should extend mesiodistally as far as the proposed implant sites. If a pronounced bony septum is present, it may be necessary to create two separate windows or use an alternative approach (see next section). The outline is preferably created with diamond-coated surgical burs using copious irrigation, with great care taken not to perforate the underlying sinus membrane.

The inferior and lateral cuts are taken completely through the bone but the superior cut may be partially perforated to allow the window to be infractured, leaving the superior aspect as a hinge. Once the cuts are complete the surgeon should be able to move the window inwards with fairly gentle pressure.

As the trapdoor is elevated, the sinus membrane is gently lifted off the surrounding bone. It is important to keep the sinus membrane intact throughout this procedure because it is exceedingly difficult or impossible to suture tears in the membrane. Small perforations may be patched with resorbable membranes or carboxymethylcellulose. Large tears may dictate that the procedure is abandoned, particularly if the intention is to graft the sinus with a particulate graft material rather than a corticocancellous block. The elevation continues until the desired size of void has been created, with the sinus membrane pushed medially and superiorly along with the trapdoor. The degree to which the sinus floor may be lifted is also dictated by the position of the osteon on the medial wall, which allows drainage of the sinus. Once the space has been created within the sinus, two different approaches may be taken. If there is enough residual alveolar bone to accept and stabilize implants (usually at least 5 mm in height), then they may be placed immediately, with any residual voids being packed with graft material. If large blocks of bone are being placed into the sinus these may be stabilized by placing the implants through both the alveolus and the graft (Figure 12.15I). In cases where there is little residual alveolar bone the void is first grafted and implants are then placed 3 months later. This latter technique is probably the preferred option, with more predictable results in all cases. The preferred graft material is autogenous bone.

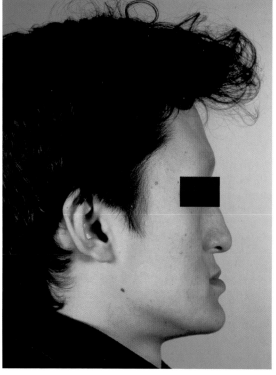

A

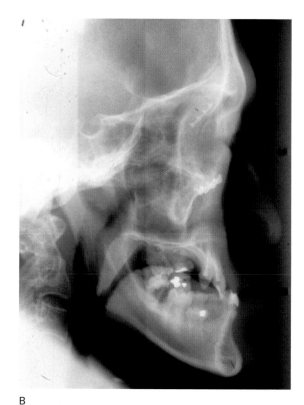

B

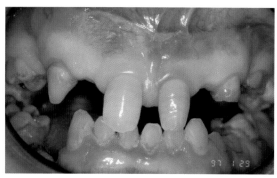

C

Figure 12.14

(A,B) This patient has a severe skeletal base discrepancy, as well as many developmentally absent teeth. A combination of bone grafting and maxillary osteotomy using a Le Fort 1 down-fracture and advancement is required to alter the skeletal relationship. Additionally, large maxillary sinuses dictate the use of short implants, unless bone grafts are placed. (C) Intraoral view showing degree of oligodontia (postosteotomy). (D) Lateral cephalogram showing the skeletal profile after Le Fort 1 osteotomy and iliac crest inlay graft. (Orthognathic surgery by Dr Paul Robinson.)

continued   D

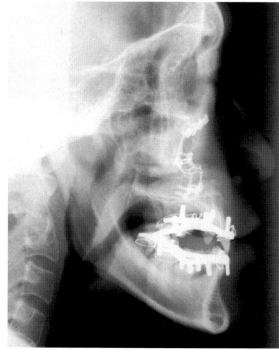

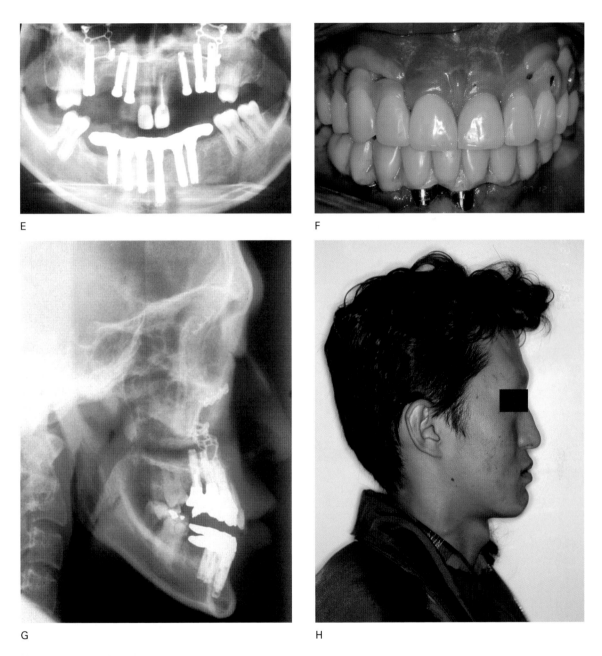

E

F

G

H

Figure 12.14 *continued*

(E) Dental panoramic tomograph showing implants in place in the maxilla with the completed implant-retained bridge in the mandible. The increased available alveolar height provided by the inlay graft allows placement of long implants with a favourable implant/prosthesis ratio. (F) The final result with bridges in place. Despite the grafting procedure, the alveolar orientation dictated the placement of labially inclined implants and buccal access holes for the bridge screws. (G) Lateral cephalogram showing the final bridgework *in situ*. Note the improved facial profile and the orientation of the maxillary implants. (H) Clinical photograph showing the final result, with good profile and facial height.

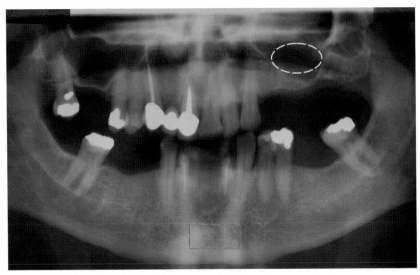

A

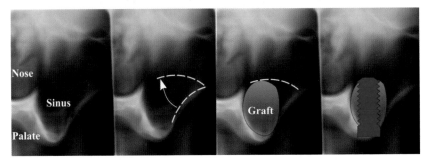

B

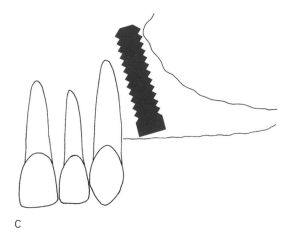

C

Figure 12.15

(A) Dental panoramic tomograph of a patient requiring implants in the posterior maxilla. The alveolar ridge has a good intraoral height but the extension of the maxillary sinus on the left side makes it impossible to place more than one implant without using a grafting procedure. There is no indication of sinus pathology or fluid levels/mucosal thickening. Additionally there would appear to be no bony septa running across the lateral wall. The proposed site for a cortico-cancellous graft from the chin is also outlined. (B) Sectional tomograms of the patient shown in Figure 15A allow evaluation of the space available to elevate the trap door (shown by the yellow line). An indication of the likely volume of graft required can be ascertained as well as the length of implant that may eventually be placed. The amount of residual alveolus in this case would not be enough to stabilise the implant at the sinus grafting stage. Implants would be placed as a separate procedure three months later. (C) Placement of a single implant into the residual alveolous distal to the upper left cuspid is possible for the patient shown in Figure 15A. This may be enough in patients with a restricted smile line or in low load situations but is rarely the treatment of choice unless solely replacing the upper second bicuspid.

continued

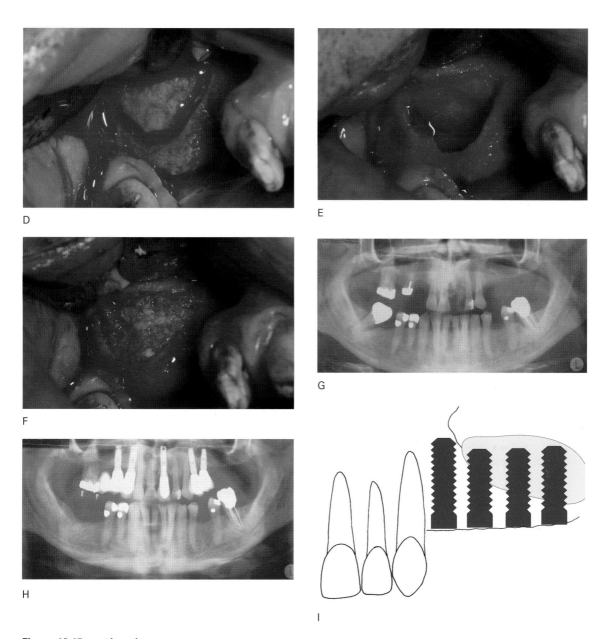

D

E

F

G

H

I

Figure 12.15 *continued*

(D) A trapdoor has been outlined in the posterior maxilla by careful bone removal with a surgical bur. (E) The trapdoor has been elevated and the sinus membrane has remained intact during this stage. There is not enough residual alveolous (5 mm) to allow simultaneous sinus lift and implant placement, therefore a graft will be placed into the void created. (F) Residual space within the cavity is packed with autogenous bone material including osseous coagulum. The graft may be covered with a resorbable membrane to ensure it remains within the void. The flap is then sutured back into place. (G) Pre-operative radiograph showing limited bone height in the posterior maxilla. (H) Post-operative radiograph after a sinus lift has been performed in the upper left quadrant. The new level of the sinus floor in relation to the installed implants can be seen. Enough residual alveolous was present in the upper right quadrant to allow implant placement without grafting. (I) Large blocks of corticocancellous graft material may be stabilised by placing implants through both the residual alveolous and the graft. Ideally the graft should be orientated so that the cortical plate is superior allowing good fixation of the apices of the implants.

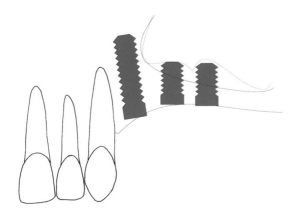

Figure 12.16

The floor of the sinus may be elevated at each osteotomy site using Summers' technique. By pushing a plug of bone apically with osteotomes, the floor may be infractured to leave the sinus membrane intact.

Care should be taken when using particulate graft materials to ensure that the membrane is intact or that any tears are well sealed and protected. Once the graft material and/or the implants are in place and the trapdoor is held in its elevated position, closure of the wound is straightforward with no need for the placement of a GBR membrane over the buccal aspect of the original trapdoor.

Transalveolar sinus floor elevation

Implants are often placed with their apices extending into the sinus cavity by a few millimetres when attempting bicortical stabilization in the maxilla without any associated problems. Attempts to lift the sinus membrane through the osteotomy site have been described and bone apposition around the apices of the implants also has been shown. A more refined technique has been described by Summers, using specific osteotomes to drive bone apically through the osteotomy site but to retain it under the sinus membrane (Figure 12.16). Implants may be inserted immediately with this technique as long as the minimum 5 mm of alveolar ridge height pre-exists to give the implants initial stability.

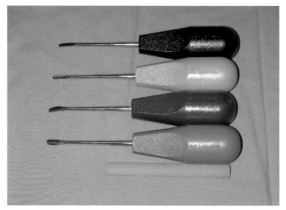

Figure 12.17

Luxators have much larger blades than the Periotome® (see Chapter 11, Figure 11.4) and tend to expand the socket more than sever the periodontal ligament. They are supplied with a sharpening stone (shown at the bottom of the picture) and if they are maintained in their original sharp-edged condition they may be used readily to extract teeth and preserve alveolar form.

Other techniques

Management of extraction sites

Teeth requiring extraction and subsequent implant placement may be dealt with in several ways. It should be remembered that the majority of extraction sites heal uneventfully with good bone fill of the socket, particularly when only one tooth is involved and there are adjacent standing teeth.

Preservation of the tooth socket is a prerequisite for predictable bone fill and this is best achieved using an atraumatic extraction method, in particular, the use of a Periotome® (Friedrichsfeld GmbH, Mannheim, Germany) or luxators can be useful in achieving this (Figure 12.17). Difficult extractions requiring bone removal and associated soft-tissue involvement may be aided in healing by good wound closure, particularly soft-tissue advancement to effect primary closure. Placing graft material into the extraction socket as well as the use of occlusive membranes have been advocated to improve bone fill. Problems may arise, however, if the socket and graft/membrane subsequently become infected, resulting in more bone loss than would have occurred without the graft procedure.

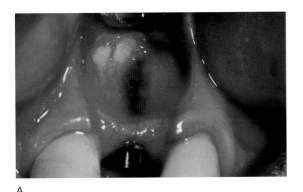

A

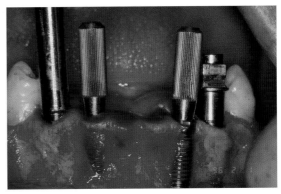

B

Figure 12.18

(A) Small fenestrations such as this are often created at the time of implant placement. The need to graft such defects or to employ GBR techniques is questionable. The implant has good initial stability and the majority of it is in good bone; placement of a membrane could lead to infection and loss of bone. (B) Larger dehiscences such as that on the lower left implant may require grafting to encourage bone coverage of the exposed threads. Because the threads are outside the labial cortex, a membrane would tend to collapse onto the threads, thus reducing the amount of bone formed. Support for the membrane to maintain volume should be sought, therefore, by the use of a titanium-reinforced membrane or preferably using bone chips under the membrane.

Dehiscences and fenestrations

Small defects created at the time of implant placement, such as marginal dehiscences or fenestrations, may require grafting, depending on their shape, size and location (Figure 12.18). The rationale for such procedures must, however, be questioned because grafts placed in such defects as well as bone created using GBR techniques are unable to contribute to the initial stability of the implant and the bone may not ever integrate with the surface of the implant. Repair of such defects may be useful in situations where the overlying mucosa is thin and there is a risk of the implant showing through the gingiva.

Crest splitting and dilation

Placement of an implant into a ridge that is slightly narrower than the implant diameter can be achieved by increasing the crest width using one of two techniques. Dilation of a site can be achieved in its simplest form by allowing the implant to expand the ridge as it is inserted. This can be achieved where the bone is thin and soft enough to allow this. Formal dilation of the ridge is achieved using osteotomes, such as Summers' osteotomes or those for specific systems, e.g.

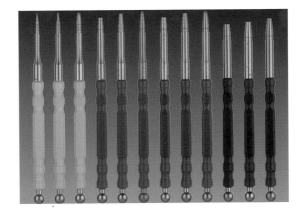

Figure 12.19

Osteotomes for dilation of implant sites have been developed and are useful particularly in the softer maxillary bone. They all have markings along their length to correspond with the different implant lengths available.

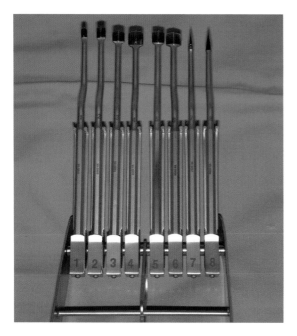

Figure 12.20

The Crestosplit® osteotomes allow a combination of dilation at specific implant sites along with ridge expansion mesially and distally. Great care is required using this technique and case selection is very important.

brittle bone, especially in older individuals and smokers. A combination of ridge splitting and individual site dilation can allow marked changes in the ridge profile. Once the ridge has been expanded, implants, bone graft or a combination of the two can be placed in the void. Immediate placement of implants into sites that have been ridge split may be complicated by an inability to achieve initial stability of the implants.

A limiting factor for these techniques is that they do not allow for any change in orientation of the ridge and therefore the implant. In areas where implant angulation is important and the ridge does not allow such orientation, other techniques are required to augment bone at the desired location.

Distraction osteogenesis

The use of bone plates secured either side of a surgically created fracture line, which are then mechanically separated incrementally on a daily basis, has been described both in orthopaedics and maxillofacial surgery to increase bone

Friatomes® (Friatec, Mannheim, Germany) (Figure 12.19). This technique is dependent on there being enough cancellous bone present between the cortical plates to allow initial site development with a surgical drill. By gentle manipulation and the use of osteotomes of slightly increasing diameters, reasonable expansion of the ridge can be achieved, enabling implant placement.

Total expansion of a ridge can be performed using bladed osteotomes or ridge splitting sets, e.g. Crestosplit® (J van Straten Medische Techniek, Nieuwegein, The Netherlands) (Figure 12.20). Again, there must be some cancellous bone present within the ridge to allow for a natural plane of cleavage. Care must be taken to limit the area of expansion by placing limiting cuts at each end of the ridge. The danger of fracturing one cortical plate from the other is not to be ignored and considerable practice is required to master this technique. In particular, caution should be exercised in sites with

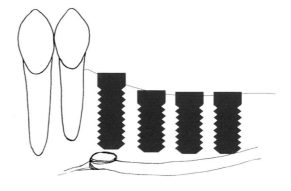

Figure 12.21

With restricted height available above the inferior dental canal, the use of multiple short implants may be advocated. Achieving initial implant stability in such situations can be difficult to achieve because there is often poor cancellous bone and it is not possible to engage the apices of the implants in cortical bone. The need to leave a safe margin of error between the length of the drills and the canal usually means leaving the implants 3 mm short of the canal, in contrast to the distal implant in the figure.

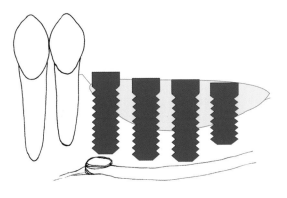

Figure 12.22

The use of an onlay graft allows the placement of longer implants and reduces the height of the prosthesis. The implants engage another layer of cortical bone and are therefore easier to make stable at implant placement.

length. Miniature distraction sets have now been developed to allow ridge height augmentation over limited spans and subsequent implant placement.

Nerve transpositioning/obliteration

Loss of alveolar height in the posterior mandible will eventually compromise implant placement unless the mandible is wide buccolingually and space exists to place an implant to one side of the nerve. In the majority of cases this is not possible and the operator is left with several options. Placement of multiple short implants may provide enough support without compromising the restoration biomechanically. Gaining stability of the implants may be difficult because the cancellous bone is often sparse (Figure 12.21). Placing implants anterior to the mental foramen and cantilevering distally has been used with great success and is appropriate in cases with well-spaced implants of good length and in the presence of a favourable occlusion. Onlay grafts also may be used in this situation and act to improve the implant/crown ratio (Figure 12.22).

The alternative is to surgically expose the inferior dental bundle and to move it buccally to allow implant placement through the bulk of the mandible and thus achieve bicortical stabilization. This is a difficult procedure and the potential morbidity, in particular anaesthesia or paraesthesia of the mental nerve should be explained fully to the patient. Good exposure of the mandible is required, with complete dissection of the mental nerve as it exits from the body of the mandible. The buccal plate is then gently removed with burs and irrigation to facilitate moving the nerve to the buccal aspect over the required distance. The implants can be placed and the nerve placed back in close proximity to them.

The only other neurovascular bundle that commonly compromises implant placement is the incisive nerve in the premaxilla. This can be very large and can limit ideal placement of an implant in either of the central incisor spaces. Removal of the bundle and packing of the canal with bone graft can render this site amenable to treatment after a 3-month healing period.

Soft-tissue grafting techniques

The soft tissues around implants serve a functional role as well as an aesthetic one. Aesthetic problems are commonly diagnosed at the planning stage of treatment and their management may be carried out alongside the implant treatment. Functional problems often appear once the implant prosthesis is *in situ* and are frequently managed as a separate entity.

Functional soft-tissue problems

The peri-implant soft tissues have the same functional demands placed upon them as those around the natural dentition. They are therefore required to withstand the trauma of oral hygiene practices and the forces placed upon them during mastication. It is therefore preferable to have implants emerging through non-mobile keratinized mucosa. The severely resorbed edentulous mandible is frequently devoid of attached mucosa, and implants in such cases are prone to soft-tissue inflammation and reactive hyperplasias. Recurrent problems associated with mobile and inflamed

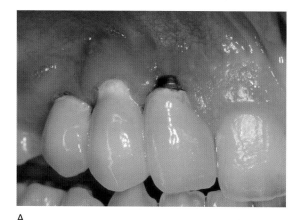

A

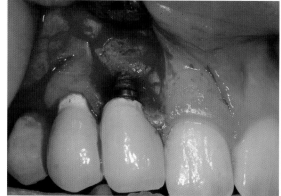

B

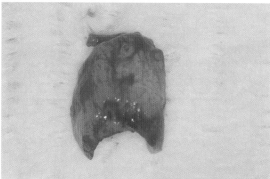

C

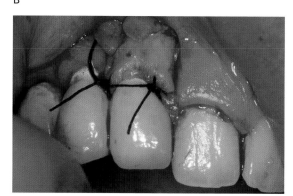

D

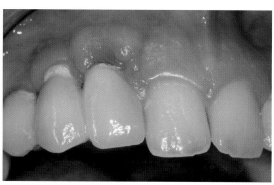

E

Figure 12.23

(A) The lack of attached gingiva around the abutment of the upper right lateral incisor presents an aesthetic problem for the patient (despite a low smile line) but also prevents good oral hygiene due to the thin friable nature of the mucosa; a soft-tissue graft is therefore indicated. (B) A split-thickness flap is raised to include a sound margin of tissue for the graft bed, leaving the papillae intact. (C) The connective-tissue graft is harvested from the palate and trimmed to the correct shape and size. Some shrinkage should be allowed for and so the graft should be kept slightly larger than is required for the final result. By harvesting via an epithelial longitudinal incision, a cuff of epithelial tissue can be incorporated into the graft. (D) The graft is laid into position and held in place with sutures, ensuring good coverage of the abutment. Note that the epithelialized cuff has been placed around the abutment, with the connective tissue extending apically. (E) Two weeks postoperatively, the increase in bulk of the tissues is obvious. The increased width of attached gingiva and coverage of the abutment has been achieved. Further maturation will result in a smoother overall gingival profile.

soft tissues are best treated by the placement of free gingival grafts taken from the palate and sutured to a prepared vascular bed around the implant in the same way as would be performed around a tooth.

Care must be taken to immobilize the graft during healing, which can be difficult to achieve in sites with a shallow sulcus. The use of interpositional connective-tissue grafts may also provide a more stable and robust gingival margin around the implant. Free gingival and connective-tissue grafts (Figure 12.23) may be used in this way at any stage of implant treatment: pre-implant placement, at abutment connection or once the prosthesis is in place. If grafting is required after the prosthetic phase is complete, it may be necessary to remove the prosthesis, bury the implant and graft the site and then bring the abutment through the attached mucosa once healing has taken place.

Aesthetic soft-tissue problems

Small soft-tissue defects, which may also have a bone deficiency, may be considered unaesthetic at the initial evaluation and treatment planning stage but it should be remembered that such defects often will be rectified once the prosthetic

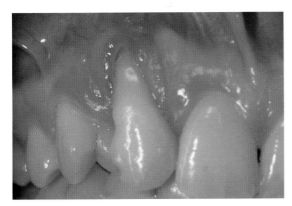

A

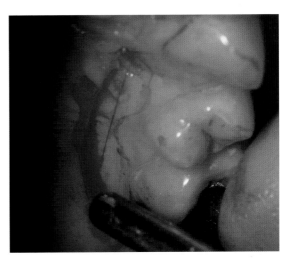

B

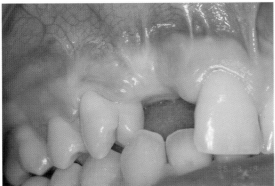

C

Figure 12.24

(A) Gross loss of buccal hard and soft tissues of the upper right canine dictates that grafting of this site is required to achieve an acceptable aesthetic result. The loss of soft tissue is the biggest problem in such cases, particularly the entire loss of the attached gingiva. Placement of a connective-tissue graft at the time of extraction will replace the lost tissues. (B) Connective-tissue grafts are readily obtained from the palatal soft tissues by employing a filleting technique via a limited incision. (C) Two months postoperatively there is a good width of attached gingiva. The height of the adjacent tissues will retain the profile during the healing phase. Once an implant is emerging through the gingival complex, further restoration of the buccal profile will be achieved.

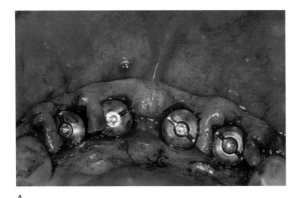

A

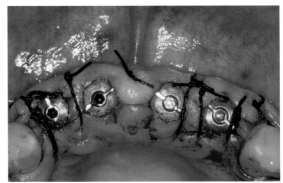

B

Figure 12.25

(A) By careful manipulation of the soft tissues at stage II surgery, the gingival morphology may be optimized and the attached gingiva preserved. (B) Suturing of the flaps allows for healing by primary intention. The use of vertical mattress sutures, as shown in the midline papilla, maintains the height of the papillary tissues.

components are emerging through the mucosa. Soft-tissue maturation occurs around implants, particularly around lone-standing single tooth implants with adjacent natural teeth. This is optimized by good implant placement, allowing a natural emergence profile of the restoration as well as careful soft-tissue handling at all stages of treatment.

Larger defects need to be rectified surgically and this can be achieved readily using free gingival grafts and interpositional connective-tissue grafts in combination with hard-tissue augmentation for the more severe defects. Such techniques are usually best performed before or at the time of implant placement in order to achieve the best results (Figure 12.24). Once again, the use of the patient's own tissue is preferable to any of the other graft materials available.

Papillary preservation or interdental papillary regeneration has been widely advocated; the degree to which this is possible is open to question, but the basis of the technique, careful soft-tissue manipulation and the preservation of as much keratinized tissue as possible, will undoubtedly maximize the soft-tissue healing potential (Figure 12.25). Healthy peri-implant soft tissues are more likely to respond favourably to good prosthetic work with anatomical emergence form.

Bibliography

Andersson B, Odman P, Widmark G, Waas A (1993). Anterior tooth replacement with implants in patients with a narrow alveolar ridge form. A clinical study using guided tissue regeneration. *Clin Oral Implants Res* **4**: 90–8.

Balshi T, Lee HY, Hernandez R (1995). The use of pterygomaxillary implants in the partially edentulous patient: a preliminary report. *Int J Oral Maxillofac Implants* **10**: 89–98.

Becker W, Becker B (1990). Guided tissue regeneration for implants placed into extraction sockets and for implant dehiscences: surgical techniques and case reports. *Int J Period and Rest Dent* **10**: 377–91.

Bloomqvist JE, Alberius P, Isaksson S (1996). Retrospective analysis of one stage maxillary sinus augmentation with endosseous implants. *Int J Oral Maxillofac Implants* **11**: 512–21.

Dahlin C, Andersson L, Linde A (1991). Bone augmentation at fenestrated implants by an osteopromotive membrane technique. A controlled clinical study. *Clin Oral Implants Res* **2**: 159–69.

Hammerle CHF, Karring T (1998). Guided bone regeneration at oral implant sites. *Periodontol 2000* **17**: 151–75.

Hammerle CHF (1999). Membranes and bone substitutes in guided bone regeneration. *Proceedings of the 3rd European Workshop on Periodontology-Implant Dentistry*. Ed. by Niklaus P Lang. Quintessence Publ. 468–99.

Kahnberg KE, Nilsson P, Rasmusson L (1999). Le Fort I osteotomy with interpositional bone grafts and implants for the rehabilitation of the severely resorbed maxilla: a 2-stage approach. *Int J Oral Maxillofac Implants* **14**: 571–8.

Lundgren S, Moy P, Johansson C, Nilsson H (1996). Augmentation of the maxillary sinus floor with particulate mandible: a histomorphometric study. *Int J Oral Maxillofac Implants* **11**: 760–6.

Nyman E, Kahnberg KE, Gunne J (1993). Bone grafts and Brånemark implants in the treatment of the severely resorbed maxilla: a 2 year longitudinal study. *Int J Oral Maxillofac Implants* **8**: 45–53.

Palmer RM, Floyd PD, Palmer PJ, Smith BJ, Johansson CB, Albrektsson T (1994). Healing of implant dehiscence defects with and without expanded polytetrafluoroethylene membranes: a controlled clinical and histological study. *Clin Oral Implants Res* **5**: 98–104.

Sigurdsson TJ, Fu E, Takakis DN, Rohrer MD, Wikesjo UME (1997). Bone morphogenetic protein-2 for peri-implant bone regeneration and osseointegration. *Clin Oral Implants Res* **8**: 367–74.

Simion M, Baldoni M, Rossi P, Zaffe D (1994). A comparative study of the effectiveness of e-PTFE membranes with and without exposure during the healing period. *Int J Period and Rest Dent* **14**: 167–80.

Tidwell JK, Blijdorp PA, Stoelinga PJW, Brouns JB, Hinderks F (1992). Composite grafting of the maxillary sinus for placement of endosteal implants—a preliminary report of 48 patients. *Int J Oral Maxillofac Surg* **21**: 204–9.

Tong DC, Rioux K, Drangsholt M, Beirne OR (1998). A review of survival rates for implants in grafted maxillary sinuses using meta-analysis. *Int J Oral Maxillofac Implants* **13**: 175–82.

Yildirim M, Spiekermann H, Biesterfeld S, Edelhoff D (2000). Maxillary sinus augmentation using xenogenic bone substitute material Bio-Oss® in combination with venous blood. A histologic and histomorphometric study in humans. *Clin Oral Implants Res* **11**: 217–29.

PART IV

Prosthodontics

13
Single tooth implant prosthodontics

Introduction

Prosthodontic treatment is not just restricted to the final stage of implant treatment. The treatment planning chapter (Chapter 2) will have demonstrated the need for the correct decision to be taken regarding the suitability of implant treatment over conventional techniques and the desirability for a clear view of the desired end result prior to implant placement. The importance of realistic diagnostic wax-ups or restorations and surgical stents cannot be overemphasized. It is also essential that provisional restorations that can function and be adapted during the stages of implant placement and exposure be provided. Whether one operator provides the implant treatment from start to finish or different dentists are undertaking the surgical and prosthodontic stages, prosthodontic input from the start is mandatory.

In many respects the prosthodontic treatment for a single tooth is straightforward if the planning and placement of the implant is correct. However, with poor implant positioning or planning, prosthodontic correction of the error to achieve an acceptable result can be impossible. Restoration of single tooth implants therefore can be the easiest and the most demanding of all implant restorations. The choice of the appropriate single tooth abutment is one of the most important prosthodontic factors and this is dealt with in subsequent sections.

Abutment types

All manufacturers produce a variety of abutments suitable for single tooth restorations. Abutments attach the crown to the implant and prevent rotation between components. Many different types are required to allow for variations in such

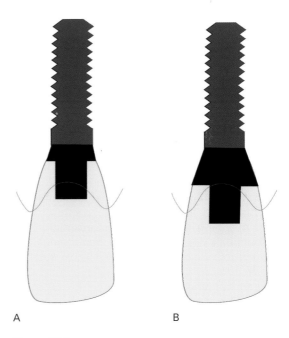

A   B

Figure 13.1

Selection of abutment height. In (A), a short abutment collar places the margin deeper in the soft tissues but allows more height for the development of a suitable emergence angle compared with a longer abutment collar height (B).

factors as implant position, angulations, depth and soft-tissue contours and still achieve an aesthetic end result. The final restoration needs the correct emergence profile in order to support and contour the soft tissue. This may require a transition from a standard 4-mm diameter implant to the 7-mm wide neck of a central incisor tooth within the vertical dimension of only a few millimetres (Figure 13.1). The abutment needs to resist conventional compressive and tensile loads and rotational forces, because it will not be joined to other implants or teeth. There

Table 13.1 Abutment types for single tooth restorations

Type	Name	Manufacturer
Standard abutment	CeraOne	Nobel Biocare
	ST abutment	AstraTech
	Abutment MH6/A0 (A15)	Frialit
	Solid abutment	Straumann
Prepable abutment	TiAdapt, CerAdapt	Nobel Biocare
	Profile BI abutment	AstraTech
	Abutment MH6/A0, CeraBase	Frialit
	Solid abutment	Straumann
Fully customized abutment	AurAdapt	Nobel Biocare
	Cast-to abutment	AstraTech
	AuroBase	Frialit
Computer-generated abutment	Procera	Nobel Biocare
Screw-retained crown abutment	Internal Hexed EsthetiCone	Nobel Biocare
	SynOcta	Straumann

AstraTech: Astra Meditec AB, Mölndal, Sweden; Frialit: Friatec AG, Mannheim, Germany; Nobel Biocare: Nobel Biocare AB, Göteborg, Sweden; Straumann: Institut Straumann AG, Waldenburg, Switzerland.

are few situations in which it is acceptable for a single tooth restoration to show metal at the gingival margin and so there must be adaptability in the abutment design to allow for an aesthetic margin placement. Most anterior single tooth restorations will be cemented onto the abutment and this will get over any problems there may be with labial paths of insertion.

Abutments for single tooth restorations fall into the following categories (see Table 13.1):

• Standard abutments
• Prepable abutments
• Fully customized abutments
• Computer-generated abutments
• Ceramic abutments
• Abutments for screw-retained crowns

Standard abutments

Most implant types have a pre-made abutment, normally made of titanium. There are usually two pieces, with an abutment that fits onto the implant head and a separate abutment screw that can be titanium alloy or gold alloy. A variety of heights are offered, with a smooth collar that extends from the implant head to the margin for the crown (see Chapter 1, Figures 1.17–1.20). Matched impression copings, temporary copings, laboratory analogues and gold and porcelain cylinders are produced to ease manufacture. The standard technique is illustrated in Figure 13.2.

For the Nobel Biocare implant the CeraOne abutment fits onto the flat top and engages the raised hexagon to give anti-rotation for the abutment. As with all flat-top implant designs, it is essential that the abutment properly seats onto the implant head and so a verification radiograph is required (Figure 13.3). The abutment is retained to the implant by a gold alloy screw that is torqued into position at 32 N.cm for a regular platform implant, once seating has been confirmed. To achieve this exact level of torque a mechanical device such as an electronic torque controller is essential and the abutment needs to be held with a counter-torque. Narrow-platform implant abutment screws are tightened to 20 N.cm and wide-platform abutment screws to 45 N.cm.

The conical-headed implant (AstraTech, Frialit and Straumann) abutments have a matched conical fit surface but also an anti-rotational

Figure 13.2

Missing central incisor tooth replaced by an AstraTech ST implant with a standard prosthodontic approach:

(A) standard ST abutment in place; (B) abutment mounted on holder prior to placement—note the conical design with hexagonal anti-rotation base; (C) abutment and holder are seated and the abutment screw is tightened; the pencil mark on the holder aligns the position of the abutment in the implant; (D) impression coping seated onto abutment; (E) impression coping picked up in an impregum impression; (F) a laboratory information sheet gives technical instructions; (G) a Polaroid clinical photograph with the chosen shade guide in position provides further information for the technician;

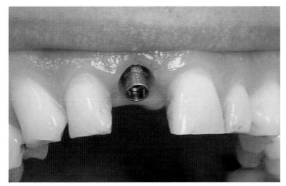

A

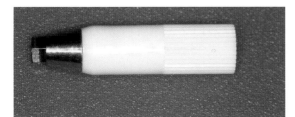

B

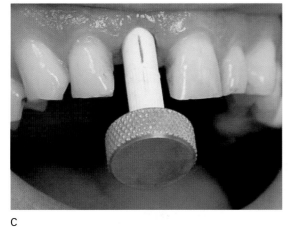

C

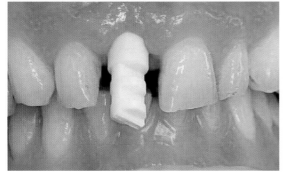

D

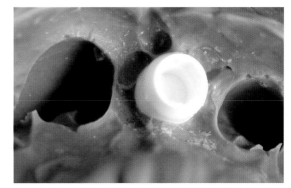

E

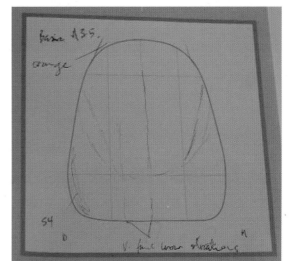

F

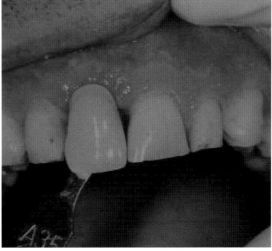

G

continued

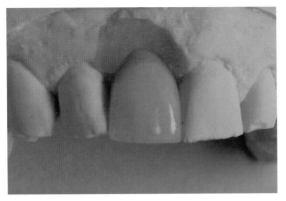

H

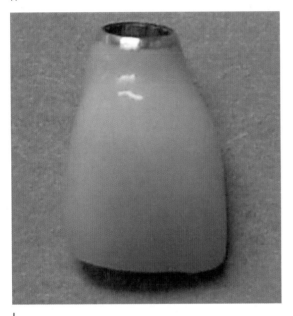

I

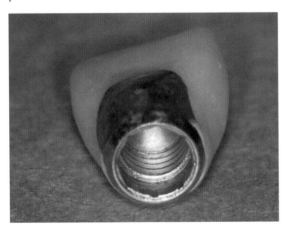

J

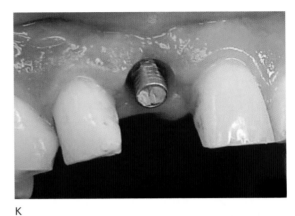

K

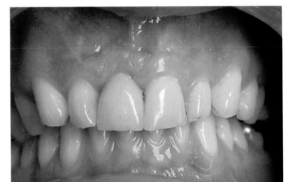

L

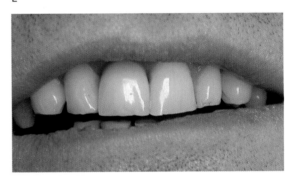

M

Figure 13.2 *continued*

(H) the completed crown on the working model—note the soft-tissue replica; (I) the completed crown, where the metal margin has been formed from the pre-made semi-burnout gold cylinder provided by the manufacturer; (J) internally the crown will have a precise, retentive and non-rotational fit; (K) the abutment screw hole is sealed with gutta percha; (L) the crown is cemented into place; (M) the end result is highly aesthetic.

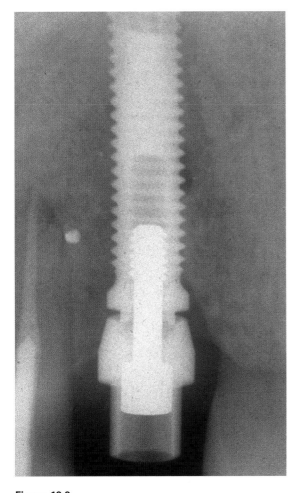

Figure 13.3

A periapical radiograph demonstrating the failure to correctly seat a CeraOne abutment onto a Nobel Biocare implant.

either parallel sided or with a slight taper. A flat facet is required to provide resistance to rotation. The Nobel Biocare CeraOne abutment is a parallel-sided hexagonal cylinder, which delivers considerable retention and stability to rotational forces to the crown. The precision of fit for these restorations, particularly when using the matched gold cylinders, is such that difficulty can be encountered when cementing them into position and cements with a low viscosity or the provision of a vent hole may be required. Other designs such as the Astra Tech ST (single tooth) have space between the abutment and crown to allow for cement release. Tapered abutment heads, such as the Straumann solid abutment or Frialit 2 abutment MH 6, should not offer as much resistance to seating as parallel-sided abutments.

The matched impression copings for all designs are simple push-fit plastic that can be picked up in an impression material. The gold cylinders provided are designed to have wax built up to a contour necessary for a conventional metal–ceramic crown. Alternatively, plastic 'burn-out' copings are available that produce a similar result. Some manufacturers produce porcelain copings onto which conventional porcelain can be fired.

Advantages/indications of standard abutments

* Simple to use.
* Minimal chairside and laboratory time.
* Predictable fit and retention for crown.
* Use in 'straightforward' cases where optimal space and implant orientation have been achieved.

Disadvantages/contraindications of standard abutments

* Margin for crown does not follow gingival contour.
* Cannot be customized for implant orientation or anatomical features—particularly not suited to very labially inclined implants.

Prepable abutments

The connection to implant with these abutments is the same as for standard abutments

element to give the abutment resistance to rotational forces. This element is found at the end of the cone in the deepest part of the implant and it is essential that the abutment is held and rotation attempted prior to tightening the screw to ensure that the abutment is fully seated. A verification radiograph is not usually required but may be used if there is any doubt that the abutment has not seated properly.

The coronal part of single tooth abutments needs to provide adequate retention and resistance form for the crown to be retained by cement to the abutment. They are usually cylindrical in shape, and an outline of the technique is illustrated in Figure 13.4. The retentive element for the crown is a block of metal that can be customized to achieve an 'ideal' preparation contour. The abutments come in a variety of diameters roughly corresponding to the dimensions of upper lateral and lower incisors (4–4.5 mm), upper central incisors, canines and premolars (5.5 mm) and molar teeth (6.5–7 mm). A smooth collar extends from the implant head to this dimension. An impression is taken of the implant head and a model is made with a silicone soft-tissue replica (see later section on laboratory techniques). The abutment is prepared using high-speed instrumentation either by the dentist or the dental technician. The metal can be cut back to achieve a preparation comparable with a conventional crown preparation. The gingival margin can follow gingival contours and be placed subgingivally on the labial and proximal sides but can be supragingival palatally. Enough space must be created to allow sufficient space for the crown.

The metal surface that will be covered by the crown can be left with a coarse finish to aid retention and does not need to be polished, but any metal that will be in contact with the soft tissue should be as smooth as possible.

A major advantage of this approach is the ability to change orientation for the crown relative to the implant (Figure 13.5). This is normally required to rectify a labial inclination of the implant. The correct transverse shape for the crown also can be achieved. With a conventional abutment the whole restoration is circular in cross-section at the implant head and through the abutment. The ideal contour is developed only from the start of the crown. With a prepable abutment, the abutment itself can be modified to resemble more accurately the cross-sectional shape of a natural tooth. For example, an upper central incisor tooth is roughly triangular in shape at the gingival level with a flat labial surface. If a circular abutment is put in position this will tend to be under-contoured mesiodistally or, if a larger size is used, it will push down

Figure 13.4

Missing central incisor tooth where an AstraTech ST implant has a minor labial angulation: (A) On presentation, the healing abutment has been cut back to preserve labial soft tissue; (B) following an impression of the implant head, a cast is prepared using an implant analogue and a soft-tissue replica; (C) the Profile BI abutment try-in kit; (D) abutment analogues can be tried on the cast to assist in the correct choice of abutment height and width; (E) the amount of preparation required and residual abutment can be visualized; (F) the prepared abutment in place—note the poorly formed gingival contour at this stage; (G) following provisional cementation of the crown the gingiva is healthy and well contoured; the abutment screw access hole has been filled with gutta percha; (H) the completed restoration; (I) a post-cementation periapical radiograph.

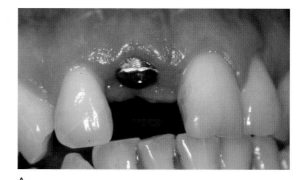

A

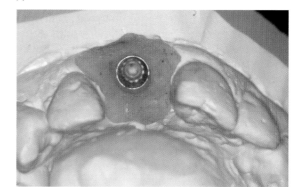

B

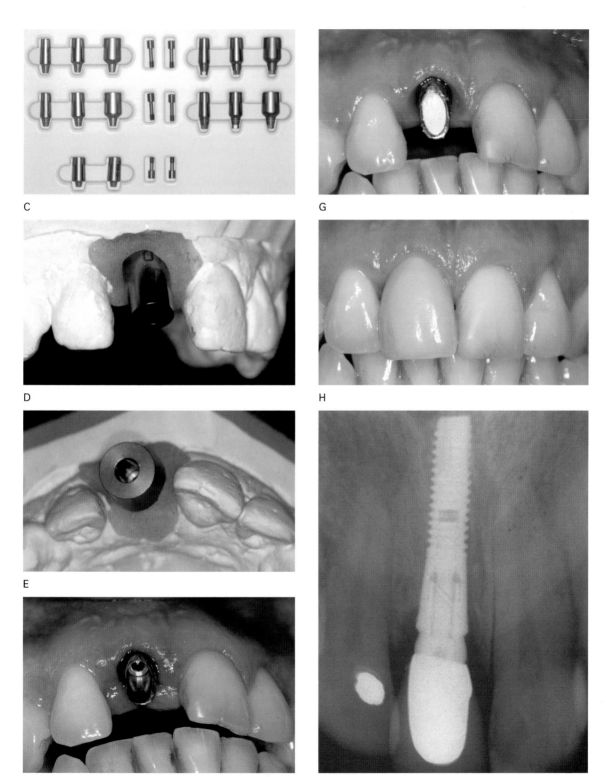

C

D

E

F

G

H

I

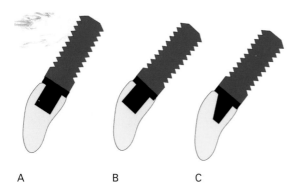

A   B   C

Figure 13.5

When the desired crown is in the same long axis as the implant, a standard abutment will achieve a good result (A). If the implant has a more labial angulation, as in (B) and (C), and the path of insertion of the crown needs to be different to that of the implant, a prepable abutment may be indicated. The crown in (B) will be too thin on the labial aspect and the prepable abutment (C) allows more space for the crown.

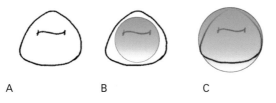

A   B   C

Figure 13.6

An upper central incisor tooth is essentially triangular in cross-section (A). Choosing an implant diameter that is narrower than the tooth (B) will allow the emergence to be developed through the contour of the abutment and crown. An oversized implant (C) will not allow a suitable emergence to be developed.

the labial gingival margin in the centre. A prepable abutment can be cut back on the labial surface in the centre but still keep adequate width mesiodistally and affect a good emergence profile with more ease (Figure 13.6).

Prepable abutments should be prepared out of the mouth. Small changes can be made intra-orally with an air-rotor under copious irrigation, but are best avoided. They can be prepared in two ways. The first way is to produce the abutment and final crown in one stage. This is acceptable for restorations where minor changes

are being made to the implant orientation and the soft tissue is healthy and will remain stable. This technique ensures a good marginal fit between abutment and crown because it does not require a second impression. There is the risk of a poor long-term result if the gingival margin is only placed just subgingivally, because if there is some recession of the gingival margin following cementation, then some metal will show. A margin for error with a slightly deeper margin placement is recommended. It is often wise to cement the crown temporarily to allow for soft-tissue resolution prior to final cementation.

The second way is to prepare the abutment and provisional crown as a first stage. Then a second impression is taken with the abutment in place and a final conventional crown made. More stages are required for this approach but a more predictable result may be obtained. However, it can be difficult to take an impression of an abutment in position and deep margins pose a problem because gingival retraction cord is hard to use. Acrylic copings can be made in advance and a pick-up technique employed. Alternatively, once the abutment has been deemed acceptable, it can be removed from the mouth and the crown frame-work can be produced directly on the abutment. Minor changes to the margin carried out in the mouth can result in gingival bleeding, so it is best to remove the abutment and place it back onto the implant head model for chairside adjustment.

This second technique is particularly useful if the emergence and profile of the soft tissue need to be modified significantly. A prepable abutment is produced with a provisional crown that partly satisfies the desired end contour. Following temporary cementation, the soft tissue will be deformed and then re-modelled to the new shape. The contour can be modified over successive visits by addition to the provisional crown until the desired contour and gingival emergence have been achieved. An impression of the abutment and adjacent soft tissue will allow for production of the final crown.

Advantages/indications of prepable abutments

- the technique will suit almost every situation
- copes with angulation changes
- allows for soft-tissue remodelling and good emergence profiles

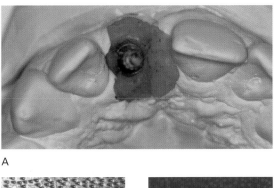

A

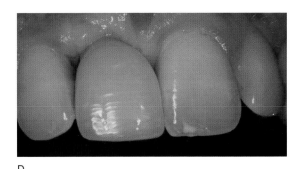

D

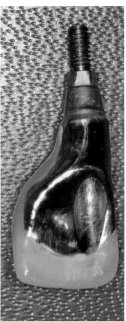

B

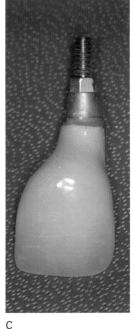

C

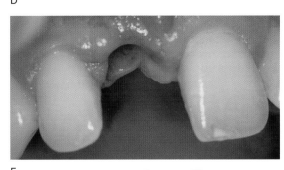

E

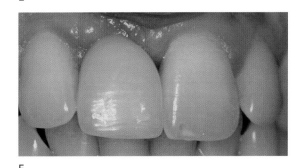

F

Figure 13.7

Restoration of an AstraTech ST implant that is close to the adjacent tooth. There was a large incisive canal that influenced implant placement. (A) From the implant head model, the lack of space between the implant head and the adjacent tooth can be seen. Use of an abutment and separate crown would therefore be difficult. (B) Using a cast-to abutment, a one-piece abutment and crown has been produced. The abutment is completely customizable using a conventional wax pattern and casting technique. (C) The resulting restoration eliminates the need for cementation and is retained by the abutment screw. (D) On initial insertion, the crown causes blanching to the soft tissues. (E) Removal of the restoration 4 weeks later demonstrates a healthy contoured gingival cuff. (F) The completed crown.

Disadvantages/contraindications of prepable abutments

- more complex laboratory technique
- may require second intraoral impression
- precision of fit of crown to abutment is less predictable

Fully customized abutments

These abutments share many properties with prepable abutments but they can be produced with even more allowances for compromised implant positioning. The basic procedure is illustrated in Figure 13.7. Following an implant head impression the abutment pattern is placed in position on the working model. Some designs have a precious metal base that provides the accuracy and detail of the fit surface to the implant; other designs reproduce the fit surface in the burn-out pattern. The abutment shape is waxed onto the pattern and then cast in precious metal. With this process it is possible for an abutment to be produced to accommodate significant changes in angulation between implant and crown and also to move the apparent long axis of the final restoration to a different position on the implant long axis, although this is limited by the need to retain adequate retentive form for the final crown.

The extra complexities of this process restrict its use to difficult situations that can be resolved only by full customization. Where the fit surface of the abutment has been cast rather than manufactured, the quality of fit may not be as good. Conventional abutment screws retain the abutments and the rest of their use is the same as for prepable abutments.

Computer-generated abutments

Using the Procera system, it is possible for customized abutments to be produced using a factory process. Head of implant impressions are taken and the working model is placed in a scanner. Readings are taken of the implant position and angulation relative to the desired restoration. Using computer software, an 'ideal' abutment shape can be generated and viewed in three dimensions. The position of the gingival margin can be superimposed on the image and the information sent to a specialized centre where the abutment is produced in titanium.

The end result of these abutments is very similar to prepable abutments. With highly skilled technicians, who are experienced in the scanning technique, the process is straightforward, but the technique is limited to laboratories with those skills. The remaining process to complete the restoration is the same as for prepable abutments.

Ceramic abutments

These are essentially the same as prepable abutments and are used in the same way (Figures 13.8 and 13.9). They are made from

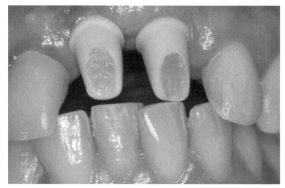

A

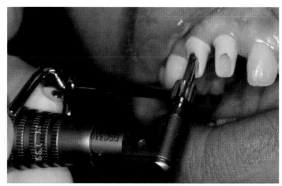

B

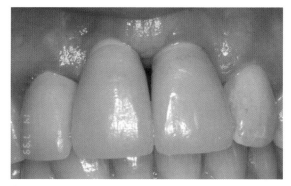

C

Figure 13.8

Nobel Biocare implants restored with porcelain CerAdapt abutments. The implant heads were close to the surface and conventional abutments could not be hidden. (A) The prepared abutments in position; the abutment screw access holes are sealed with a tooth-coloured material. (B) The abutment screws are torqued carefully into place using an electronic torque controller and a counter-torque to prevent overstressing the implant. (C) The completed Procera crowns cemented with a tooth-coloured composite resin cement.

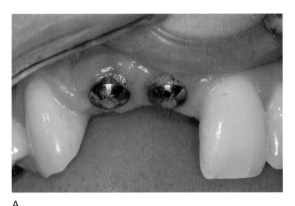

A

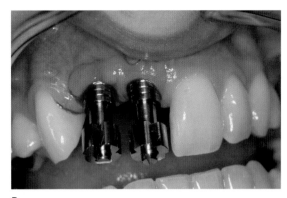

B

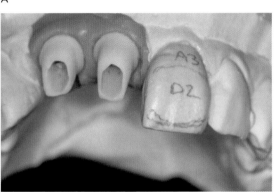

C

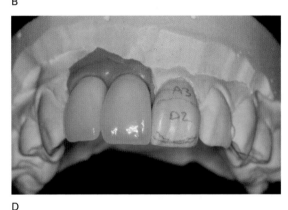

D

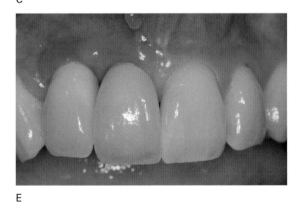

E

Figure 13.9

Two Nobel Biocare implants restored with CerAdapt abutments. The gingival tissues were thin and, to prevent shine-through of the metal abutments, porcelain abutments were chosen. (A) Healing abutments in place. (B) Implant head impression copings in position prior to impression taking. (C) On the cast, the abutments are prepared. (D) All porcelain crowns are produced directly on the abutments. (E) The completed restorations.

dense porcelain and clinical trials have demonstrated good success rates, although the number of trials is limited in number and there is little long-term data. The restorations can be highly aesthetic; the final crown should be all-porcelain in construction and cemented with a tooth-coloured lute to achieve optimal results. Ceramic abutments are not suitable for situations where significant angulation changes need to be made,

because the porcelain remaining following preparation will be at risk of fracture if it is too thin.

Abutments for screw-retained crowns

The desirability for screw retention has already been discussed. The normal way to achieve a screw-retained crown is to use an abutment designed for bridges (EsthetiCone from Nobel Biocare or Octa from Straumann) but to use a gold cylinder that has an internal surface with facets that engage the abutment (Figures 13.10 and 13.11). If the abutment does not have this type of surface, such as the Uni-abutment (AstraTech), then there will be nothing to resist rotational forces other than the gold screw.

Systems such as the Frialit have components specifically for screw retention where the screw does not seat into the abutment in the long axis, but has a lateral retaining screw that can be positioned on the palatal or lingual aspect of the crown. As long as there is sufficient space for this, it can produce an aesthetic retrievable crown with no screw hole on the occlusal surface.

Generally, screw-retained crowns are more applicable to premolar and molar regions where occlusal screw access may be less of an aesthetic problem and in situations where there may be more of a need to remove restorations (e.g. to tighten the abutment screw) or join implants to further implants in the future.

Impressions and abutment selection

The previous section described in detail the various abutments and techniques available. However, before an abutment is selected, a choice needs to be made between two alternative

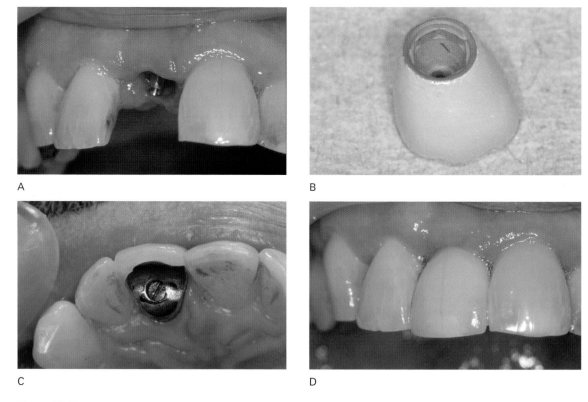

A

B

C

D

Figure 13.10

A missing central incisor tooth with a Nobel Biocare implant in place. (A) An EsthetiCone abutment has been placed. The patient expressed a desire for the restoration to be easily retrievable, so a screw-retained crown has been chosen. (B) The internal contour of the gold cylinder used will engage the anti-rotational features of the abutment. (C) Palatal view of the final restoration in place shows the position of the retaining screw in the cingulum of the crown. (D) The completed restoration.

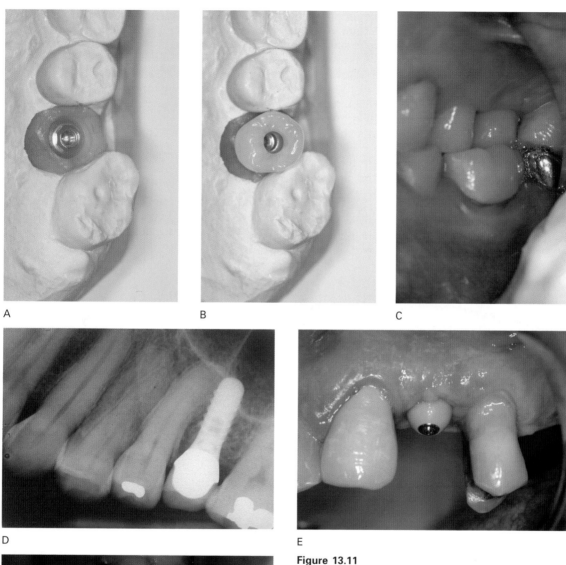

A

B

C

D

E

Figure 13.11

A single Straumann implant placed for a missing upper second premolar tooth: (A) the working cast with a replica of the implant; (B) completed crown – the screw access hole is centrally placed; (C) buccal view of the crown in position—the upper teeth are in cross bite with the lower teeth; (D) periapical radiograph of the completed restoration; (E) a similar case of a missing first premolar tooth also with a Straumann implant; the abutment is protected with a healing cap; (F) occlusal view of the implant prior to abutment connection;

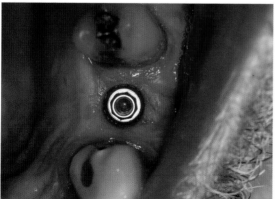

F

continued

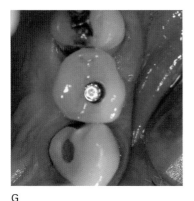

G

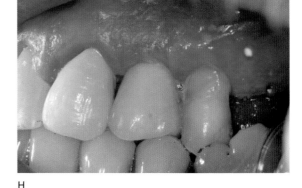

H

Figure 13.11 *continued*

(G) the completed crown, occlusal view; (H) the completed restoration.

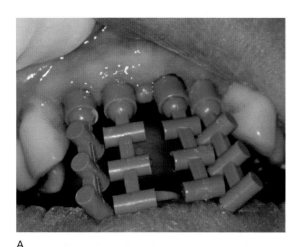

A

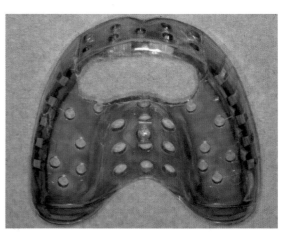

B

C

Figure 13.12

Four Nobel Biocare implants to be restored in single restorations: (A) CeraOne abutment impression copings in place; (B) a stock tray has been modified to allow the copings to project; (C) an impression taken in Impregum—note the finger marks over the copings due to the operator holding the copings down to prevent their movement while the impression material sets.

techniques: abutment impressions or implant head impressions.

Abutment impressions

The conventional approach for single tooth restorations using standard manufacturer-made components is to choose the abutment and place it into position. An impression is made of the abutment and a working model is produced using ready-made components (Figure 13.12). The abutment can be left in position and covered with a temporary cover or a temporary crown can be built up using conventional crown and bridge techniques (with a temporary component from the manufacturer).

Alternatively, the abutment can be removed following impression taking and stored for use at the next appointment. The healing abutment is therefore replaced. This technique requires less chairside time and the original provisional restoration (denture or resin bonded bridge) can be re-fitted. It is important that the abutment is stored in a sterile container and care must be taken to ensure that it will go back into exactly the same position next time. With the CeraOne system, for example, the abutment will seat back onto the implant in a reproducible way each time because the components are symmetrical and matched. With some systems, such as the AstraTech ST, there is a difference between the number of facets on components, i.e. the abutment could reseat into a different position next time. Many components are made in this way because it allows more positions of the abutment on first seating. If the abutment is to be removed, it needs to re-orientate in the correct position. Marking the abutment holder prior to removal of the abutment and leaving it in the holder until the next appointment will achieve this (see Figure 13.2C). Whichever of these alternatives is followed, this technique requires that the abutment is chosen in the mouth and an error in choice can be costly.

Implant head impressions

This technique is mandatory for all abutment types other than conventional abutments and

has much to recommend it as the approach of choice. An impression is recorded of the implant head using an impression coping (see Chapter 14 for more detail), which is cast with an analogue of the implant head to produce a working model (Figure 13.13). The abutment can be selected and seated onto the model. Choice of the abutment outside of the mouth ensures that the correct decision can be made more easily without taking up clinical time. Any of the abutment types can be used in this way. Care must be taken not to damage the abutment assembly, particularly the screw, and therefore a laboratory screw should be used and the clinical screw stored until the abutment is seated into the mouth. The abutment should be sterilized before placement in the mouth.

Some prosthodontists prefer to choose the abutment using this technique but then place the abutment into the mouth and re-take the impression.

Choosing the abutment

Abutment selection is based on several features.

Depth of soft tissue

The vertical height from implant head to the gingival margin is measured at the shallowest point on the labial surface. This can be measured intraorally with a periodontal measuring probe or with various devices provided by manufacturers that fit onto the implant head and indicate the depth. To ensure that the metal collar of the abutment does not show, the abutment is chosen so that the labial margin is at least 1 mm subgingival. Care must be taken to ensure that choosing abutments to suit the labial margin does not result in an excessively deep margin elsewhere. The authors find that margins more than 3 mm deep result in restorations that are difficult to seat and removal of excess cement may be impossible. In situations where there is a marked discrepancy between the gingival heights around the margin, a prepable abutment is indicated because it allows the margin to be placed in relation to the gingival contour. This technique assumes that the chosen abutment

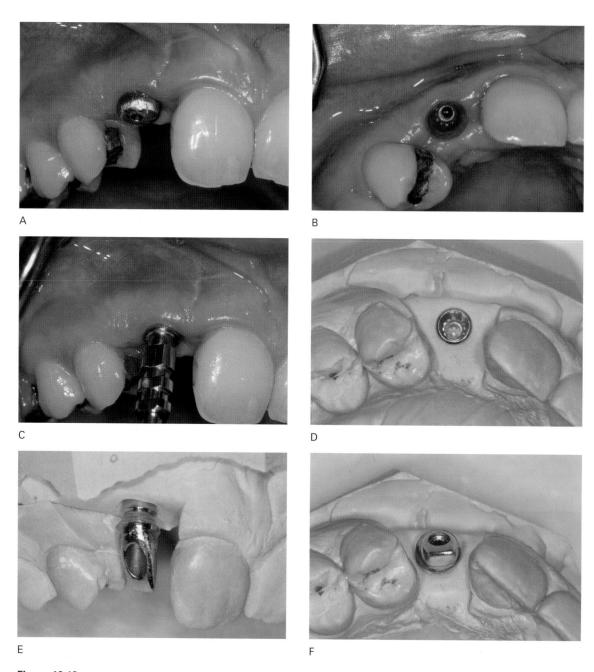

A

B

C

D

E

F

Figure 13.13

Restoration of an AstraTech ST implant with a Profile BI abutment: (A) Missing upper lateral incisor tooth; (B) healing abutment removed; (C) implant head impression coping in place; (D) the working cast—the gingival replica has been removed; (E) the prepared abutment; (F) there has been more labial reduction to allow for the desired crown contours;

continued

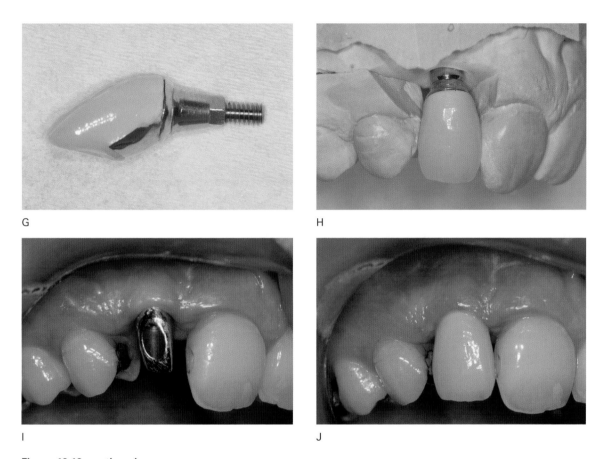

G

H

I

J

Figure 13.13 *continued*

(G) the completed crown and abutment—note the contour that has been achieved; (H) the completed restoration on the master cast; (I) the abutment in place; the gingival blanching is normal due to the difference in contour between the healing abutment and the definitive abutment; (J) the completed restoration.

has a diameter close to that of the cervical margin of the tooth to be replaced.

Emergence profile

It is easier to create a good emergence profile if there is at least 3 mm of vertical space from implant head to gingival margin (Figure 13.14). This allows a transition from an implant head, which is often at least 2–3 mm less in diameter than the cervical margin of the proposed restoration. If it is necessary to flare from the implant head to a wide-necked restoration in a short vertical space, it is most readily achieved using a wide-diameter prepable abutment. This can

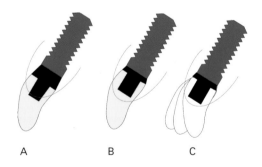

A   B   C

Figure 13.14

Selection of a shorter abutment (B,C) allows more vertical space for possible alterations in labial angulation with standard abutments compared with a normal selection (A) where the crown margin has been placed just subgingival.

create a dramatic change in little vertical space, but care must be taken not to excessively overcontour this region, which then may be difficult to maintain. There may be a desire to create a final restoration with a wide gingival dimension especially where the interdental gingival papillae have been lost to leave 'black triangles', which will spoil the final appearance.

Orientation

Ideally the implant will have been placed close to the long axis of the missing tooth crown and adjacent clinical crowns. Implant placement with the long axis of the implant through the incisal tip or just to the palatal surface is easiest to restore and any of the abutments can work in this situation. It is a common scenario, however, for the implant to have a slight or even pronounced labial inclination. There are several reasons why this may be the case, including:

* The bony contour following resorption from tooth loss often results in an alveolus which dictates implant placement in a more labial inclination.
* As a result of the natural curvature of the original and adjacent teeth, the roots may be orientated at a different angle to the clinical crown.

Small degrees of labial angulation (see Chapters 3, 4 and 9) can therefore be desirable and easily accommodated by standard abutments. If standard abutments are used in situations with more labial angulation, they may result in either an excessively overcontoured labial surface or a porcelain surface that is too thin to mask the metal structure underneath. Starting the restoration more apical by using a shorter abutment will help (Figure 13.14). A better result can be achieved by using prepable abutments or fully customized abutments, because the path of insertion of the crown can be different to the long axis of the implant. Changes of between 30° and 40° can be made; the limiting factors are normally the need to retain some abutment structure around the abutment screw hole and the need to provide adequate retention for the crown. To assist with the correct abutment choice, the best approach is to determine the

correct labial contour using either the provisional restoration or from a diagnostic wax-up. A silicone putty labial mask can be produced from this and placed either in the mouth or, ideally, on a working implant head model. The true orientation of the implant relative to the labial surface is then clear and the correct abutment choice can be made.

Interocclusal space

The space from implant head to the opposing tooth needs to be assessed. The shortest standard abutments require a minimum vertical space of 6–7 mm. If less space exists a prepable abutment may be indicated, although vertical spaces less than 5 mm are difficult to restore and alternative conventional dental techniques, such as increasing the vertical dimension of the occlusion or the use of 'Dahl' appliances, should have been considered. Once again, correct planning and a deeper implant placement can avoid this problem. Excessive vertical dimensions can be restored using any of the abutment types. Standard abutments are available in various heights and they have adequate retention and resistance form to support restorations with considerable vertical height. The implant crown needs to be made so that the porcelain is correctly supported by the metal work.

Retrievability

A screw-retained restoration will be easier to remove at a later stage if it is envisaged that this will be required. A cemented crown, even placed on a standard abutment with a temporary cement, can be very difficult to remove. In general, a restoration can only be made screw retained if the path of insertion for the screw will be on the palatal or occlusal aspect. Specific abutments for single teeth are available or a standard abutment can have the crown cemented onto the abutment out of the mouth and a larger access hole made through the crown to fit the restoration onto the implant with the abutment screw. Screw retention can be useful in situations where there is limited space between adjacent teeth. Access for the cementation process can be limited and the space needed for the abutment, cement lute and crown takes up more space than a one-piece screw-retained restoration (see Figure 13.7).

Special aesthetic requirements

The techniques already outlined aim to provide an aesthetic restoration with no metal showing. Problems can arise if the implant head is close to the surface or if the labial gingival tissue is thin so that the metal abutment shows through the gingiva, causing greying and a poor appearance. This can be determined by attaching an implant head impression coping and looking for a colour change. A porcelain abutment such as the CerAdapt from Nobel Biocare can allow for an aesthetic restoration to be achieved.

Final restoration

Before a single tooth implant abutment is chosen, the type of final restoration required must be considered because this will have a bearing on the abutment selection. When using metal abutments there is little reason for avoiding the use of metal ceramic restorations. All porcelain restorations cemented onto metal abutments need to be quite thick to avoid the metal showing through and resulting in a grey restoration. Problems can arise when single tooth implants are being matched to adjacent teeth that are already restored with porcelain crowns or porcelain veneers. It is often best to replace adjacent restorations so that they can be reconstructed together in the same materials. Alternatively, more space needs to be created in the abutment to accommodate the all-ceramic crown.

Abutment selection kits

Several manufacturers produce abutment selection kits that are exact replicas of the different abutments available (Figure 13.4C). They are normally used on an implant head cast but can also be used intraorally. Because it can be difficult to visualize an abutment in position and an incorrect choice can be very costly, their use is

highly recommended (see Chapter 14 for more detail).

Having chosen the abutment and decided upon the final restoration, the clinical techniques can now be outlined.

Abutment connection

Deep soft-tissue tunnels will make abutment seating a purely tactile process. It may also be an uncomfortable process for the patient, particularly if the soft tissue is still in a fragile state. It is essential that healing abutments are not left out for any length of time because the soft tissue will quickly collapse into the space and will be painful to push back. Local anaesthetic may therefore be required. A degree of soft-tissue blanching is to be expected, but patients should feel the area return to normal within a few minutes.

If the abutment is to be placed in the mouth and left in place, the abutment screw will need to be tightened to the manufacturer's recommendations. Electronic and hand torque devices are available, with and without counter-torques. It is essential that the abutment is fully seated and in the correct position before torquing the screw because the fit surfaces will be damaged and it can be difficult to remove if incorrect, or the screw may fracture.

The complications of removing abutments once impressions have been taken and reseating them in the same position have been discussed already.

Impressions

For standard abutments, plastic push-on impression copings are seated onto the abutment (Figure 13.15). These are often a tight fit and hydrostatic pressure can build up inside such that they tend to lift up from the abutment if seating pressure is released. If it is obvious that the coping is not stable, it should be left untrimmed and a hole cut in the impression tray so that finger pressure can be exerted on the coping while the impression material is setting. A retentive impression coping is trimmed so that

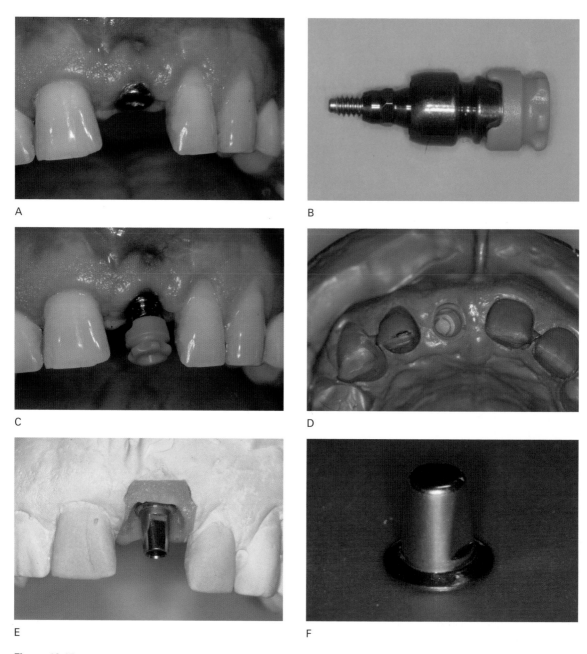

A

B

C

D

E

F

Figure 13.15

A Frialit 2 implant placed to replace a missing upper central incisor tooth: (A) healing abutment in position; (B) the impression coping; (C) the coping is seated into the implant—the metal part will stay in the implant following removal of the impression; (D) the blue plastic component is picked up in the impregum impression; the metal coping that remained attached to the implant will reseat accurately back into this; (E) working cast with abutment in position; (F) the metal coping for crown manufacture;

continued

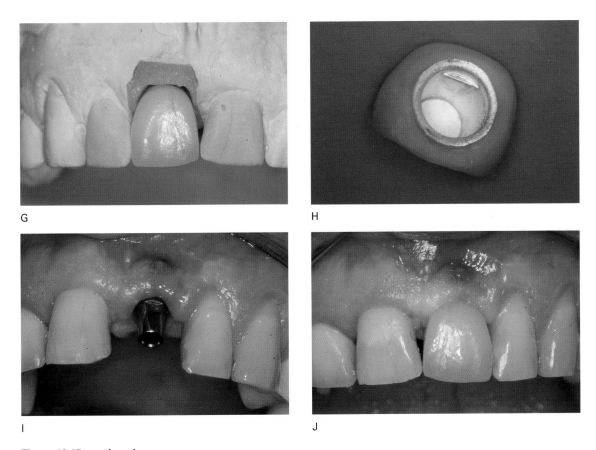

Figure 13.15 *continued*

(G) completed crown on cast; (H) internally, the use of a pre-made coping ensures an accurate fit; (I) abutment seated; (J) the crown immediately after cementation; the gingival blanching will resolve in a short time.

it does not interfere with an impression tray. Conventional crown and bridge techniques can be employed. A stock tray that is rigid enough to support medium- or heavy-bodied impression material is used. The impression material used needs to be rigid enough when set to hold the impression coping without tearing. Light-bodied materials are therefore not suitable. Putty consistency materials alone are also not suitable, because they will not flow around the copings. Single-phase materials such as polyethers and addition-cured silicones (medium- or heavy-bodied pastes) are recommended.

Impression material is syringed around the coping and the tray is seated. A full-arch impression is recommended. Once set, the impression should retain the coping and it should be tested carefully for looseness with tweezers. If there is any doubt that the coping may have moved in the impression, it is best to re-take the impression. The impression should also record the adjacent teeth and their gingival margins, as well as the articular surfaces of all the teeth in the arch. The abutment analogue needs to be attached to the impression coping ready for the laboratory to cast the impression.

Good quality opposing impressions and occlusal records are required. For a single tooth restoration it is normally not necessary for models to be fully articulated, but similar requirements to conventional crown work should be followed and a complex occlusal relationship that needs to be copied may indicate full articulation on a suitable articulator.

For a prepable abutment to be used, an impression of the implant head is required to allow the abutment to be modified on a model in the laboratory. A 'pick up' impression technique is followed, with an impression coping held into position with a guide pin. The pin needs to be unscrewed before the impression is removed from the mouth (see Chapter 14 for more detail). Once a prepable abutment has been placed, a secondary impression of the abutment in position and the gingival contour may be required. If the gingival margin of the abutment is only just subgingival, it may be possible to record the margin using a conventional impression technique, syringing light-bodied material into the gingival crevice. Deeper margins or situations where there is some gingival bleeding make the use of a gingival retraction cord necessary (Figure 13.16). This needs to be packed with care because it must not be pushed below the widest contour of the abutment, otherwise it will be difficult to remove. It is important that the margin of the abutment is checked after the impression has been removed to ensure that fragments of material have not torn from the impression and remain trapped under the

convexity of the abutment. If an impression is proving difficult to take, it is better to replace a well-fitting provisional restoration and allow the soft tissue to improve and then try again, or alternatively to consider removing the abutment and directly waxing up the framework on the abutment or to construct an acrylic coping of the abutment that can be picked up in a secondary impression.

Temporary restorations

Short-term temporary crowns can be constructed at the chairside using plastic copings supplied to fit on conventional single tooth abutments. These can be time consuming to make and often it is best to remove the abutment and replace the provisional restoration. Temporary crowns can be constructed from the diagnostic wax-up using either a putty or vacuum-formed mould in crown and bridge temporary acrylic materials. The temporary crown will need to extend down to the margin of the coping and the material will not flow subgingivally. The temporary restoration needs to be contoured carefully to have an acceptable emergence profile and this is best completed out of the mouth using light-cured composite.

Longer term provisional crowns to be placed on prepable abutments or to be used for soft-tissue moulding techniques (see earlier) are best constructed in the laboratory in advance. Temporary crowns can be cemented using conventional materials such as zinc oxide/ eugenol or temporary cements.

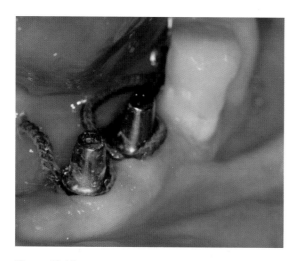

Figure 13.16

Gingival retraction cord placed around prepable abutments to assist in an accurate impression being taken of the subgingival margins.

Shade taking and laboratory procedures

Ideally the shade should be taken with agreement of the dentist, patient and technician. The design of the abutment also should be a joint responsibility between dentist and technician. For single tooth restorations, the expectations of the patient are often very high and only the highest quality aesthetics will be acceptable.

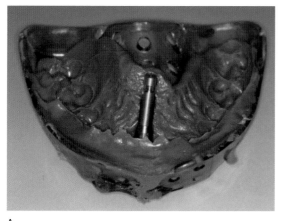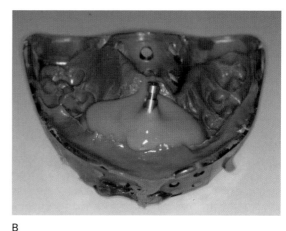

A   B

Figure 13.17

(A) An impregum impression of an abutment with the laboratory replica attached. (B) The soft gingival replica is poured into the impression

Laboratory techniques

Analogues for either the abutment or the implant head are attached to the coping in the impression (Figure 13.17). A soft-tissue replica in a flexible material needs to be incorporated into the working model, because a hard model would not allow the restoration to extend subgingivally and create a good emergence. Several silicone materials are available and they are placed into the impression around the laboratory replica before dental stone is poured. The soft-tissue replica is removable to allow access to the margin area.

Conventional techniques are followed for crown construction, as already outlined.

Fitting the completed restoration

Try-in

The restoration can be tried in prior to completion. Straightforward cases can go to completion from the initial impression but where significant changes have to be made to orientation or soft-tissue contours, a try-in is advised. The crown can be seated with finger pressure but will often rise up due to the gingiva being displaced. It is often difficult for patients to see the exact result at this time unless the crown is being firmly held in. The contact points are checked with dental floss, as for conventional crowns.

Occlusion

The occlusal contacts should be checked prior to and after cementation. The ideal arrangement is for the implant restoration to be in very light contact when the patient gently holds their teeth together and to be in full contact only when heavy load is applied. The best test is for the implant restoration not to hold shimstock on light contact, whereas the adjacent teeth do. As more pressure is exerted, the implant restoration can start to hold shimstock.

This can be difficult to determine until the restoration is finally cemented. Prior to cementation it is probably best to adjust and check the occlusion with occlusal indicator papers for gross overcontact. The crown should be adjusted so that it lightly marks and so that heavier marks are visible on adjacent teeth. The implant crown should not be placed without occlusal contact because this could result in movement of the opposing teeth.

The occlusal contacts are first checked in the intercuspal position (the position of maximum intercuspation). This may not be in the retruded arc of closure and so the crown should be checked in this position to ensure that it will not create an occlusal interference.

Next the crown is checked for protrusive and lateral contacts. In protrusive movement, if the crown is to be in contact it should be shared with other teeth and not be the sole point of contact. In lateral movement, the crown should conform to the existing occlusal scheme: either a group contact or canine-guided. It is not desirable for the implant restoration to act as the only guiding surface for lateral movement.

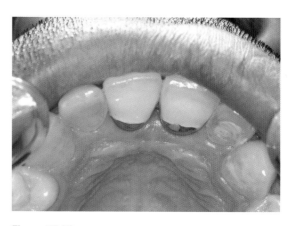

Figure 13.18

Two single tooth implant-supported crowns with cement venting holes just visible above the gingival margin on the palatal aspect. These have been restored with composite resin.

Cementation

It may be prudent for the final restoration to be cemented provisionally while the patient accommodates to it, and to give time for the soft tissue to mature around the new shape. A modified temporary cement should be used because well-fitting crowns can be difficult to remove later, especially as the smooth shape and lack of an accessible margin can make it difficult to hold the crown to remove it.

Prior to finally cementing the crown the abutment screw should be checked for tightness and some gutta percha or similar soft material placed over the screw head so that it can be found easily and the head remain undamaged if the crown ever needs to be removed and the abutment taken out in the future.

Traditional cements such as zinc phosphate are often recommended but care has to be taken to ensure that the viscosity of the cement is low enough for the crown to be fully seated. The quality of fit between abutment and restoration means that softer cements designed for temporary cementation are adequate as the definitive cement.

Whatever cement is used, the crown does not need to be filled completely with cement because excess cement extending down below the margin can be difficult to detect and remove. Ideally, exactly the right amount of cement to produce no excess should be aimed for and there are few complications to having an incomplete cement lute compared with conventional crown and bridgework. Many operators prefer to create a vent hole in the back of the crown to ensure that excess cement comes out in a controlled position. The hole can be sealed later with composite filling material (Figure 13.18).

It can often be difficult to seat the crown into position due to the deep position of the implant, the need to recontour the soft tissue by overbuilding the proximal areas or due to bleeding from the soft tissues. Do not try to force the crown down with permanent cement. Place it provisionally first with a temporary cement and remove it and re-cement at a later stage once the gingiva have recontoured and matured.

Following cementation, a long cone periapical radiograph should be taken to:

- verify seating of the restoration
- check that no excess cement is present
- act as a record of the marginal bone height for comparison with follow-up images

Instructions to the patient

The patient must be armed with the knowledge and ability to maintain the restoration. For single tooth restorations no special oral hygiene techniques are required and the patient should be able to follow the same cleaning techniques that they follow for their other teeth. Patients should be warned that the new implant restoration might feel 'hard' and 'heavy' to bite on for a few days, a feeling that soon passes. It is not normal for patients to feel any discomfort from single tooth restorations and they should be encouraged to return if they have any symptoms. The complications of single tooth restorations are covered in Chapter 16.

Additional considerations

Multiple single tooth restorations

The process of providing multiple single tooth restorations next to each other raises the following issues:

- Is there adequate space, not just to place the implants but also to place abutments and crowns and to allow for adequate space for interdental gingivae to develop? It is

sometimes better to place fewer implants and restore the region with a bridge.
- A single tooth space normally has some interdental papillae left due to the presence of adjacent teeth. If several teeth are lost, the ridge often heals with a flat contour. Placement of individual crowns can result in triangular dark spaces interdentally. This can be overcome to some extent by overcontouring the crowns (see Figure 13.19) but it may be remedied better by placing linked crowns. Soft-tissue augmentation techniques are considered in Chapter 12.

Restorations from impressions at implant placement

It is possible to provide an implant-supported crown from impressions taken at implant placement and to insert the abutment and a provisional crown at implant exposure. This will speed up the process of provision of a restoration and, in particular, dispense with the need to adjust a temporary restoration to allow for

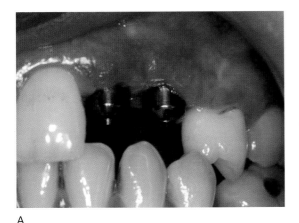

A

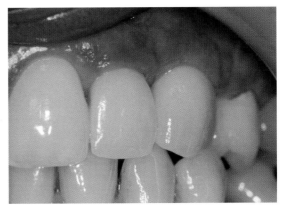

B

Figure 13.19

(A) Missing lateral incisor and canine teeth. The gingival contour, particularly between the two implants, is evident. (B) An acceptable aesthetic result has been obtained by producing crowns with a long contact area and overcontouring interdentally.

healing abutments. This may be a particular advantage where a temporary partial denture is thin due to the occlusal contacts. Further thinning of the denture to accommodate healing abutments can make the denture unusable. It is also proposed that the soft-tissue contours form to the correct shape more speedily, although this will depend upon achieving a correct emergence profile and margin placement from the limited information available from the first impression. On the whole, the disadvantages and extra complexity of this technique make it only worth considering in exceptional situations.

An impression is taken at implant placement. Because the implant is not integrated at this stage, care must be taken not to compromise the implant. An impression coping is placed onto the implant head and, rather than take a conventional impression, the coping is linked to a rigid surgical stent using acrylic. The study model is then adjusted to accept the stent, which is replaced with the impression coping attached to an implant analogue. A new working model is created that will give a reasonably accurate representation of the implant position but will not reproduce the gingival contour around the implant. A prepable abutment is adjusted to give an ideal emergence, and margin placement is dictated by the contours of adjacent teeth. A standard abutment also can be used. An acrylic provisional crown is made on the abutment. At implant exposure the abutment is seated, and this can be verified visually. The provisional crown is cemented with temporary cement and the soft tissue sutured around the crown. Following healing, a prepable abutment can be adjusted to ensure that the margins are in the correct position and an impression is taken for the final crown.

Bibliography

Andersson B, Odman P, Carlsson L, Brånemark PI (1992). A new Brånemark single tooth abutment: handling and early clinical experiences. *Int J Oral Maxillofac Implants* **7**: 105–11.

Andersson B, Odman P, Lindvall AM, Brånemark PI (1998). Cemented single crowns on osseointegrated implants after 5 years: results from a prospective study on CeraOne. *Int J Prosthod* **11**: 212–8.

Balfour A, O'Brien GR (1995). Comparative study of antirotational single tooth abutments. *J Prosth Dent* **73**: 36–43.

Belser UC, Bernard JP, Buser D (1996). Implant supported restorations in the anterior region. Prosthetic considerations, *Pract Period Aesth Dent* **8**: 875–83.

Jemt T (1998). Customized titanium single-implant abutments: 2 year follow-up pilot study. *Int J Prosthod* **11**: 312–6.

Jemt T, Laney W, Harris D, Henry PJ, Krogh PHJ, Polizzi G, Zarb GA, Herrmann I (1991). Osseointegrated implants for single tooth replacement: a 1-year report from a multicenter prospective study. *Int J Oral Maxillofac Implants* **6**: 29–36.

Jorneus L, Jemt T, Carlsson L (1992). Loads and designs of screw joints for single crowns supported by osseointegrated implants. *Int J Oral Maxillofac Implants* **7**: 353–9.

Laney W, Jemt T, Harris D, Henry PJ, Krogh PHJ, Polizzi G, Zarb GA, Herrmann I (1994). Osseointegrated implants for single tooth replacement: progress report from a multicenter prospective study after 3 years. *Int J Oral Maxillofac Implants* **6**: 29–36.

Lewis S (1995). Anterior single-tooth implant restorations. *Int J Period Rest Dent* **15**: 30–41.

Palmer RM, Smith BJ, Palmer PJ, Floyd PD (1997). A prospective study of Astra single tooth implants. *Clin Oral Implants Res* **8**: 173–9.

14
Fixed bridge prosthodontics

Introduction

The chapters on treatment planning and surgery have emphasized the role of prosthodontic planning prior to embarking on treatment. For fixed bridges, it is essential that thorough planning has been undertaken to determine the end result required. From this, a surgical stent can be produced to guide the surgery and good provisional restorations made that will be able to function during the stages of treatment until the final restoration is achieved.

A further complication of constructing bridges on implants is the need for exact clinical and technical control to take impressions and construct the restoration so that it will fit with a high level of accuracy. With conventional bridge-work supported by teeth the displacement of the abutment teeth within the periodontal ligament can compensate for small errors in the fit of a bridge. Placing a bridge onto implants demands a higher level of accuracy in fit because the bridge needs to seat passively onto the rigid implants. This requirement is increased if the bridge is to be screwed to the abutments rather than cemented.

Principles

Short-span and long-span bridges

The abutments and techniques used to construct implant-supported bridges are the same whether the bridge just involves two implants linked together or if the full jaw is to be restored with six or more implants supporting one fixed bridge (Figure 14.1). The complexity of achieving an acceptable fit is, however, increased when multiple implants are used. Linking implants in a fixed bridge has the following benefits:

- Shorter implants (under 10 mm) can be protected from overload by the other implants, because the rigid structure will distribute the load over the combined surface areas of the implants.
- Implants placed in areas of high potential stress can be protected by linked structures. For example, linking to other implants can protect the most distal implant in a posterior reconstruction.
- Linked implants allow cantilever pontics to be incorporated into a bridge. This is particularly useful with distal extension bridges. It is often difficult to place adequate length implants in distal positions due to lack of bone and anatomical features. By linking implants placed anteriorly, the patient can be provided with teeth in these regions.

Where several implants are available of adequate dimensions it may be advisable to divide the restoration into separate bridges so that it is easier to construct and maintain in the future if complications arise. Much debate has arisen regarding the desirability of bridges extending across the midline due to the potential flexure (particularly of the mandible) during loading. However, clinical trials have not demonstrated this to be a clinical problem and the authors do not see this as a potential complication.

Distal cantilevers

Distal cantilevers may be indicated with free end saddle restorations where it has not been

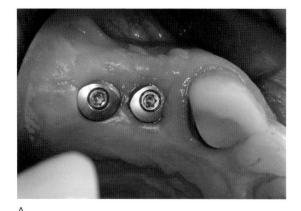

A

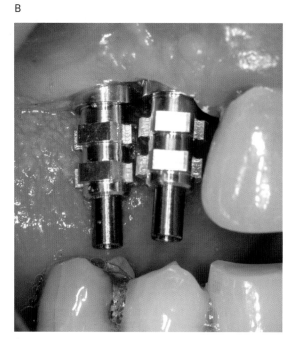

B

C

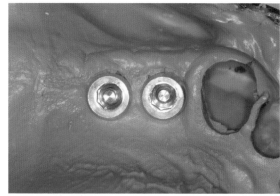

D

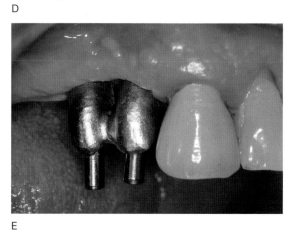

E

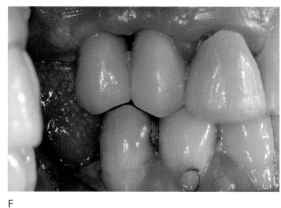

F

Figure 14.1

Two Straumann implants have been placed in the missing premolar teeth sites: (A) healing caps in position; (B) SynOcta bridge abutments have been placed; (C) impression copings attached to the abutments; (D) impression copings removed in the impression; (E) metal framework tried in with guide pins; (F) completed bridge—note the subgingival margin placement for optimum aesthetics.

possible to place an implant as far distal as required for appearance and function. The ability to provide a cantilever depends upon several factors (see also Chapter 5):

- The potential load that might be placed on the extension. Natural opposing teeth or a patient with a previous history of parafunction requires caution compared with a cantilever opposed by a removable restoration or pontic.
- The length and width of the most distal implant, which will take the greatest compressive load.
- The length and position of the most anterior implant, which will take the greatest tensile load.
- The antero-posterior dimension measured from a line drawn between the most distal implant on either side, to the most anterior implant. The greater this distance the longer the potential cantilever that can be placed as the anterior implant will not be subject to as much stress as if the implants are placed in a straight line.

Some authorities have suggested that cantilevers as long as 20 mm can be constructed safely. The authors would recommend that this figure be treated with caution and ideally distal cantilevers, even with several long implants in a good arch shape, should be restricted to 10–15 mm (two premolar-sized pontics).

Screw-retained or cemented bridges

Attaching bridges to implants with screws allows the possibility of making the restoration easily retrievable and free from the potential problems of cementation, a concept that can offer considerable advantages over conventional bridgework based on teeth. In the Brånemark system, abutments are chosen that locate onto the implant head and are held into position with an abutment screw. The abutment is designed to accept a smaller 'bridge' screw that will retain the bridge. This screw passes through a machined gold cylinder that is incorporated into the bridge structure and seats accurately onto

the abutment (Figure 14.2). The small bridge screw that retains the restoration is designed to be the weakest link in the implant assembly and should be the part to fail if the restoration is overloaded or subjected to trauma.

Variations exist with the other systems. AstraTech Uni-abutments (AstraTech: Astra Meditec AB, Mölndal, Sweden) and Straumann SynOcta abutments (ITI/Straumann: Institut Straumann AG, Waldenburg, Switzerland) are one-piece. Frialit abutments have a single screw that acts as the bridge screw and the abutment screw.

The screw-retained bridge needs to be a passive fit onto the abutments, confirming that it is in the same path of insertion and plane as the abutment head. If a bridge screw is tightened into an abutment and the gold cylinder is not seating evenly, the screw will be put under tension and not only will the bridge not be seating down properly and marginal gaps exist, but there is a high chance of the screw loosening or fracturing with time. Each bridge gold cylinder needs to be in this exact relationship and the complication of constructing a bridge with multiple abutments lies in achieving this degree of accuracy. For many dentists, the advantage of ease of removal of the bridge is outweighed by these potential difficulties.

Cemented bridges do not necessarily demand such high standards of precision, because the cement lute will allow a bridge to seat without putting the structure under tension. This is not a justification for poor technical or clinical standards but reflects a reality that perfection is not reliably achieved. Cemented bridges are constructed on abutments that are prepared in the laboratory to resemble prepared teeth as required for conventional bridges (Figure 14.3). More laboratory time is often required than for techniques that use standard manufacturer-made components. The retrievability of cemented bridges can be controlled to some extent by the use of temporary cements because these may allow removal of bridges if required. The potential for dissolution of cement from margins will not result in caries as it can with conventional bridges. Cemented bridges do not require an access hole for the gold screw through the bridge. Although this is rarely a problem for most patients, it can present complications if the screw hole has to be positioned in a visible area or at

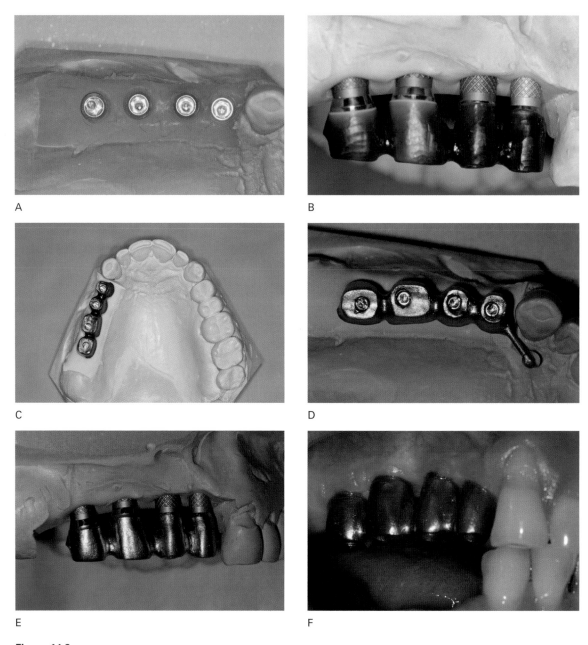

Figure 14.2

Four Frialit implants have been placed to replace the missing premolar and molar teeth: (A) master cast produced following implant head impressions—the different coloured implant analogues correspond to the diameter of implant placed; (B) bridge cylinders are linked in a wax pattern ready for casting; (C) occlusal view showing access for abutment/bridge screws; (D) completed casting—the mesial handle is for production purposes and will be removed before final insertion; (E) casting from buccal side—note the precise fit; (F) the casting is tried in prior to porcelain placement to verify the fit;

continued

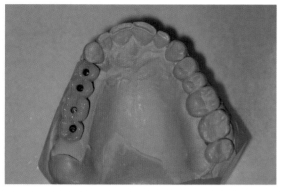

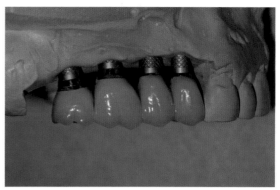

G

H

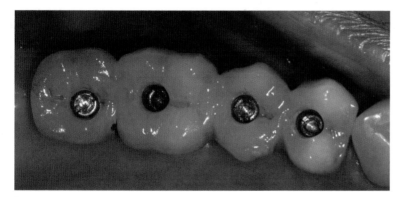

I

Figure 14.2 *continued*

(G) the completed bridge; (H) adequate embrasure space has been provided for oral hygiene measures; (I) completed bridge from the occlusal surface; the retaining screws eventually will be covered with a tooth-coloured restoration; (J) the metal collars of the abutments are visible only where the patient's lip line will cover the gingival margin on smiling.

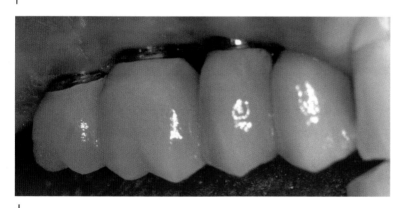

J

a point of essential occlusal contact. Cemented bridges therefore are often indicated if implants have not been placed in the long axis of the desired restoration. For many dentists, the major advantage of cemented bridges is the similarity to conventional crown and bridge techniques.

The decision between screw-retained and cemented bridges also depends upon the ability of the dental laboratory to construct an acceptable restoration. The decision should be based on the clinical situation and articulated working models prior to abutment selection, and the technique most suited to the individual situation is chosen. Often the choice has been made at the treatment planning stage following discussion with the patient.

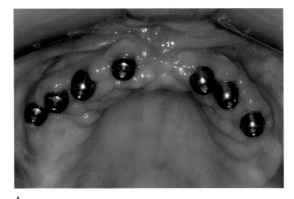

A

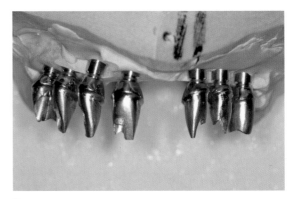

B

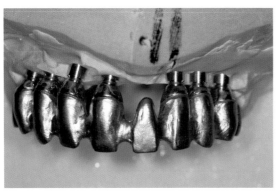

C

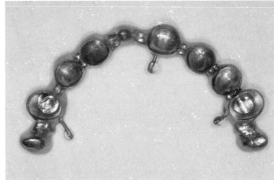

D

Figure 14.3

A cemented full-arch bridge constructed on AstraTech implants and Profile BI abutments: (A) seven implants have been placed; (B) following head of implant impressions, the prepable abutments have been prepared to ensure parallelism, adequate retention and the ideal bridge contours; in this case there has been more labial reduction of the anterior abutments to compensate for a slight labial angulation of the implants; (C) the metal superstructure for the bridge; (D) the fit surface of the superstructure;

Advantages of screw-retained bridges

- easily retrieved
- complete seating of the restoration is more readily ensured
- utilizes manufactured components for all fitting surfaces
- no risk of cement retained at margin—allows deep margin placement

Disadvantages of screw-retained bridges

- implant needs to be in long axis of restoration so screw hole is on occlusal surface or angled abutments need to be used
- screw hole may be visible or in an important area of the occlusal surface

- requires a 'passive fit' for each gold cylinder onto the abutments
- risk of bridge screw loosening or fracture

Advantages of cemented bridges

- 'passive fit' not as critical but is desirable
- no screw access holes
- similar to conventional bridge techniques
- can easily overcome differences in angulation between implants and restore implants with adverse angulations

Disadvantages of cemented bridges

- retrievability more difficult

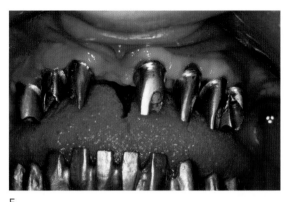

E

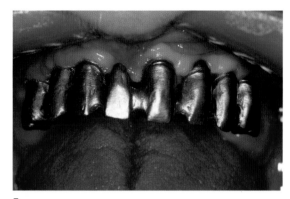

F

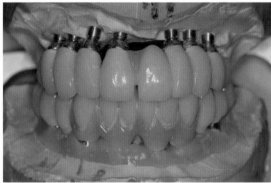

G

H

Figure 14.3 *continued*

(E) the abutments are in position; (F) the bridge superstructure is tried in to ensure the fit; (G) the bridge is completed; in the lower jaw a full-arch screw-retained bridge has also been constructed; (H) the completed restoration in the mouth.

- more laboratory time required to produce prepared abutments and temporary bridges if required
- cementation needs to be controlled, especially with subgingival margins
- difficult to ensure full seating of the bridge, especially with tight or deep gingival 'collars' or if there is bleeding
- increased technical costs and chairside time if temporary bridges are required

Abutment types

As with single tooth restorations, there are several types of abutments and the manufacturers versions are listed in Table 14.1.

Table 14.1 Abutment types for fixed bridge restorations

Manufacturer	Type	Name
Nobel Biocare	Screwed	Standard abutment
		EsthetiCone
		MirasCone
		Multi-abutment
		Angled abutment
	Cemented	TiAdapt
		AurAdapt
AstraTech	Screwed	Uni-abutment
		Angled abutment
	Cemented	Profile BI abutment
		Cast-to abutment
Frialit	Screwed	MH2 abutment
	Cemented	Telescopic abutment
		AuroBase
Straumann	Screwed	SynOcta abutment
	Cemented	SynOcta solid abutments

Nobel Biocare: Nobel Biocare AB, Göteborg, Sweden
Frialit: Friatec AG, Mannheim, Germany

For screw-retained bridges

Bridge abutments can be either one-piece or two-piece. As the abutments are to be linked, there is no need for the bridge cylinders to have individual anti-rotational features, because the whole bridge structure will not be able to rotate. The individual abutments, however, may engage into anti-rotational features in the implant if present. For example, the Nobel Biocare EsthetiCone abutment engages the external hexagon on the top of the implant so

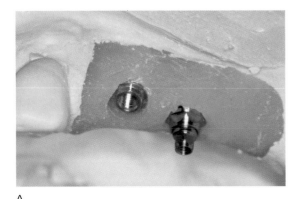

A

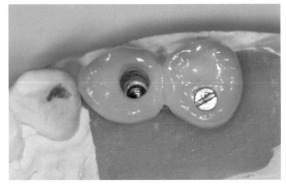

D

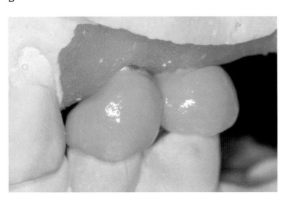

B

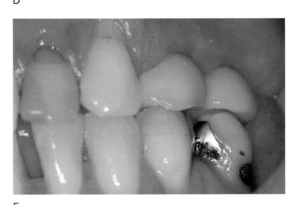

E

Figure 14.4

Two Nobel Biocare implants have been placed to replace missing premolar teeth. The mesial implant head is very superficial. (A) Working cast of implant heads. The distal implant can receive a conventional bridge abutment (EsthetiCone). Mesially, the implant head is level with the gingival margin. (B) A fully customizable UCLA abutment (similar to AurAdapt) in place. This will allow the mesial abutment to be customized to allow for extension of the porcelain to the implant head without the metal collar required for conventional abutments. (C) The customized abutment has been incorporated into the bridge casting. (D) The completed bridge shows a conventional bridge screw for the distal abutment. The mesial abutment requires a larger access hole for the abutment screw, which will directly retain the bridge/abutment to the implant. (E) The completed bridge in place; minimal metal is visible.

that the abutment is stable and cannot rotate. The abutment is in two parts and the separate abutment screw is tightened to 20 N.cm to prevent it from loosening. The top of the abutment is conical in contour with flat facets, on the side. By using a gold bridge cylinder that does not engage the facets, the cylinders can be linked together without each abutment having to be parallel to each other. The facets can be engaged with a hexed gold cylinder for a single tooth restoration where anti-rotation is required. Bridge abutments are designed to cope with differences in angulation between implants. The EsthetiCone abutment has a 20° taper so that angulations up to 40° between implants can be compensated for. The bridge abutments with the Straumann SynOcta and Frialit MH2 systems are similar to the Nobel Biocare design. The new multi-abutment from Nobel Biocare dispenses with the abutment engaging the external hexagon of the implant (no anti-rotational feature) and this aids seating of the abutments.

The bridge abutment for the AstraTech system is a one-piece abutment (Uni-abutment) so it does not have an anti-rotational component in its attachment to the implant, although once the abutment is fully seated in the internal cone of the implant it has a high level of stability. The smooth-sided abutment head has a matched bridge cylinder and the anti-rotational element for the system relies upon the linkage of the components. Abutments are made with 20° and 40° tapered tops to allow compensation for even severe angulation differences (40° and 80°).

The original Nobel Biocare standard abutment is a simple parallel-sided abutment with a flat top. The bridge construction starts at the top of the abutment and this design lends itself to reconstructions, particularly in the lower jaw, where considerable resorption has occurred and aesthetics are not demanding. In areas with higher aesthetic demands, the designs already discussed allow the bridge framework to cover the abutment so that it is, in effect, hidden under the bridge. Abutments come in a variety of collar heights to allow for different soft tissue thickness. The collar height is chosen to allow for a subgingival margin placement if required (Figure 14.4). Variations in design also allow for different abutment head

heights. In a situation where there may be little intraocclusal space between the head of the implant and the opposing tooth, a shorter abutment will be required. It is not normally possible to restore an implant with a screw-retained bridge if there is less than 5–6 mm of interocclusal space. Ideally there needs to be at least 2 mm of space beyond the bridge screw so that it can be covered with an aesthetic restoration. Cases with reduced intraocclusal space are often better restored with a cemented restoration, especially if appearance is paramount.

Angled abutments

The access hole for the bridge screw ideally needs to emerge through the centre of the occlusal surface of the restoration. Angled abutments are designed to compensate for a different path of insertion for the bridge and bridge screw compared with the implant (Figure 14.5). Angled abutments are available in the range 15–35°. Depending upon the position in which the abutment is seated on the implant it is also possible to use this angulation change to 'move' the bridge screw access in a mesial or distal direction. Angled abutments still have the same top as conventional screw abutments and accept the same gold bridge cylinders. The angled design is therefore dependent upon a variation in the height of the metal collar at the implant end of the abutment. Care should be taken therefore, to check if this higher metal collar will compromise the appearance, because angled abutments are not suited to situations with a superficial implant head. Although it is possible for the margin to be altered and the gold cylinder modified to cover the metal collar, this will decrease the quality of fit of the restoration.

When angled abutments are used, it is normally necessary for the laboratory to provide an acrylic jig to allow the clinician to orientate the abutment to the correct position. This can relate either to adjacent teeth or other abutments. The jig should be kept for the future in case the abutments ever need to be removed and replaced.

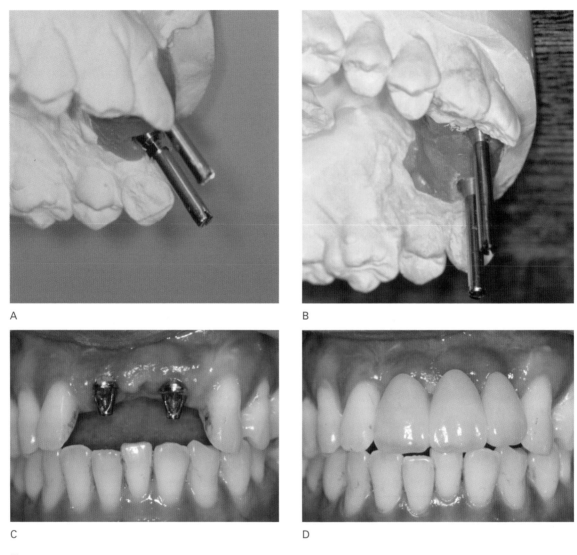

Figure 14.5

Two Nobel Biocare implants supporting an anterior bridge: (A) guide pins have been placed in the implant analogues following head of implant impressions; the path of insertion of the implants would dictate labial screw access holes if convention screw-retained abutments are used; (B) using angled abutments the screw access can be realigned to an acceptable position; (C) angled abutments in position—note the metal collar, which is just visible above the gingival margin; (D) the completed bridge; the bridge structure has been extended in front of the abutments to disguise the visible metal;

continued

For cemented bridges

Prepable abutments

These abutments are the same as those already discussed in Chapter 13. They are abutments with a solid head that can be prepared in the laboratory so that they are retentive, have margins in an aesthetic position and have an acceptable degree of parallelism to each other to be able to have a conventional bridge cemented onto them. To construct a bridge using this approach, a head of

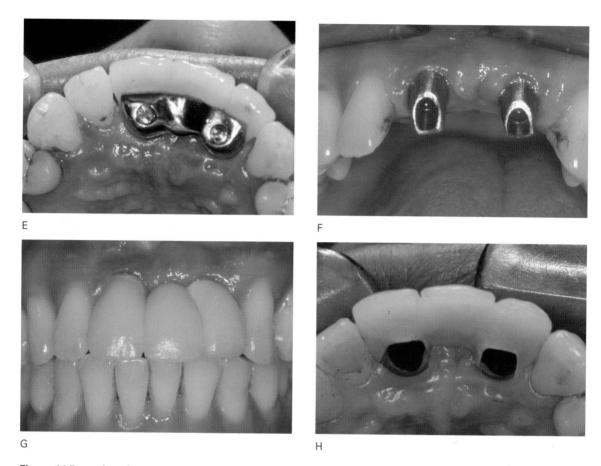

Figure 14.5 *continued*

(E) the palatal screw access results in a bulky contour; (F) the same case restored with prepable (TiAdapt) abutments; the angulation change has been achieved by heavily preparing the abutments labially; (G) the bridge cemented to the abutments; it has not been possible to completely disguise the metal abutment margin; (H) the resulting palatal contour more closely resembles natural contours than the previous screw-retained bridge.

implant impression should be taken and the abutments chosen to correspond to the tooth being replaced. Manufacturers produce abutments in a variety of widths, normally in the range of 4.5 mm corresponding to lower incisor and upper lateral incisor teeth, 5.5 mm corresponding to upper central incisors, canine and premolar teeth and 7.0 mm for molars. Abutments also come in a variety of heights and some manufacturers also produce angled prepable abutments.

Abutments are best chosen using a trial kit of abutment analogues placed onto the working model (see Figure 13.4C). They should be chosen so that:

- the dimension and height of the abutment as it sits on the implant allows for the planned emergence of the restoration through the gingiva;
- there is adequate bulk of metal just below the gingival margin to allow for the abutment to be prepared to accept an adequate thickness of bridge margin subgingivally;
- there is adequate height of the abutment to allow it to support properly the bridge framework;
- there is adequate bulk of metal in regions where there may need to be significant reduction of the abutment to allow for changes in

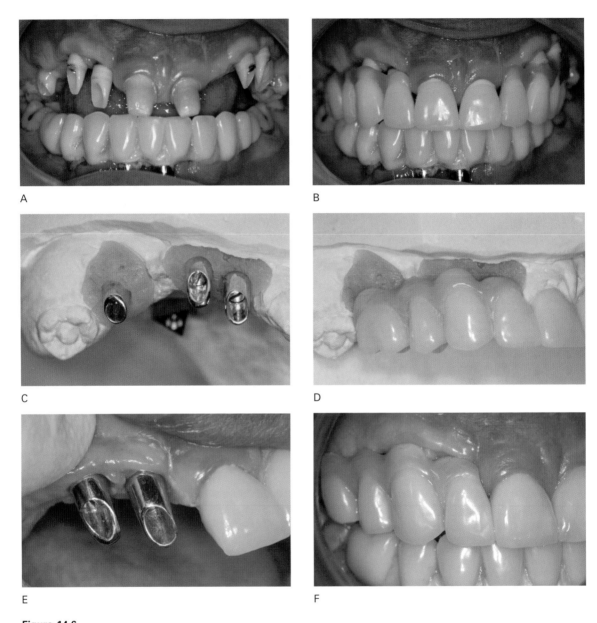

Figure 14.6

A complex case where implant placement was only possible in potentially compromised positions due to skeletal malformation. A lower bridge supported by implants has already been placed. Nobel Biocare implants have been placed. (A) Fully customizable abutments have been prepared and are tried in prior to finalization to ensure that the correct shape has been achieved. (B) A try-in of the proposed bridge in wax to confirm an acceptable result can be achieved. (C) The abutments are cast and finished prior to placement. (D) A cemented bridge is produced to restore the missing teeth and soft tissue. Space has been left for access to the implants for cleaning. (E) The abutments in place. (F) The completed cemented bridge. Surgical aspects of this case are illustrated in Figure 12.14.

angulation and orientation between implants; it is sometimes better to choose a larger abutment

Implants that have a feature in the design that allows the abutment to seat into a predictable position each time by engaging a hexagon or an internal facet (Nobel Biocare, Frialit 2, AstraTech ST and Straumann solid screw) can have the abutments prepared and the definitive bridge constructed from one original working model. However, if there is any degree of gingival re-contouring required or if implants do not have an indexing feature (standard AstraTech implant), the abutment needs to be seated with a jig, although exact positioning cannot be guaranteed. It is best to place a provisional bridge following insertion of the abutments and then take a further impression of the abutments in position for construction of the definitive bridge.

Fully customized and computer-generated abutments

Just as for single tooth applications, abutments for cemented restorations can be produced using castable abutments or the computer-generated Procera system. Cast abutments are indicated when significant re-orientation of abutments is required, because they can be waxed up and then cast to the desired angulation and dimension (Figure 14.6). It is often a matter of familiarity and experience of the dental technician when choosing between cast abutments or prepable abutments, because both can achieve similar results.

The Procera system can provide correctly orientated abutments for cemented bridge construction from one master impression of the Nobel Biocare implant heads, without significant laboratory time. The technician uses guide pins placed in the implant replicas and the model is mounted into a scanner. Using three–dimensional imaging, the desired abutment shape can be developed and the information sent to a factory facility that will construct the abutment in titanium. The abutments need final finishing of the margin position and occlusal surfaces in the laboratory prior to use.

Abutment selection and impressions

Abutments can be selected either directly in the mouth or an impression can be taken of the implant head and the abutments chosen from the resulting model (Figure 14.7). Quite commonly, it is not clear exactly which abutment will be required from a clinical examination. The incorrect choice of abutment can be costly, especially if the error is not determined until after the restoration has been made. Before the abutment is finally chosen however, it is essential that there is adequate information available to know exactly what the shape and position the final restoration should be, so that the correct abutment is chosen to achieve that result. This can be just as relevant for short-span bridges with only two or three implants as for extensive full-arch reconstructions.

Implant head impressions

An impression of the implant head to produce a laboratory cast can be used to choose the abutment, allow preparation of prepable abutments and often to act as the working model for complete bridge construction. Impressions copings are placed onto the implant head (Figure 14.8). With a flat-top implant a verification radiograph will be required to ensure that the impression coping is fully seated over the external hexagon. The impression coping is secured to the implant by a guide pin that screws into the abutment screw hole. The top of the guide pin projects beyond the coping and should be longer than adjacent teeth. An impression tray is modified so that the guide pin projects through the tray without touching it (for more detail, see later in this chapter). The coping is picked up in an impression material that sets rigid and the guide pin is unscrewed. The coping should not move in the impression and an analogue of the implant is attached to the coping prior to pouring a cast. The cast should be produced with a soft tissue replica because the implant head will normally be subgingival and a rigid replica of the gingiva will not allow access to the implant head. Using this model, the abutments can be selected.

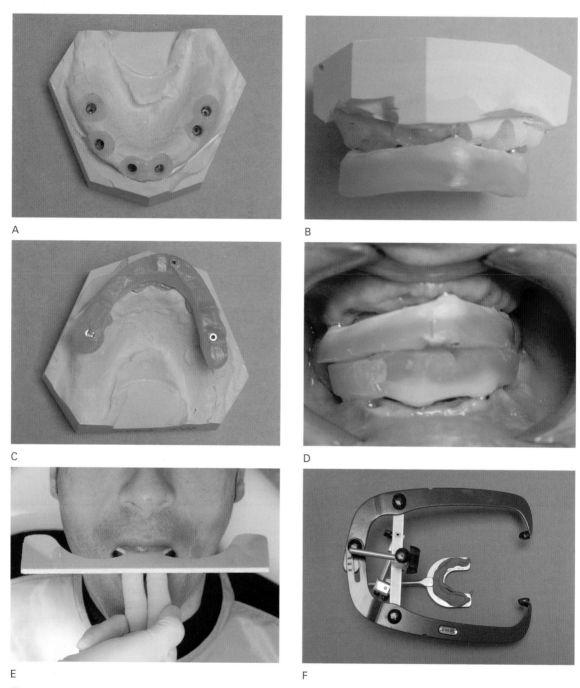

Figure 14.7

Upper and lower full-arch bridges constructed on AstraTech implants. (A) Upper cast following implant head impressions, implant analogues and soft tissue replicas are required. (B) By linking three impression copings in a rigid laboratory composite beam, a wax rim can be constructed. (C) The wax rim is trimmed and indexed to facilitate accurate jaw relations. (D) Trimmed occlusal rims are stable in the mouth. (E) The occlusal plane is checked. (F) A facebow record can be taken.   *continued*

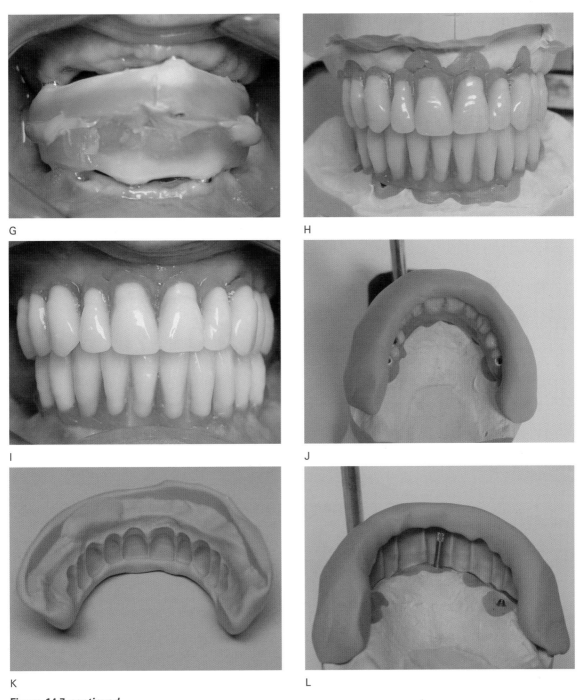

Figure 14.7 *continued*

(G) A final interocclusal record is taken. (H) A full diagnostic set-up of tooth position is produced, supported by the composite beams. (I) The set-up is tried in. The jaw relations and appearance are assessed and altered as required. The patient can see the result and changes can be made easily at this stage. (J) Following approval of the tooth position a putty mask is made of the try-in. (K) The putty mask records tooth position. (L) It can be located onto the working model and the correct abutment chosen to achieve the desired tooth position. continued

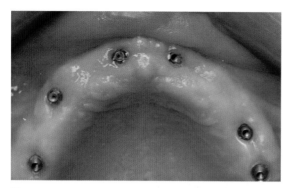

M

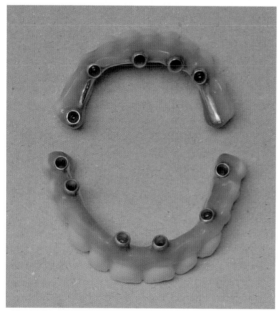

N

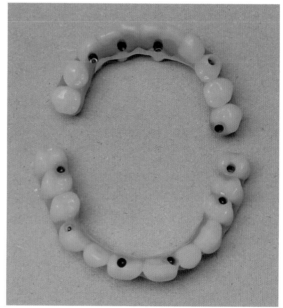

O

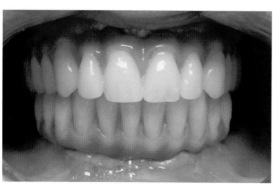

P

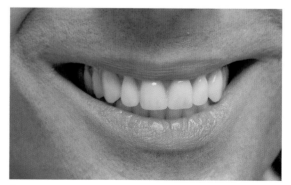

Q

Figure 14.7 *continued*

(M) The chosen abutments (Uni-abutments) in place. (N) The completed bridges from the fit surface. The gold bridge cylinders can be seen clearly. The underside of the bridge is carefully contoured and polished to aid cleaning. (O) Occlusal view of the bridges showing the bridge screw access holes. (P) The completed bridges. (Q) On smiling, the appearance is excellent.

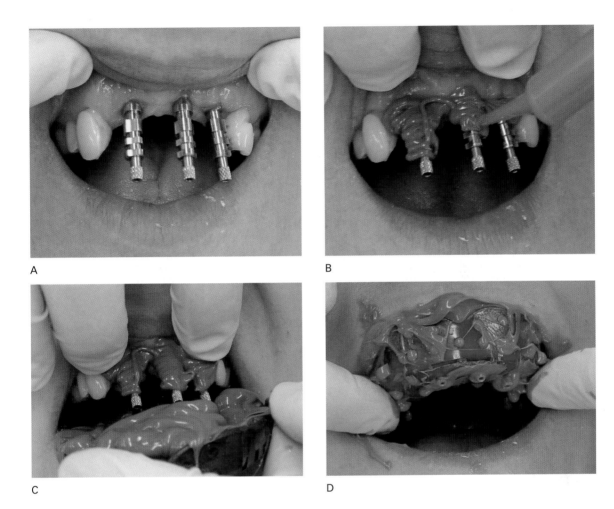

Figure 14.8

(A) AstraTech implant head pick-up impression copings have been screwed to the implants. (B) Impregum impression material is syringed around the copings. (C) The tray is seated over the copings. (D) The end of the copings is identified with the fingers and the tray is stabilized until set. The screws are undone prior to removal of the impression.

Evaluation using a diagnostic work-up

A guide is needed of the required tooth position to relate the implant head model to the new restoration. If the patient has a satisfactory existing denture or bridge that is to be copied, an impression can be taken of it and a putty mask made of the labial and incisal surfaces (Figures 14.7J–L). This can be tried against the implant head model and will demonstrate the relationship between the tooth and implant. Alternatively, if a diagnostic wax-up has been carried out, from

which a surgical stent was provided, this can be related to the new working model.

If no accurate guide is available and there is any doubt as to the orientation of the implants, it is advisable to produce a new diagnostic tooth set-up that can be tried into the mouth and agreed with the patient before the abutments are chosen. This can be produced as a denture type set-up or ideally as a fixed set-up. Temporary bridge cylinders are linked together with acrylic or laboratory composite resin on the working model and a diagnostic set-up is produced in wax or with denture teeth, which can be tried into the mouth secured to the implants. It can give an exact idea as to the possible complications that may be encountered before expensive abutments and laboratory work have been undertaken. This information can be transferred into a provisional bridge and the patient allowed to live with the restoration for a period of time to ensure that it is satisfactory before the final restoration is made.

Abutment try-in kits

Many manufacturers produce replicas of the abutment types that can greatly assist abutment

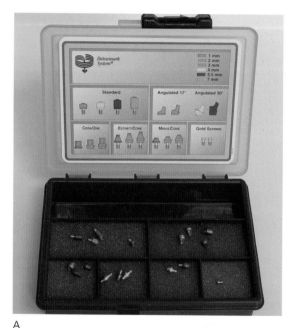

A

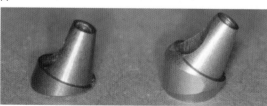

B

Figure 14.9

(A) The Nobel Biocare abutment try-in kit. Replicas of the abutments can be tried on a cast or intraorally. (B) Examples of the analogues. The 17° and 30° angled abutments can be compared.

selection (Figure 14.9). They can be used in the mouth or more commonly, on an implant head cast. Made of aluminium they will not damage the implant or implant replica and for ease of recognition they are often colour coded so that different sizes can be easily recognized. The implant head cast is related to the putty mask. Abutments can be tried in to get the best possible screw access position, marginal height and emergence. The selected abutment then should be related to the opposing model to check for interocclusal clearance. Try-in kits are also produced for prepable abutments.

Selection and seating for screw-retained bridges

In a straightforward situation where a short-span screw-retained bridge is to be constructed and it can be certain that the implant is orientated such that the bridge screw will emerge through the occlusal surface (placement of a guide pin into the implant will give a clearer view of the implant's orientation), the following steps can be followed:

- Determine the distance from the implant head to the opposing tooth using a periodontal probe or dividers. If there is going to be insufficient space to allow coverage of the bridge screw, reconsider a cemented approach.
- Using a periodontal measuring probe or a manufacturer's depth-measuring device, determine the abutment gingival collar height. The planned margin should be 1–2 mm below the gingival margin at its lowest point on the visible surfaces.
- Place the abutment but do not tighten it. Check the orientation and the occlusal clearance. Seating may need to be verified radiographically.
- If the abutment is going to be left in position and the temporary restoration can be placed over it, the abutment screw can be tightened. If the abutment is to be removed to allow the healing abutment to be replaced between appointments, it should only be hand tightened.
- A transfer impression of the abutment can be taken.

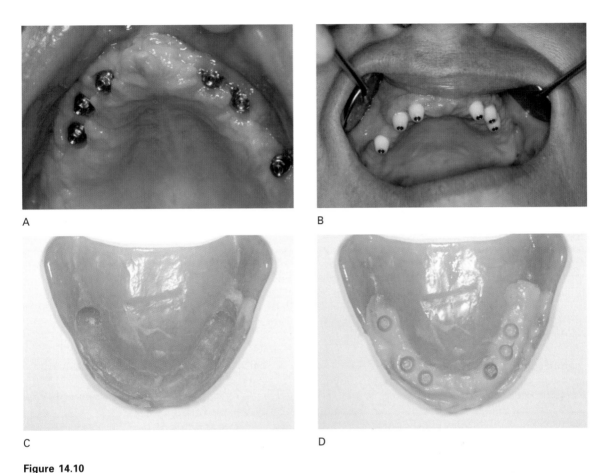

Figure 14.10

(A) Nobel Biocare EsthetiCone bridge abutments in place. (B) Abutment protection caps used as the abutments will be left in the mouth between appointments. (C) The complete denture is adjusted to accommodate the abutments and caps. (D) Soft re-line material is used to adapt the denture for use while the bridge is being constructed.

• A protective cap can be placed on the abutment if it is to be left *in situ* (Figure 14.10) and the temporary restoration can be modified to accommodate the resulting dimensions.

If it is not possible for the abutment to be chosen from a clinical examination, an implant head impression should be taken and the abutment selected on the model as already outlined. The implant head model can be used as the working model for the final bridge as long as it is accurate and shows sufficient detail of the rest of the arch. Many operators have proposed that for large bridges it is better to choose the abutments from the implant head model and then re-take an impression with the abutments seated in the mouth. The authors find that this is not necessary if the implant head impression is accurate. The chosen abutments are therefore seated onto the implant head model and hand tightened using laboratory screws (because the gold or titanium screws used in the mouth might be damaged in the stainless-steel implant analogues). The bridge is therefore constructed on the actual abutments, which will need to be cleaned and sterilized before placement in the mouth.

Abutment seating for flat-top implants involves ensuring that the abutment is fully seated over the external hexagon by holding the abutment with the correct placement tools to feel that it cannot rotate before the abutment screw is hand tightened. This can be difficult if the gingiva is thick, tight or bleeding and a verification radiograph is essential to ensure that the hexagon is properly engaged and no soft tissue is trapped. This potential problem has been reduced with the Nobel Biocare multi-abutments, which are easier to seat fully because the external hexagon is not engaged. Care should always be taken not to leave the healing abutment out for any length of time because the gingiva will quickly contract and it will be painful for the patient when it is pushed back. If the abutment is to be left on the implant, it can be tightened into position following verification of seating. With the Nobel Biocare EsthetiCone this involves torquing to 20 N.cm and counter-torquing to prevent stressing of the implant. Straumann however, recommend the SynOcta abutment be torqued to 32 N.cm without counter-torquing. The manufacturer's recommendations should be followed. A ready-made protection cap covers the abutment.

Abutments that are to be removed following impression-taking to allow the provisional restoration to be replaced should only be hand tightened until the final stage of bridge construction.

Implant systems with an internal conical design (Straumann/AstraTech) allow seating of the abutment in a more predictable way and a verification radiograph is not usually required.

Impression trays

Custom-made trays are useful in a mouth with difficult access or a complex or outsize shape or in cases with multiple implants where the chair-side time in modifying a stock tray is longer (Figure 14.11). They should be rigid in design and should be formed to support the impression coping along its full height. Spacing of at least 2 mm is recommended.

Stock trays should be of a good quality so that they will still be rigid following cutting of an access hole for the guide pin. The stock tray size is chosen in the normal manner and the position of emergence of the guide pin is marked. Access holes are prepared to ensure

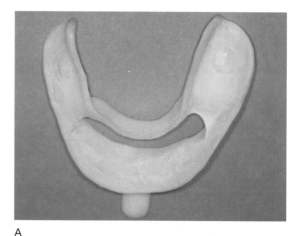

A

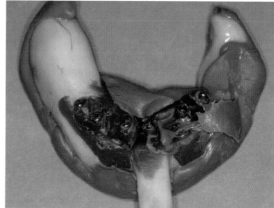

B

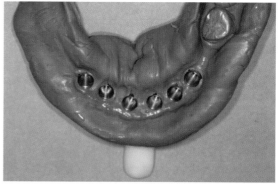

C

Figure 14.11

(A) A special tray constructed for impressions for a full-arch bridge. (B) The impression coping securing pins are visible through the tray. (C) The EsthetiCone abutment impression copings are securely held in the impression material using this pick-up technique.

that the tray does not encroach on the impression coping, because they should not touch the tray.

The access holes for the guide pins are covered in wax to prevent the impression material flowing out through the hole (Figure 14.8D).

Impression materials

Polyethers and silicone impression materials have physical properties that make them suitable for implant impressions:

- The material should set rigid enough to support the coping and prevent movement of the coping on removal from the mouth and casting of the model.
- It should record enough fine detail to identify properly the gingival contours and other teeth in the mouth.
- It should be dimensionally stable and not react with materials used in model production, such as the gingival replica.
- It should accept disinfection techniques.

For these reasons it is not recommended that light-bodied impression materials be used around the impression copings because they will not be strong enough and heavy putty materials will not flow around the copings or record fine details. One-phase medium-bodied paste systems are preferred.

Some operators recommend splinting impression copings together with acrylic prior to impression-taking to ensure that the copings are stable relative to each other. There is nothing to recommend such extra complexity.

Pick-up impressions

The most reliable impression technique to follow is the pick-up technique (Figure 14.12). As described already, the impression coping is secured to the abutment with a guide pin. These are available in a variety of lengths to ensure the correct projection through the impression tray while still having access with a screwdriver to the pin. The impression material is syringed around the coping and the tray is filled. As the tray is seated in the mouth, the guide pins can be felt by the operators' fingers through the wax over the access holes. If the pins are not felt, the tray should be seated further while the impression material is still fluid. The tray is stabilized until the full set is reached and the guide pins are then fully unscrewed. The impression copings will be removed with the tray and so remain fully seated in the impression material at all times. The guide pins are used to locate and retain the abutment analogues for cast production.

Reseating impressions

The reseating technique can be used in areas of difficult access where locating and unscrewing the guide pins with an impression tray in the mouth may be difficult. Impression copings, which have a retentive and distinctive pattern on the surface, are fully screwed onto the abutment (Figures 14.13 and 14.14). They do not project beyond adjacent teeth and a tray should be used with stops so that it will not touch the copings when seated in the mouth. Access holes are not cut in the tray. Impression material is syringed around the coping and the tray is seated. Once set, the tray is removed and an impression will have been made of the coping shape. The coping will stay in the mouth following impression removal. The coping is then unscrewed from the abutment and the abutment analogue is attached for model production. The impression coping is reseated into the impression and its stability is checked. It is important that adequate material extends around the coping or it will not locate and remain stable.

For cemented restorations

Prepable abutments need to be selected and produced on implant head casts and the technique described already should be followed. Once again, abutment selection kits are available from some manufacturers. The prepared abutments need to be re-tried in the mouth with the aid of a transfer jig to assist with correct

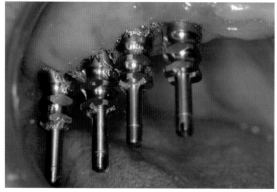

A

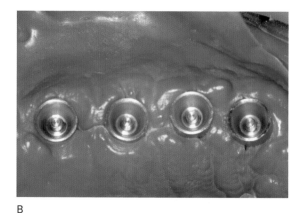

B

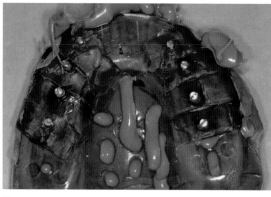

C

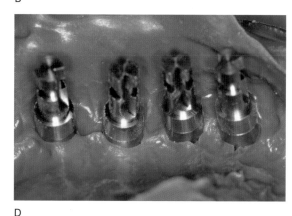

D

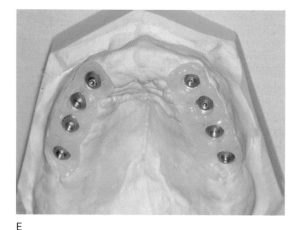

E

Figure 14.12

(A) MirasCone abutment impression copings have been secured to the abutments. (B) The impression copings record the position of the abutment as well as the soft tissue contours. (C) A stock tray was used because access was straightforward. (D) Abutment replicas are secured to the impression copings prior to cast construction. (E) The working model.

orientation. If a further impression of the abutments in position is required, conventional bridge impression techniques are employed. Light-bodied materials are syringed around the abutment and a heavy-bodied material is used for the bulk of the impression. Recording the fine detail of deep margins can be difficult. A gingival retraction cord does not retain well in the sulcus and care must be taken not to push it down below the bulbosity of the abutment where

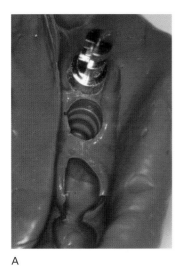

A

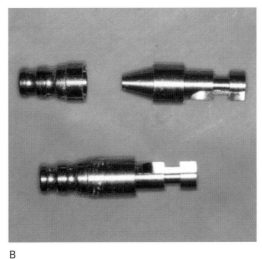

B

Figure 14.13

(A) A reseating impression using Nobel Biocare EsthetiCone impression copings. The ribbed contour of the coping can be seen clearly in the impression. The distal coping and abutment replica have been re-inserted into the impression. (B) The impression coping (top left) and the abutment analogue (top right). When screwed together, the coping can be reseated into the impression.

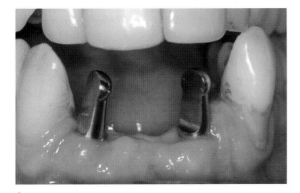

A

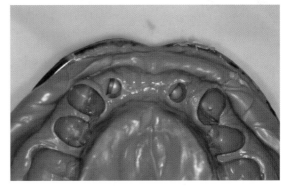

B

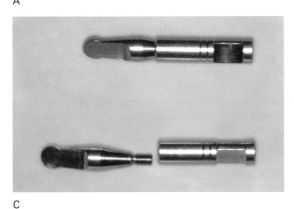

C

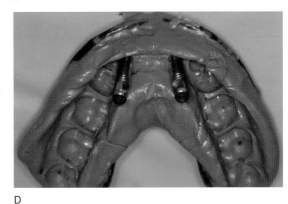

D

Figure 14.14

(A) AstraTech implant head reseating impression copings in place. (B) The impression of the copings. (C) The impression coping and analogue—the impression coping has a flat facet to ensure that it can be re-orientated correctly in the impression. (D) The coping and analogue are reseated into the impression together.

it may be difficult to remove (see Figure 13.16). Electrosurgery is completely contraindicated. The best results are achieved by careful removal of temporary restorations and treating the soft tissue with great care so that marginal bleeding is avoided. Acrylic transfer copings can be made in advance in the laboratory at the time of abutment preparation. These can be picked up in a new impression but are only useful if the gingival margins have not needed to be altered intraorally.

Impression verification for all techniques

The impression is checked for:

- coping stability: each coping should be tested with tweezers to ensure that no more than very limited movement occurs;
- adequate record of immediate gingival contours: at least 4–5 mm beyond the coping so that a proper gingival replica can be made;
- full record of adjacent teeth: to ensure proper contact point construction and harmonious emergence profiles;
- full record of articular surfaces of whole arch: for accurate articulation of casts

Occlusal records

Good quality opposing casts are essential and it is recommended that these are made using rubber base impression materials rather than alginate. As for conventional bridgework, there are no exact rules to follow but it is recommended that a semi-adjustable articulator be used as a minimum for all full-arch bridges and shorter span bridges where the occlusal scheme is likely to be changed by the bridge. This includes all posterior extension designs and anterior bridges where incisal guidance may be altered. If a short-span bridge is to be constructed where adjacent teeth are present and a conformative occlusal scheme is to be adopted, it may be acceptable for full articulation to be avoided. Unlike complete denture jaw relations where the stability of a wax rim can be difficult, this is greatly simplified by construction of a wax rim that is secured to the implants

(Figures 14.7B–G). The rim then can be trimmed to the correct vertical height of occlusion and an interocclusal record taken. It is also useful to mark such features as the centreline and smile line.

Full information needs to be sent to the laboratory including occlusal registration (with the abutments in position), records of provisional restorations if they need to be reproduced in the final bridgework and shade registration. If gingival-coloured material is to be used to mask long crowns or interdental areas, this should also be shade matched.

Provisional bridges

The use of provisional bridges to ensure an acceptable appearance has been discussed already. Manufacturers produce temporary components that attach directly to the implant head or can fit onto the abutments. These components are either made of acrylic or metal. Although a provisional bridge is not usually indicated for long periods of time, it is still essential that it has an accurate fit. A provisional structure can damage implants if it is screwed down tightly when it does not fit properly. Provisional bridges also can be used to determine tooth position and speech patterns before final bridge construction. Patients who have worn dentures, particularly for missing maxillary anterior teeth, for many years may have problems in adapting their speech. Placement and subsequent adaptation and modification of a provisional bridge that can be copied in the permanent restoration smoothes this process.

Provisional bridges are commonly used with cemented bridges, where removal of the customized abutments between appointments can lead to errors occurring. Replicating the position of the abutments is difficult if there is no anti-rotational (indexing) element in the implant/abutment junction, e.g. AstraTech standard implant and Uni-abutment. A provisional bridge is therefore produced at the same time as the abutments are prepared. Following placement of the abutments, the provisional bridge is used to form the ideal gingival emergence and margin position and, if necessary, the bridge can be altered to change gradually the emergence contour. Once the ideal contour has been achieved, a conventional crown and bridge impression is taken of the abutments in position.

Laboratory procedures

The material chosen for the bridge construction has a significant effect on the design and clinical techniques followed. Original designs favoured rigid cast gold beams produced by waxing together manufactured gold cylinders supporting acrylic denture teeth embedded in pressure-cured pink denture acrylic. This had the great advantage of being a familiar technique and as the superstructures were removable the problem of acrylic wear was not an issue as the bridge could be refurbished easily. In a desire to make restorations more aesthetic, clinicians moved towards the use of porcelain on bonding gold or even titanium frameworks. When constructing large bridges this involves a high level of technical expertise, particularly to achieve a good fit as well as good appearance. Some clinicians prefer to undertake post-ceramic soldering or welding to ensure that the porcelain firing process does not distort the metal substructure. Large metal ceramic bridges are subject to a high incidence of long-term porcelain fractures and so are sometimes divided into smaller units and made easily retrievable where possible.

The development of laboratory composite materials has allowed the production of extensive bridges with a customized, durable and aesthetic surface similar to porcelain, without the need for firing and possible distortion. These materials are highly suitable for implant-supported bridges, because they are more resilient than porcelain and can be more easily repaired. They are not as resistant to wear as porcelain, although evidence suggests that they will wear at a rate similar to natural teeth and are particularly indicated if the opposing restoration is made of the same material. They will not retain their appearance as well as porcelain but for longer span bridges they are clinically acceptable. Patients who are provided with extensive implant-supported fixed bridges in opposing jaws may report problems with 'noise' and the very hard feeling from the porcelain surfaces contacting.

Titanium frameworks may offer considerable advantages over the use of gold from the cost and weight aspects. Titanium cannot be cast in the conventional way but manufacturing processes can be employed to produce machined frameworks.

The technical procedures for implant bridges are similar to conventional crown and bridge techniques, but the following features are of note:

- A soft gingival replica is essential to allow for access to subgingival implant heads and abutment margins. The gingival replica is removable to check the marginal fit.
- The highest possible standard of metal framework production is required to achieve a passive fit.
- Care must be taken to ensure that no distortion of the framework occurs during firing of the porcelain. Damage to the framework fit has been reported following acrylic polishing of full-arch bridges if handled roughly.
- Frameworks should be cast in a high-gold-content metal compatible with the gold bridge cylinders provided by the manufacturers. Several laboratories are able to produce titanium frameworks that may offer advantages over conventional gold frameworks.
- The importance of relating the implant position to the desired tooth position before choosing the abutment has been discussed already. Of equal importance in the laboratory is the relationship of the abutment to the final tooth position so that the framework is the correct contour to support the aesthetic portion of the bridge and the correct occlusal form. Many dental technicians prefer to wax-up the whole bridge and then cut the wax-up back to allow space for the porcelain or resin to ensure this contour (Figure 14.2B).

Trying and fitting the restoration

Try-in

Larger span or short-span bridges should be tried in before fit. Try-in can be carried out at the following times:

- Before framework construction: the gold cylinders are linked together with a rigid material such as laboratory composite resin. The accuracy of the impression can be verified by seating this in the mouth. There should be no displacement of the frame when screwed down at either end and the resin connection will normally crack if the structure is tried in and there is a poor fit. If this occurs it is best to retake the impression. The linked gold cylinders can be used for occlusal records by attaching a wax rim, and they can also support a trial set-up of teeth if required.
- Following framework construction but before placement of teeth: try-in at this time will allow for full evaluation of the fit of the frame and detection of errors before time is wasted completing a bridge that does not fit. The frame is first seated down with finger pressure and any gross error in fit is detected by rocking of the framework. The bridge screws are then tried in one at a time to see if tightening a screw results in movement of the frame away from another abutment. Tight gingival cuffs or a framework pressing on soft tissues can make this difficult. Finally, all of the screws are tightened and a misfit may be revealed as discomfort and a tight feeling by the patient. An error in fit detected at this stage is remedied either by retaking the impression or by sectioning the frame and splinting it in the mouth for it to be soldered or welded. A frame that has to be sectioned should be tried in again before proceeding further.
- Finally a bridge can be tried in prior to polishing or at a biscuit bake if porcelain. This will allow for checks to be made on the appearance and the occlusion prior to completion.

Placing the bridge

If the definitive abutments have been removed between appointments they should be seated and tightened as recommended, normally using a torque device. The bridge is seated onto the abutments and the fit is verified as discussed above. There is little point in trying to verify marginal fit visually unless the margins are supragingival. It is quite normal for there to be some gingival blanching due to pressure on the soft tissues from the new profile of the bridge. Patients should be reassured that this is a temporary problem. If the fit is acceptable, the occlusion is checked.

Occlusion

If the bridge is being placed as a conformative restoration (in a partially dentate patient), it should be checked firstly in the retruded arc of closure to ensure that it does not create an occlusal interference. Next, the intercuspal position should be checked. Ideally, the bridge should be only just in contact when the patient closes lightly and should come fully into contact when the patient exerts heavy force. This will obviously depend upon how many natural teeth remain and how good their occlusal contacts are. This degree of contact is difficult to quantify but the best way of proceeding is to use occlusal indicator paper to get even contact between teeth and implants (Figure 14.15). Shimstock should then be used and on light contact the implant bridge should not hold the shimstock, but the teeth should. As the patient exerts more force so the implant bridge should hold the shimstock as well as the teeth. Ideally, the areas of contact should be located as close to the centre of the implants as possible so that forces are transmitted down the long axis of the implant under loading. Cantilever pontics should be loaded as little as possible.

The bridge is then checked in lateral and protrusive movements. If a natural canine guidance is present, this will protect the bridge from lateral loading. If a group function occlusion exists, the implant bridge should be harmonious with this. If the canine tooth is being replaced as part of the bridge, it is normal practice for the occlusion to be reorganized as a group function occlusion if this can be achieved without sacrificing appearance. If lateral guidance has to be provided, this should be shallow, shared over several teeth if possible and be centred on the strongest implant.

Protrusive guidance should have been determined prior to construction because the anterior tooth position will dramatically alter this. The protrusive movement should be smooth and

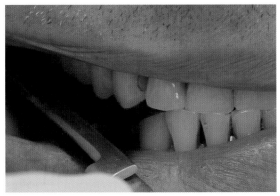

A

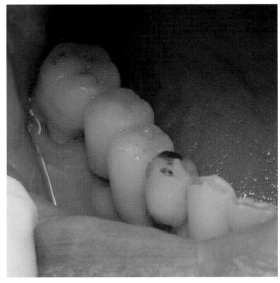

B

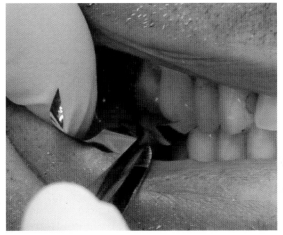

C

spread over as many teeth as possible, once again ideally centred over the implants rather than on pontics.

If a reorganised occlusal scheme is to be adopted, such as a full-arch bridge, this would follow normal crown and bridge and complete denture prosthodontics without the need for a balanced occlusion. The intercuspal occlusion should be provided at the ideal vertical dimension in the retruded arc of closure (retruded contact position), there should be an even and flat forwards movement of 1–2 mm, the lateral movement should be a group function with multiple contacts and the protrusive movement should be shallow and even.

Bridge screw tightening

With short-span bridges the screws can be tightened to 10 N.cm of torque, either manually or with a torquing device. Large implant-supported bridges should be seated progressively to assist with complete seating and prevent overtorquing the bridge screws. The screws in the centre should be hand-tightened first, moving distally and alternating from side to side. When the bridge is first placed, the screw access holes should be sealed with some cotton wool and temporary filling material. There is a significant incidence of early screw loosening, particularly with long bridges. The bridge therefore should be checked after 1–2 weeks and the bridge screws checked for tightness. Movement of a screw by 90° or less is considered acceptable. Any screws more loose than this must be checked a further 1–2 weeks later. It is unusual for a screw not to retain its tightness for the second time and if this occurs it should be checked carefully because it may indicate a poor

Figure 14.15

The occlusion is checked on a lower implant-supported bridge: (A) Articulating paper is used to mark initial contacts under light pressure. (B) The heaviest marks are present on the natural teeth, and the implant bridge (the second and third from the back) is only lightly touching. (C) Shimstock is used to confirm that the implant restorations are in contact under loading.

fit for the framework or that the bridge is being overloaded.

Once the screws have remained tight and the patient has approved all aspects of the bridge, the screw access holes can be sealed permanently. In order to allow access in the future without possible damage to the screw heads, they should be covered first with a layer of softened gutta percha or similar material, which will seal the space but not set hard so it can be removed easily if required. The occlusal portion of the screw access hole is best restored with a colour-matched light-cured composite resin filling material and the occlusion re-checked afterwards.

Bridge cementation

On completion of a cemented bridge a decision needs to be made regarding the type of cementation required. With multiple parallel abutments the restoration does not require a hard (permanent) cement because this will make the bridge difficult to seat fully and will make it impossible to retrieve in the future. Implant bridges therefore can be 'permanently' cemented with provisional cements as long as they demonstrate good retention and stability at the try-in.

When the bridge is first completed, it is prudent to cement it provisionally to allow the patient to 'live with' the bridge for a short while and check on contour, appearance and speech before final cementation. Weakened or modified temporary cement is all that will be required. Provisional seating also allows the gingiva to adapt to the new contour and will make final cementation an easier technique, because the bridge will not be prevented from seating by a tight gingival collar.

Prior to final cementation, the abutment screws are checked for tightness and the screw slots sealed with gutta percha. The chosen cement is mixed and placed in the bridge, only a thin layer will be necessary and the excess cement should be kept to a minimum to ease its removal. If hard cement such as zinc phosphate has been chosen, this should not be mixed as a viscous material or the bridge will not fully seat. The margins must be checked very carefully to ensure complete excess cement removal. The occlusion must be re-checked following cementation.

Instructions to the patient

On completion, long-cone periapical radiographs should be taken for all implants to confirm seating and act as a future guide for marginal bone levels (Figure 14.16). If a cemented bridge has been placed, excess cement should also be checked for. The patient is given specific hygiene instructions, particularly on how to access the areas between implants. They should be warned to be careful with the new bridge during function, because they are more likely to bite their inner cheek, lips or tongue as they get used to having a fixed structure rather than a denture. Patients who have worn a denture long term prior to implant treatment experience more problems at the start, and these are best discussed before problems arise in order to prevent the patient from becoming dissatisfied.

In particular, speech may be affected when restoring the upper anterior teeth. The perception of speech change is often more apparent to the patient than to anyone else and usually returns to normal after 1–2 weeks. Longer accommodation times are, however, sometimes needed.

Follow-up

Following final completion of the new restoration it is wise to arrange for a review within 6 months, particularly to check home maintenance. The marginal bone levels should be checked for stability with new long-cone periapical radiographs after 1 year and then approximately every 2 years.

Additional considerations

Joining teeth and implants

Ideally, implants should not be linked to natural teeth due to differential mobility. In particular, it

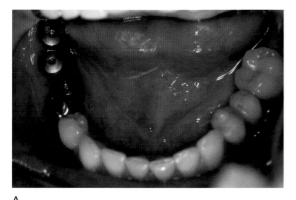

A

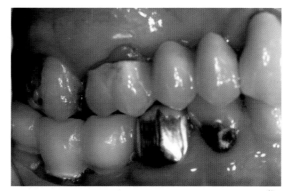

B

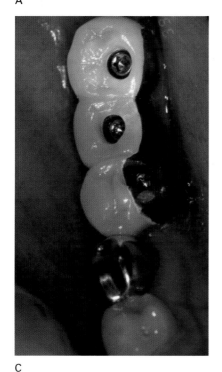

C

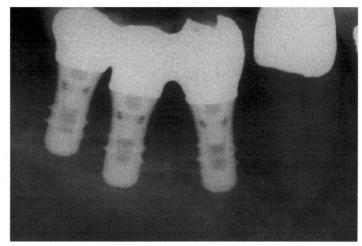

D

Figure 14.16

A posterior bridge supported by Straumann implants: (A) three healing abutments are visible; (B) the completed bridge; (C) occlusal view—screw retention has been used; (D) a periapical radiograph taken at the end of treatment.

is not advisable for a tooth to be linked into a bridge that is supported by several implants. In this situation, the bridge will be supported purely by the implants and the tooth will be superfluous. With time, the tooth may unseat from the bridge and intrude into the alveolus. If design or other factors dictate retention of a tooth, it is advisable that the tooth be protected by a gold coping so that movement of the tooth from the bridge will not result in an unprotected tooth becoming carious.

Success in linking teeth and implants can be achieved if a single sound and non-mobile tooth is linked to a single implant (Figure 14.17). Although there is still the differential in properties between the two abutments, clinical trials have shown high levels of success with no increased bone loss or technical complications. Once again, it is advisable for the tooth to be protected with a sub-bridge gold coping, which should be cemented with hard cement and the bridge with a weaker material. In the event of

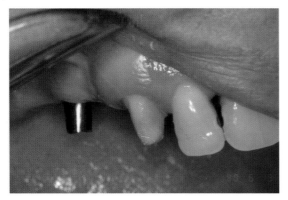

A

B

Figure 14.17

A three-unit bridge supported by a natural tooth and an AstraTech ST implant: (A) a Profile BI abutment (prepable) has been placed and the natural tooth prepared; (B) the tooth is protected with a gold coping; (C) the cemented bridge at completion.

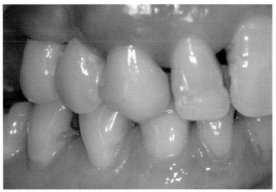

C

bridge cementation failure, the tooth will not be exposed to the potential of caries at the failed margin. Such linked bridges are useful if there is only enough bone volume for one implant to be placed but the patient requires the provision of two extra teeth. Linking the implant to the adjacent tooth will allow for either a single-unit cantilever bridge or a fixed-fixed design with a tooth and implant separated by a single missing unit. Provision of a joint as in conventional bridgework is not advised, because the joint will still allow the tooth to intrude from the bridge.

Bibliography

Arvidson K, Bystedt H, Frykholm A, von Konow L, Lothigius E (1992). A 3-year clinical study of Astra dental implants in the treatment of edentulous mandibles. *Int J Oral Maxillofac Implants* **7**: 321–9.

Arvidson K, Bystedt H, Frykholm A, von Konow L, Lothigius E (1998). Five year prospective follow up report of the AstraTech implant system in the treatment of edentulous mandibles. *Clin Oral Implants Res* **9**: 225–34.

Cameron SM, Joyce A, Brosseau JS (1998). Radiographic verification of implant abutment seating. *J Prosth Dent* **79**: 298–303.

Cheshire PD, Hobkirk JA (1996). An in vivo quantitative analysis of the fit of Nobel Biocare implant superstructures. *J Oral Rehab* **23**: 782–9.

Hellden LB, Derand T (1998). Description and evaluation of a simplified method to achieve passive fit between cast titanium frameworks and implants. *Int J Oral Maxillofac Implants* **13**: 190–6.

Hobkirk JA, Psarros KJ (1992). The influence of occlusal surface material on peak masticatory forces using ossointegrated implant supported prostheses. *Int J Oral Maxillofac Implants* **7**: 345–52.

Jemt T (1994). Fixed implant supported prostheses in

the edentulous maxilla. *Clin Oral Implants Res* **5**: 142–7.

Jemt T (1995). Three dimensional distortion of gold alloy castings and welded titanium frameworks. Measurements of the precision of fit between completed implant prostheses and the master casts in routine edentulous situations. *J Oral Rehab* **22**: 557–64.

Jemt T, Lekholm U (1993). Oral implant treatment in posterior partially edentulous jaws: a 5-year, follow-up report. *Int J Oral Maxillofac Implants* **8**: 635–40.

Jemt T, Book K (1996). Prosthesis misfit and marginal bone loss in edentulous implant patients. *Int J Oral Maxillofac Implants* **11**: 620–5.

Lundgren D, Laurell L (1994). Occlusal aspects of fixed bridgework supported by endosseous implants. In: *Proceedings of the 1st European Workshop on Periodontology*, eds Lang NP and Karring T, pp. 326–44. London: Quintessence Publishing.

McAlarney ME, Stavropoulos DN (1996). Determination of cantilever length to anterior–posterior spread ratio assuming failure criteria to be the compromise of the prosthesis retaining screw–prosthesis joint. *Int J Oral Maxillofac Implants* **11**: 331–9.

Olsson M, Gunne J, Astrand P, Borg K (1995). Bridges supported by free standing implants versus bridges supported by tooth and implant: a five year prospective study. *Clin Oral Implants Res* **6**: 114–21.

Schlumberger T, Bowley JF, Maze GI (1998). Intrusion phenomena in combination tooth implant restorations: a review of the literature. *J Prosthet Dent* **80**: 190–203.

15
Implant denture prosthodontics

Introduction

This chapter will describe the clinical procedures involved in the construction of implant dentures. Many of them are identical in principle to those used in the construction of conventional complete dentures. It is assumed that the reader will have a basic understanding of these latter procedures and it is not intended that this chapter will cover every stage in great detail. For a more detailed description of generic procedures, the reader is referred to textbooks covering complete denture prosthodontics.

Manufacturers are constantly developing their products and it is inevitable that some of them might not be included in this edition. Readers are referred to the individual manufacturers' catalogues for detailed descriptions of their products.

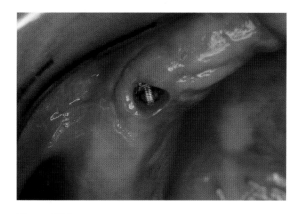

Figure 15.1

A healing abutment over a Nobel Biocare implant has been removed. The distance from the top of the implant (excluding the external hex) to the mucosa can be measured with a periodontal probe.

Selection of abutments or ball attachments

When a two-stage procedure has been carried out, the patient should be seen about 4 weeks after second-stage surgery for selection of abutments or ball attachments and primary impressions. When a one-stage procedure has been carried out, this prosthodontic stage would normally be carried out about 3 months after mandibular implant placement (6 months after maxillary implant placement with Nobel Biocare implants).

The healing abutments are removed and the distance from the top of the implant to the mucosal surface can be measured with, for example, a periodontal probe (Figure 15.1). The aim is to achieve the lowest possible profile when selecting a transmucosal abutment for a

bar or magnet, or selecting a ball attachment so that the prosthodontic components are within the intended contour of the denture. A general idea of what is required should be apparent from the treatment planning and stent construction. However, it is necessary to make the final selection after the mucosa has healed around the implants.

Most manufacturers supply a range of abutments in lengths up to 7 mm. The ITI/Straumann implant has the transmucosal element already incorporated into the implant so no choice is possible at this stage: the decision has already been made at the time of placing the implant. There is only one size of bar abutment (Figure 15.2) or ball attachment. The original Nobel Biocare standard abutment for bars and the large ball attachment (Figure 15.3) had a minimum sleeve length of 3 mm so there was a

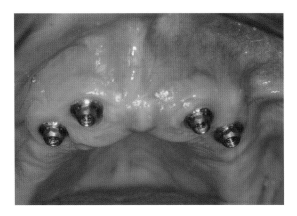

Figure 15.2

Octa abutments (SynOcta®: Institut Straumann, Walden-burg, Switzerland) in place on ITI/Straumann implants inserted at correct depth. Lowest profile for bar can be achieved.

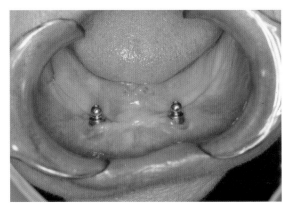

Figure 15.3

Nobel Biocare standard ball attachments with sleeve length selected to give lowest profile.

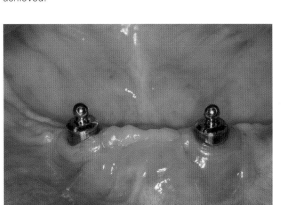

Figure 15.4

Nobel Biocare 2.25-mm ball attachments with sleeve length selected to give lowest profile.

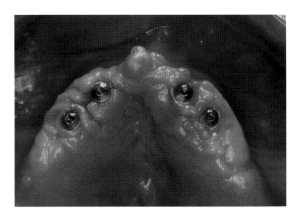

Figure 15.5

AstraTech 20° uni-abutments with appropriate cuff length to achieve lowest profile for bar or magnets.

potential shortage of space with superficially placed implants. The later Nobel Biocare 2.25-mm ball attachment has a minimum abutment sleeve length of 1 mm (Figure 15.4). The Nobel Biocare fixture-head gold coping, which fits directly onto the implant, can be reduced in height to allow the construction of a bar very close to the mucosa. The AstraTech uni-abutments for bars or magnets range in length up to 6 mm (Figure 15.5) and the ball attach-

ments have a similar range. The range of components is described more fully in Chapter 6.

Primary impressions

Once the measurements for abutments or ball attachments have been made, the healing abutments should be replaced and primary

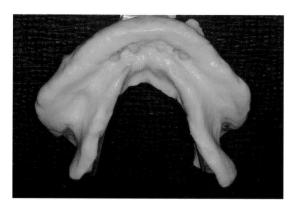

Figure 15.6

Mandibular preliminary impression in alginate material recording major landmarks. Nobel Biocare standard abutments are already in place. The intended retention system is a bar and clips.

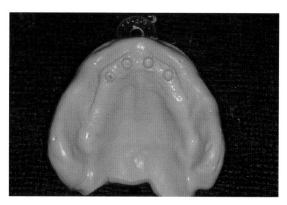

Figure 15.7

Maxillary preliminary impression in alginate material. Healing abutments are in place.

impressions made. The purpose of these impressions, usually made with alginate impression material, is to produce casts upon which custom trays can be made.

A suitable stock impression tray is selected that will allow a minimum thickness of 3 mm of alginate material and that extends to cover the major landmark areas. In the mandible these are the buccal, labial and lingual sulci, the retromolar pads and the retromylohyoid fossae; in the maxilla these are the buccal and labial sulci, the hamular notches and the palate. The imprints of the healing abutments are required for the custom tray design.

The container of alginate impression material should be shaken to homogenize the powder particles. The water and powder are dispensed using the manufacturer's measures and a thermometer should be used to adjust the temperature of the water. Warmer water can be used to accelerate the setting time for patients who have a strong gag reflex. Once a satisfactory impression has been made (Figures 15.6 and 15.7), it should be rinsed, disinfected, wrapped in damp gauze or tissue and placed in an airtight box. A polythene sandwich box is ideal because it prevents the impression from drying out and is rigid to prevent the impression from being crushed during transportation to the dental laboratory.

Custom tray construction and final impressions

A custom tray is made on the primary cast from acrylic resin tray material or light-curing tray material. Polyether impression material is used for the final impressions because it is sufficiently rigid to hold the various prosthodontic components that will be used during the impres-

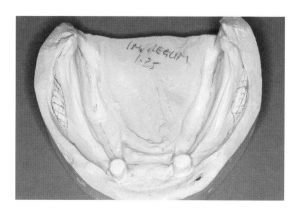

Figure 15.8

Primary mandibular cast showing prescription for dental technician: spacer thickness, extent and buccal shelf stops, window areas (healing abutment areas have had plaster added to indicate eventual height of studs).

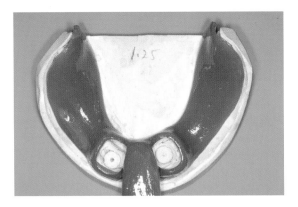

Figure 15.9

Typical mandibular custom tray with windows with sufficient clearance around implant.

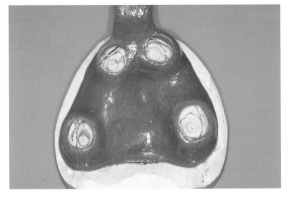

Figure 15.10

Typical maxillary custom tray.

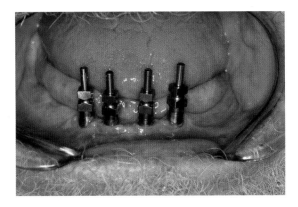

Figure 15.11

Standard bar impression technique: standard Nobel Biocare abutments have been attached to the implants and standard impression copings have been attached to the abutments.

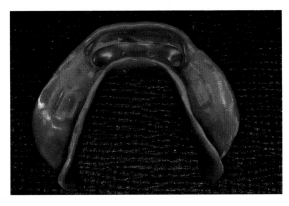

Figures 15.12

Standard bar impression technique: the custom tray has a window area through which the impression coping pins can be accessed. The window is a single large window because the implants are relatively close. A wax sheet has been added over the window and the tray has been tried in the mouth. The imprints of the tops of the pins can be seen clearly on the underside of the wax sheet. The stops on the posterior part of the tray are visible.

sion procedure. This material requires a 1.25-mm spacer, so a single sheet of baseplate wax is placed on the primary cast to the desired outline and areas are cut out for the tray stops (Figures 15.8). Extra wax or plaster is placed around the abutments to ensure adequate clearance and the tray is constructed with windows over the abutments; tray material is brought vertically to enclose the intended impression copings or ball attachments (Figures 15.9 and 15.10).

The various manufacturers' implant systems have similar principles involved in making the final impressions for implant dentures. The original standard method for bar-retained implant dentures (and for AstraTech magnets) is shown in Figures 15.11–15.20 and involves the attachment of irregularly shaped impression copings

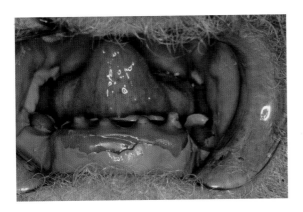

Figure 15.13

Standard bar impression technique: the impression is made using Impregum (Espe, D-82229 Seefeld, Germany) material. The tray has been placed so that the pins fit into the imprints on the underside of the wax sheet.

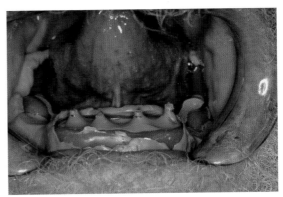

Figure 15.14

Standard bar impression technique: the impression material has set and the wax sheet has been removed, revealing the tops of the impression coping pins. These pins can now be unscrewed so that the impression can be removed from the mouth.

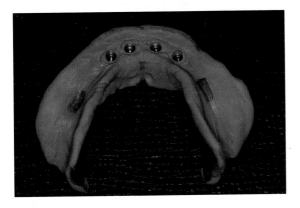

Figure 15.15

Standard bar impression technique: the final impression showing well-formed borders and impression copings securely held in material. The stops on the posterior ridge areas are clearly demarcated – these areas will be adjusted when the denture is fitted.

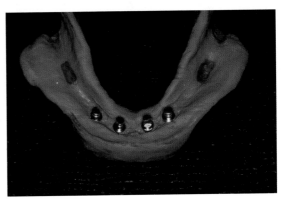

Figure 15.16

Standard bar impression technique: the laboratory replicas of abutments have been attached to the impression copings with the impression coping pins.

by long pins to the selected abutments that have been attached to the implants. The custom tray has a window through which the pins protrude when the impression is made. Once the material has set, the pins are loosened and the impression is removed from the mouth with the impression copings now firmly held in the impression. Then, laboratory replicas of the abutments are attached to the impression copings via the long

pins prior to boxing the impression and pouring the cast. In the standard method, the position of the abutment is recorded via the coping rather than an impression being made of it.

With ball attachment systems, the abutment screw has a ball head and this is screwed into the implant with the appropriate screwdriver. The large Nobel Biocare ball attachment is large enough to have the screwdriver hole in the ball

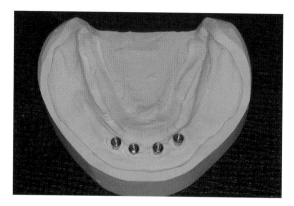

Figure 15.17

Standard bar impression technique: the working cast with stainless-steel abutment replicas.

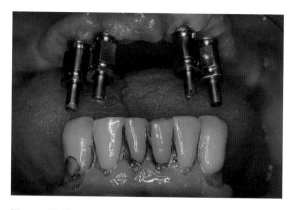

Figure 15.18

Standard bar impression technique: AstraTech impression coping, 20° squared.

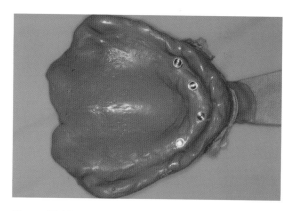

Figure 15.19

Standard bar impression technique: final maxillary impression with AstraTech impression copings.

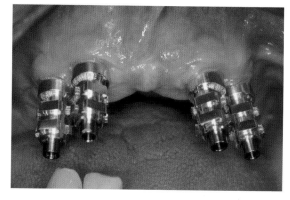

Figure 15.20

Standard bar impression technique: ITI/Straumann Octa transfer copings.

head but all the others have drivers that enclose the ball and engage suitable flats on the collar. The final impression is made of the ball attachments and laboratory replicas of them are placed in the impression prior to pouring the cast (Figures 15.21–15.29). The AstraTech ball attachment system has plastic impression copings that are placed over the ball (Figure 15.30) prior to the impression and remain in the impression

when it is removed from the mouth. The advantage of this coping is that the fit between it and the laboratory replica is more precise than with the small ball attachments of other manufacturers.

A later type of impression coping has been developed for bar-retained implant dentures – the bar impression coping. Bar impression copings are attached to the abutment already

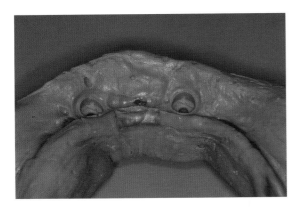

Figure 15.21

Final impression of Nobel Biocare 2.25-mm ball attachments (detail) showing driver flats.

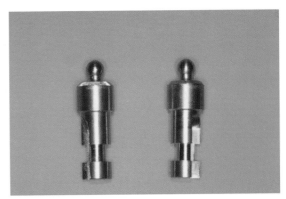

Figure 15.22

Nobel Biocare 2.25-mm ball attachment replicas.

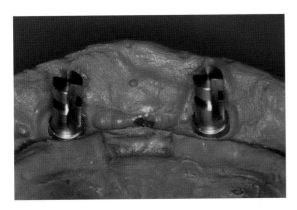

Figure 15.23

Final impression with the laboratory replicas placed into imprints of ball attachments.

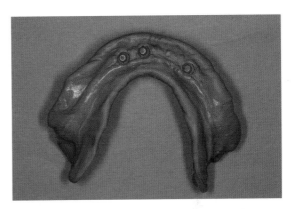

Figure 15.24

Final impression of three Nobel Biocare standard ball attachments.

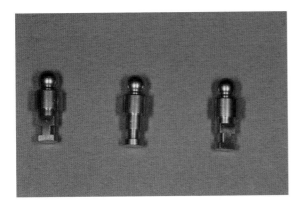

Figure 15.25

Nobel Biocare standard ball attachment replicas in brass. Also available in stainless steel.

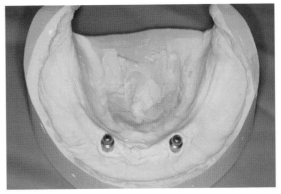

Figure 15.26

Working cast with two replicas of ball attachments. Spacers are supplied, which are inserted into the hole on the top of the ball. These spacers ensure that the retention cap is correctly aligned vertically.

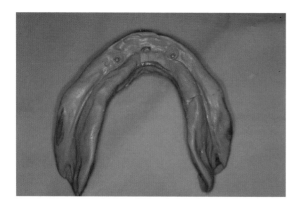

Figure 15.27

Final impression of ITI/Straumann retentive anchors with anterior and buccal shelf stops demarcated.

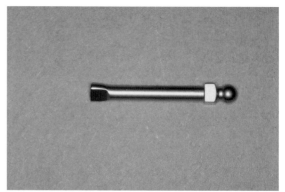

Figure 15.28

ITI/Straumann transfer pin for retentive anchor.

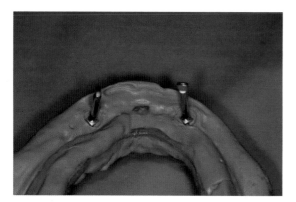

Figure 15.29

Final impression with transfer pins placed into imprints of retentive anchors.

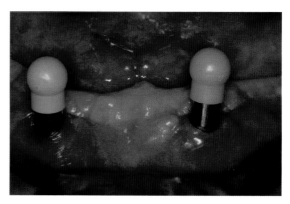

Figure 15.30

AstraTech ball impression copings. These are picked up with the final impression.

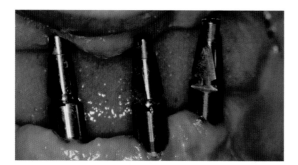

Figure 15.31

Nobel Biocare fixture head impression copings. These can be used with slot-head pins in the standard bar impression technique shown in Figures 15.11–15.17 except that a replica of the implant is attached to the copings before the cast is poured. They can also be used with round-headed pins in the bar impression coping method shown in Chapter 17, Figures 17.24–17.28.

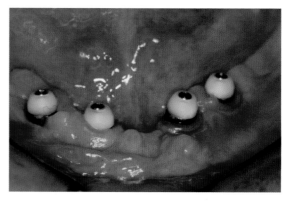

Figure 15.32

Protection caps on standard Nobel Biocare abutments.

attached to the implant and remain in the mouth when the impression is removed. The bar impression copings are then unscrewed from the abutment, attached to laboratory replicas of the abutments and then re-inserted into the impression prior to pouring the cast (see Chapter 17, Figures 17.24–17.28).

Nobel Biocare have introduced fixture head impression copings to complement the fixture head copings mentioned earlier (Figure 15.31). These impression copings can be used with slot-headed pins in the standard method shown in Figures 15.11–15.20 or as bar impression copings that remain in the mouth after the impression has been removed (see Chapter 17, Figures 17.24–17.28).

Once the final impressions have been made, the abutments or ball attachments can be left in place on the implants but protection caps are essential for the former to prevent food debris and calculus from entering the screw hole for the gold cylinders (Figure 15.32). The temporary soft lining on the base of any denture that is being worn will, of course, need to be changed to accommodate the abutments and protection caps or ball attachments. Alternatively, the abutments or ball attachments can be removed and the healing abutments replaced until the next stage. In this case, the temporary lining does not need to be changed.

Verification of final cast

It can be helpful to verify the accuracy of the final cast, especially for intended bar-retained implant dentures, to avoid discovering errors late on in the treatment. This can be done by linking impression copings with composite resin in exactly the same way as for extensive fixed restorations (see Chapter 14).

Recording the maxillomandibular relationship

For the construction of implant dentures, just as with conventional complete dentures, the spatial relationship between the maxilla and the mandible is recorded by the use of occlusion

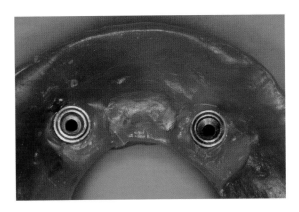

Figure 15.33

Nobel Biocare impression copings in wax occlusion rim.

rims on temporary or processed bases. The rims are shaped to prescribe the intended position of the anterior teeth and the occlusal plane, and are adjusted to meet evenly when the patient closes in the retruded position at a vertical relationship that allows for sufficient interocclusal distance (freeway space). A setting material is then introduced between the occlusal surfaces of the two rims to record their relationship.

The base of the occlusion rim can incorporate all or part of the impression coping to stabilize the rim during the recording procedure for a bar-retained denture (Figure 15.33). For a ball-attachment-retained denture, the base of the rim can incorporate the actual retention caps. The small retention caps of Nobel Biocare, AstraTech or ITI/Staumann ball attachments are best incorporated into a heat-cured acrylic resin base because they can be pulled out of a wax base (Figures 15.34). The large Nobel Biocare retention caps have sufficient surface area to remain within a wax base.

The intended vertical relationship is determined by establishing the resting vertical relationship via a sliding calliper in almost universal use (a Willis gauge) or by the use of dividers measuring between marks on the patient's nose and chin. By convention, 4 mm are subtracted from the measurement of the resting vertical relationship to arrive at a proposed occluding vertical relationship. This equates to about 2 mm of interocclusal distance (freeway space) at the first molar region. Whatever

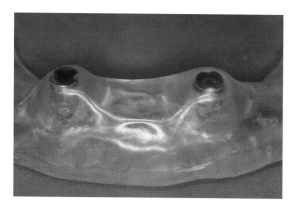

Figure 15.34

Nobel Biocare 2.25-mm gold alloy retention caps processed into heat-cured acrylic resin base.

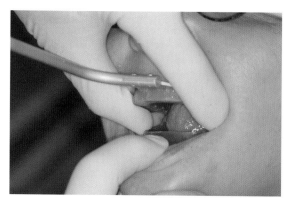

Figure 15.35

Basic hand position for making interocclusal records: the left index finger and thumb are stabilizing the maxillary occlusion rim and posterior part of the mandibular rim; the right index finger is placed in front of the mandibular occlusion rim; the right second finger and thumb are placed below the chin. The right hand guides the mandible into the retruded position. The facebow fork is in place to facilitate the facebow transfer record when the interocclusal record material has set.

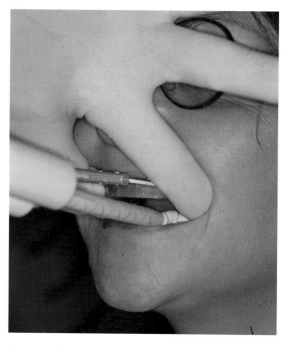

Figure 15.36

Automixed record material is injected onto the occlusal surface of the mandibular rim. The left hand remains in position to stabilize both rims and to prevent patient closing.

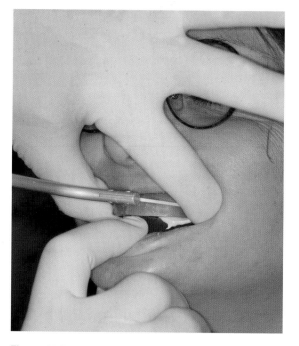

Figure 15.37

Mandibular closure is guided until the occlusion rims touch gently. The operator's fingers remain in position until the material has set.

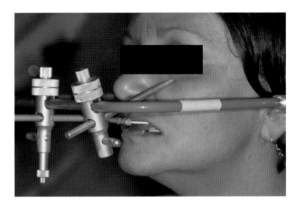

Figure 15.38

When the material has set, the facebow calliper is slid over the fork and the locking device is tightened. The orbital pointer is located and its locking device is tightened.

method is used to assess these dimensions, it has always been considered essential to have sufficient interocclusal distance for maximum comfort for conventional complete dentures. It is not clear whether or not the presence of implants alters this requirement.

The method of locating the relative position of one occlusion rim to the other is shown in Figures 15.35–15.37: a fluid-setting material is introduced between the occlusal surfaces of the occlusion rims, with a working time sufficiently long to allow an unhurried guided mandibular closure into the retruded position, a setting time sufficiently short for the material to set soon after this closure and sufficient durability for the material to remain intact after the occlusion rims are removed from the mouth. A facebow transfer record can be made conveniently at the same time as the interocclusal record by placing the facebow fork into the maxillary rim before the record is made. Once the interocclusal record material has set, the rims are then stabilized by the patient keeping the rims together while the facebow calliper is positioned over the fork and the infraorbital pointer is adjusted (Figure 15.38).

After the facebow transfer record has been made, the entire assembly is removed from the patient and disinfected. The maxillary cast is then mounted on the upper member of a semi-adjustable articulator with low expansion mounting plaster and with the use of a facebow

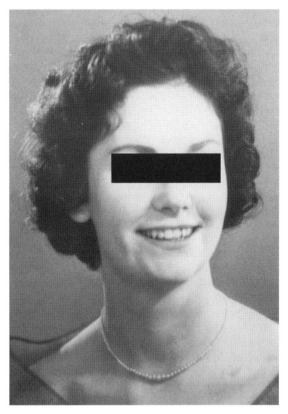

Figure 15.39

Photograph of patient with natural teeth.

support. The mandibular cast is mounted once the maxillary mounting plaster has set.

Selection of denture teeth

In general, the aim should be to select denture teeth that resemble the original natural teeth and to arrange them in a similar way. This will usually produce the most natural-looking dentures and the patient will adapt to them more quickly. Photographs (Figures 15.39 and 15.40) of the patient's original teeth will help in this procedure but the denture teeth may need the incisal edges adjusted to simulate wear (Figure 15.41).

Posterior teeth should be selected with as much care as anterior teeth. For the mandibular denture, the space available is from the distal

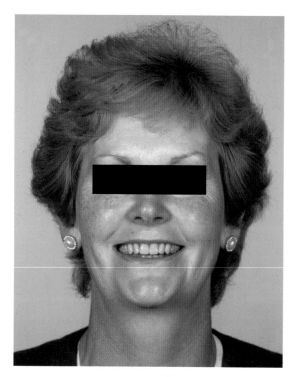

Figure 15.40

Denture teeth of implant denture have been selected and arranged to resemble those of pre-extraction photograph.

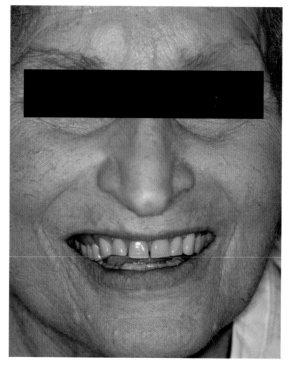

Figure 15.41

Denture teeth of maxillary implant denture have had incisal edges ground to simulate wear.

surface of the proposed canine to the commencement of any slope up to the retromolar pad. It may be possible to fit two premolars and two molars into this space, but occasionally a second molar or a premolar may need to be omitted, especially in a patient with a Class 2 jaw relationship. In general, narrow occlusal surfaces are desirable to increase masticatory efficiency, but in patients with Class 2 or Class 3 skeletal relationships wider occlusal surfaces may be necessary to develop and maintain occlusal contact in a range of mandibular positions.

Confirmation of cast relationship on articulator

The relationship of the casts on the articulator is confirmed by setting up denture teeth (on temporary wax or acrylic resin bases, or on heat-cured acrylic resin bases) in tight intercuspation and in the position prescribed by the occlusion rims (Figure 15.42). The trial dentures are then placed in the patient's mouth and, using the hand position shown in Figure 15.35, the patient is guided into closure in the retruded position (Figure 15.43). If the denture teeth come together evenly with no movement of the trial denture base, then the horizontal relationship of the casts can be considered confirmed. If this occlusion occurs at an occluding vertical relationship with a demonstrable interocclusal distance, then the vertical relationship of the casts can be considered confirmed.

If the denture teeth do not meet evenly when the patient closes in the retruded position (Figure 15.44), the occlusion should be examined with the trial dentures back on the articulator. If the teeth are not in tight intercuspation, they should

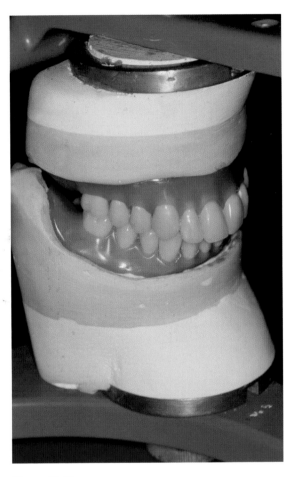

Figure 15.42

Working casts have been mounted on a semi-adjustable articulator and denture teeth have been set in tight intercuspation.

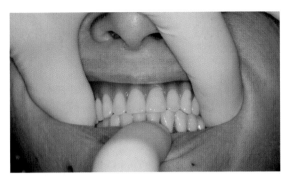

Figure 15.43

Patient is guided into retruded closure with trial dentures.

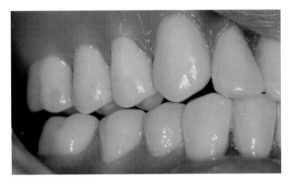

Figure 15.44

These posterior teeth do not meet evenly when the patient is guided into retruded position. A new interocclusal record will be necessary.

be reset and the trial dentures again placed in the mouth. If the teeth still do not meet evenly, the cast relationship is incorrect and a new interocclusal record will be necessary. This is carried out by removing one set of posterior teeth, marking the mandibular incisors with the degree of overlap required when the new record is being made (Figure 15.45) and then making a new record as described above. The mandibular cast is remounted using the new record, the posterior teeth are reset and the trial dentures are then replaced in the mouth to test the veracity of the cast relationship.

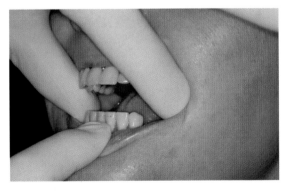

Figure 15.45

A pencil mark can be made on the mandibular teeth prior to any new record, to indicate the amount of closure required: the right index finger can be placed so that during closure the maxillary teeth will touch the gloved fingernail and prevent further closure. Thus, the new record can be made at the intended vertical relationship.

Occasionally, the denture teeth may meet evenly in the patient's mouth but at a vertical relationship that has insufficient or excessive interocclusal distance. If the amount is small, the necessary adjustment can be made on the articulator because a facebow record has been made. If the error is large, it is better to make a new interocclusal record at the correct vertical relationship because an arbitrary facebow record (as opposed to a hinge axis record) becomes less accurate with larger changes in vertical dimension.

Confirmation of anterior tooth position is accomplished by reference to anatomical landmarks such as the incisive papilla, pre-extraction records such as casts or photographs, speech sounds and direct patient feedback.

A protrusive interocclusal record is made to adjust the horizontal condylar guidance of semi-adjustable articulators but the lateral condylar guidance is usually adjusted arbitrarily because such instruments do not accept all lateral interocclusal records.

The final step at this stage is to decide on the posterior limit of the maxillary denture if this has not already been done.

Completion of the implant dentures

Where a bar and clip retention system is being used, the bar is now constructed with reference to anterior tooth position and the contour of the denture (Figures 15.46 and 15.47). The bar should be tried in the mouth prior to completion of the dentures. If the bar does not fit the abutments in the mouth (Figure 15.48), it should be examined carefully on the cast (Figure 15.49). If the bar does not fit the cast, it should be cut and resoldered or remade so that it does fit. Then it can again be tried in the mouth. If the bar demonstrates a passive fit on the abutments (Figure 15.50), then the denture can be finished. If the bar does not demonstrate a passive fit, the final impression must be at fault and will need to be repeated. If, however, the composite try-in mentioned earlier has been carried out, this can be avoided.

Ideally, the posterior teeth should be set in a bilateral balanced occlusion. Much has been

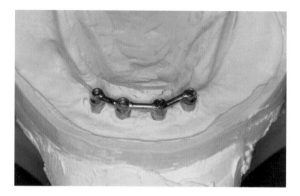

Figure 15.46

Once the final tooth position is confirmed, the bar can be constructed.

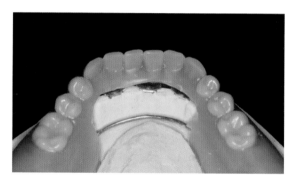

Figure 15.47

The bar is in position on the working cast and has been covered with plaster to block out all but the retentive elements of the clips. The entire assembly is within the contour of the denture after the tooth position has been confirmed.

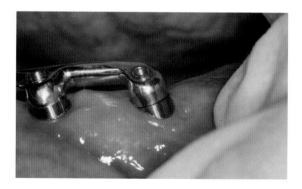

Figure 15.48

The bar has been tried in mouth. There is a gap between the gold cylinder and the standard abutment.

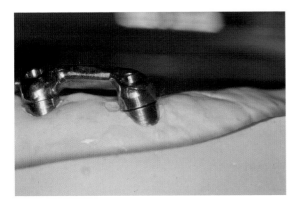

Figure 15.49

The bar is back on the cast; the gap is present on the cast. The bar will need to be cut and resoldered.

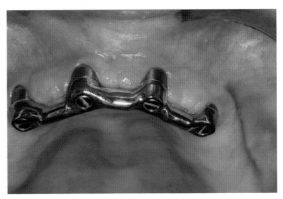

Figure 15.50

The bar on maxillary standard abutments with passive fit.

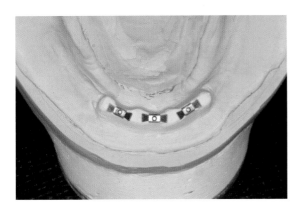

Figure 15.51

Nobel Biocare clips attached to round bar, with spacers and all but retention tags covered with plaster. AstraTech bar and riders are similar.

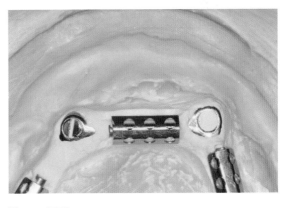

Figure 15.52

ITI/Straumann Dolder bar and clips in place with spacers. Clips should be clear of gold cylinders to avoid any impingement during denture movement. In view of the long bar, the denture is also supported on anterior gold cylinders.

written about the advantages and disadvantages of such an occlusion. It is certainly difficult to achieve with some manufacturers' teeth. My own experience over 30 years in prosthodontic practice is that dentures seem to be more stable with a balanced occlusion but it is not clear whether or not such an occlusion has any effect on implant success. However, where there is evidence of overloading of implants, it would

seem sensible to reduce the loading by reducing the anterior guidance.

The implant dentures should now be finished with any clips attached to the bar over appropriate spacers and all but the retention elements of the clips blocked out with plaster prior to flasking, packing and processing in the usual way (Figures 15.51–15.57). Where ball attachments are being used, the retention caps are attached

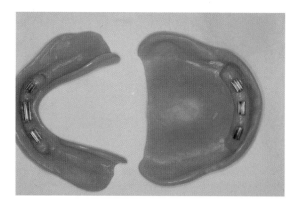

Figure 15.53

Completed dentures showing Nobel Biocare Macro-Ovoid bar clips.

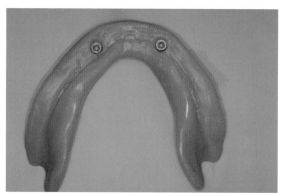

Figure 15.54

Completed mandibular denture showing ITI/Straumann titanium alloy matrices.

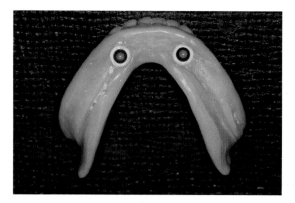

Figure 15.55

Complete mandibular denture showing Nobel Biocare standard ball attachment matrices.

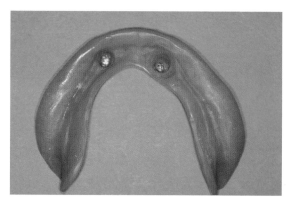

Figure 15.56

Completed mandibular denture showing ITI/Straumann gold alloy matrices (similar to AstraTech and Nobel Biocare 2.25-mm matrices). ITI/Straumann and AstraTech matrices have four tines and Nobel Biocare matrices have six tines.

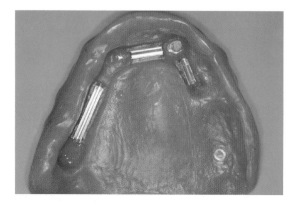

Figure 15.57

Completed maxillary denture with ITI/Straumann Dolder bar clips.

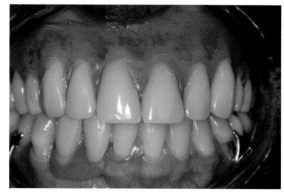

Figure 15.58

Completed maxillary implant denture with tinted gingival acrylic resin to simulate melanin pigmentation.

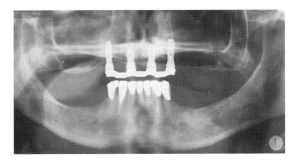

Figure 15.59

Radiograph of fitted maxillary Nobel Biocare Macro-Ovoid gold alloy bar (patient with onlay bone graft illustrated in Figure 6.9 of Chapter 6 and in Figure 15.50 above).

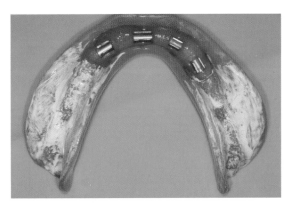

Figure 15.60

Pressure indicator paste applied to mandibular denture, showing posterior tray stop areas.

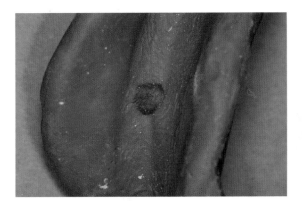

Figure 15.61

Pressure area over tray stop in original final impression.

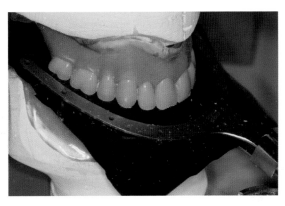

Figure 15.62

Completed dentures have been remounted with new interocclusal record and occlusion is adjusted using an extra-wide sheet of articulating paper in the forceps.

to the laboratory replicas and again blocked out with plaster. Where magnets are being used, the magnets are attached to the replicas with cyanoacrylate glue. Occasionally, gingival tinting will be required where the patient has melanin pigmentation (Figure 15.58).

Insertion of the implant dentures

Healing abutments that have been left in place in-between clinical stages should be unscrewed

and the definitive abutments for bars, magnets or ball attachments should be placed. A torque driver can be used, but hand tightening has usually been sufficient for the components under implant dentures. Bars should now be attached with appropriate screws (Figure 15.59).

The dentures should be coated with pressure indicator paste to identify pressure areas, especially those created by the tray stops. These areas should be adjusted with an acrylic resin bur, as well as any obvious sharp edges (Figures 15.60 and 15.61).

A new interocclusal record and remounting of the dentures on an articulator for final occlusal adjustments are always recommended for best results (Figure 15.62). Any small clinical errors or processing changes can be corrected by use of this procedure.

Once the dentures have been fitted, the patient should ideally be seen within 48 h for any necessary adjustments. The patient should be warned that some soreness is likely. This may be caused by pressure areas in the final impression, overextension or faults in the occlusion. Use of pressure indicator paste and the remounting procedure will reduce the prevalence of post-insertion discomfort. Occasionally, overextension will be caused by the viscous nature of the polyether impression material if the custom tray was not extended correctly. In addition, it is very difficult to make impressions for implant dentures by any other method than a static method: materials suitable for functional impressions are not really suitable for picking up the components of implant dentures or rigid enough to hold the laboratory replicas.

The patient should be seen regularly until the dentures are comfortable, and then reviewed at least annually as part of a regular maintenance programme.

PART V

Complications and Maintenance

16
Single tooth and fixed bridge

Introduction

In order to measure treatment success and the incidence of complications, it has been suggested that longitudinal studies of implant systems should be a minimum of 5 years (preferably prospective studies rather than retrospective), with adequate radiographic and clinical supporting data. Complications should be rare and in most cases avoidable by careful attention to diagnosis, treatment planning, good surgical and prosthodontic training and experience and by following well-established protocols that demonstrate high success and predictability. However, complications can occur in the early treatment phases, either surgical or prosthodontic, or following completion of treatment during the maintenance phase. Failure of osseointegration of individual implants should be relatively rare, with most failures occurring during the initial healing period or following abutment connection and initial loading. Longer term complications may be associated with:

- general wear and tear
- inadequate attention to oral hygiene
- poorly controlled occlusal forces
- poor design of prostheses
- utilization of an inadequately tested implant system
- soft-tissue deficiencies

The complications relating to surgery are common to all types of implant treatment and systems and are considered together. Prosthetic and late complications and maintenance are dealt with under separate sections for single tooth replacement and fixed bridges. Chapter 17 deals with implant dentures.

Surgical sequelae and complications

It is important to warn patients about the most common surgical/postoperative complications. Patients may experience some postoperative swelling, bruising and discomfort, even with straightforward single implant surgery. However, these sequelae are much more likely in cases involving placement of a large number of implants or grafting. These complications can be minimized with:

- gentle surgical manipulation of the hard and soft tissues
- avoidance of over-reflection of flaps
- preoperative and postoperative analgesics (preferably those with anti-inflammatory properties such as the non-steroidal anti-inflammatory drugs, e.g. ibuprofen)
- recommendations to use ice packs to reduce swelling
- intravenous steroids in more major cases
- pressure applied to the wound postoperatively to control haemostasis and avoid haematoma formation

In our experience the majority of patients have little or no postoperative swelling/bruising/pain (Figure 16.1). The success of osseointegration is dependent on minimal mechanical and thermal trauma to the bone and therefore the patient should not experience pain in the bone sites. Severe pain may suggest poor technique and may coincide with early failure of the implant. A more controversial topic is whether pre- and postoperative antibiotics are required to prevent infection and subsequent

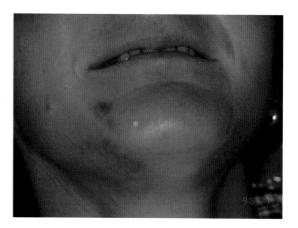

Figure 16.1

Bruising near the chin and submandibular region 1 week following implant surgery to place six implants in the upper jaw.

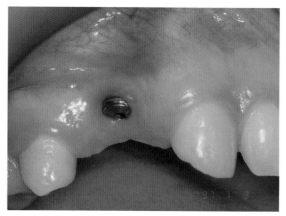

Figure 16.2

Spontaneous exposure of a previously submerged implant. There is little or no inflammation of the soft tissue. The implant position is poor, having been placed in the middle of a two-tooth space.

failure of the implant. It was once routine to prescribe antibiotics. However, as implant surgery is carried out under good surgical conditions and a sterile implant is delivered carefully into the prepared site, the chance of infection should be low. It would be prudent to use antibiotics if:

- There has been a recent infection at the site.
- Immediate replacement techniques are used.
- Multiple implants are placed where flaps have been raised extensively or for a long period of time.
- Augmentation and grafting are performed, including guided bone regeneration (GBR) membranes.
- The patient has a medical history that suggests a susceptibility to infection.
- The patient is a smoker.
- The patient has hard bone (Type 1) that has been difficult to cut and cool.
- The implant placement has breached the maxillary sinus floor.

In some cases patients experience infection in the soft tissue if the surgeon has left debris under the flap margins or a large clot has become infected. These cases are largely avoidable.

Wound dehiscence

The soft tissue wound may break down in the first week following implant installation (e.g. particularly in the severely atrophic mandible). This used to concern clinicians when it led to implant head exposure in submerged implant systems, but because it has now been shown that these implants work in non-submerged protocols it is not thought to be significant (Figure 16.2). If an implant head becomes exposed in a case that was planned to be submerged, it is important to keep the area clean with antiseptic rinses (such as 0.2/0.12% chlorhexidine) to prevent inflammation and marginal bone loss. This situation may be improved by changing the cover screw on the implant for a healing abutment. Any breakdown of the soft tissue wound can lead to inflammation/bone loss and is most critical in grafting procedures where graft vitality and success can be severely compromised.

Early implant failure

Most early surgical failures of osseointegration are due to poor surgical technique or placement of implants into bone of very poor density, or in areas with a lack of bone volume that has only allowed

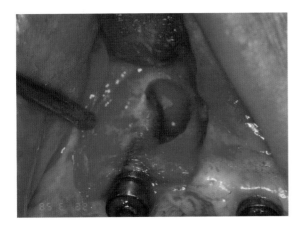

Figure 16.3

Surgical exposure of an apical lesion of bone loss, probably caused by inadequate cooling of the end of the drill during preparation of the site. The patient experienced pain and infection for several months after the implant placement.

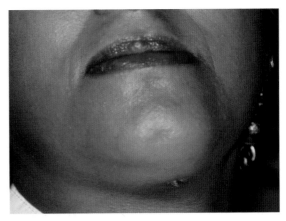

Figure 16.4

A sinus tract appearing on the skin at the lower border of the mandible. Inadequate cooling of an 18-mm implant site in hard bone was the likely cause.

utilization of very short implants (7 mm or less). Failure of osseointegration may not be obvious until the surgeon carries out abutment connection surgery or when the prosthodontist tries to load the implant. It is sometimes difficult for the clinician to assess implant stability and occasionally a loose abutment may be misinterpreted as a failed implant. The suspect abutment should be tightened and the stability reassessed. Tightening of the abutment should not elicit discomfort/pain unless there is inflammation within the bone (consistent with failure) or trapping of soft tissue between abutment and implant head. In most cases mild discomfort soon resolves and there is no long-term complication. In other cases the discomfort is a sign that there is a problem, and more obvious failure of the osseointegration is revealed some days or weeks later.

Damage to the bone resulting in necrosis, pain and subsequent infection is more likely where hard bone has been prepared with inadequate cooling and/or blunt drills (Figure 16.3). This is more likely at deep preparation sites (e.g. > 13 mm). Such deep preparations are not usually necessary in good-quality bone and should be avoided. The resultant pain can be severe and an infection that is likely to be deep seated can track through the soft tissues. In the anterior region of the mandible the infection may track to the external skin surface, producing a disfiguring sinus tract, fibrosis and scarring (Figure 16.4).

Damage to neurovascular structures

Loss of sensation to the lower lip caused by trauma to the inferior dental or mental nerve is a serious injury (Figure 16.5). Surgery close to

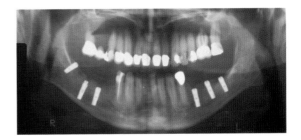

Figure 16.5

A panoral radiograph showing placement of implants in the posterior mandible with little or no regard to the position of the inferior dental canal. The implants on the patient's right breached the canal and resulted in mental anaesthesia; the implants on the left were placed so close to the nerve that paraesthesia resulted. (The clinician involved in this case is not known to the authors.)

these structures is hazardous and great care should be taken and the patient warned of the possible consequences. The following points should be appreciated to avoid this complication:

1. Avoid making relieving incisions in the area of the mental nerve.
2. Do not place crestal incisions over the region of a superficially located mental foramen in the severely resorbed mandible.
3. Adequately expose, identify and protect the nerve when operating close to it.
4. Check for anterior loops of the inferior dental nerve anterior to the mental foramen by radiography or by gentle probing of the foramen if utilizing this site.
5. Plan carefully with good tomographic or computed tomography (CT) images that allow good visualization of the inferior dental canal and the superficial ridge.
6. Take careful measurements of the available height and width of the bone above the canal.
7. In some circumstances it may be possible to place an implant in a plane that safely avoids the canal, which could not be appreciated using two-dimensional radiography.
8. Use transparent transfers of the appropriate implants at the correct magnification to overlay on the radiographic images, or a computer software program if this is available to you.
9. Avoid thermal damage to the bone that is left between the implant tip and the nerve canal.
10. Allow a safety margin for:
    - measurement error
    - a margin of bone between implant tip and and canal, which we would suggest to be no less than 2 mm (although some surgeons will place implants very close to the canal)
    - drill length at the cutting tip (different drills have various profiles and may overcut 1–2 mm longer than the planned implant length)
    - difficulty of surgical access, vision and control of cutting pressure at the depth of the site

Patients are unlikely to complain following damage to the incisive nerve in the midline of the anterior maxilla. Damage to the incisive branch of the inferior dental nerve may go unnoticed in patients with no teeth in the anterior mandible. However in dentate patients, an implant placed in the canine or first premolar region can sever or damage the incisive nerve supply to the remaining lower incisors. The patient may complain of paraesthesia or anaesthesia of the lateral incisor periodontium and this can be distressing. The central incisor is not usually affected because of dual innervation across the midline. Therefore it is wise to avoid violation of the mandibular incisive canal in dentate subjects.

A related problem can also occur when bone grafts are taken from the chin in dentate subjects. An osteotomy cut to close to the incisor or canine apices can result in alterations of sensation or, worse, loss of pulp vitality. A safety margin of 3 mm is recommended between the osteotomy cut and the apices (see Chapter 12).

Fractures

The severely resorbed mandible can be compromised by implant placement such that a fracture occurs at surgery or a short time following this. Sectional tomograms should be taken to assess adequately the profile of the severely resorbed mandible and to avoid the placement of too many implants within zones of low bone volume (e.g. mandibular first premolar region).

Prosthetic complications and maintenance

Complications and maintenance requirements vary widely between patients, depending on:

- susceptibility to caries and periodontal disease in the dentate patients
- complexity and type of implant-supported prostheses
- functional demands
- the patient's ability to maintain an adequate standard of oral hygiene

It is generally recommended that patients treated with implant prostheses are seen at least on an annual basis, but in many cases they will also require routine hygienist treatment at 3-, 4- or 6-month intervals, according to individual requirements.

Single tooth units

Single tooth units should require little maintenance. The majority of single units are cemented and the integrity of the cementation should be checked. Crown decementation of single tooth units is unusual, even in cases where a relatively weak temporary cement has been used. This is because of the close fit of the abutment to the crown, and in some cases a high degree of parallelism between them, which may make separation difficult or impossible. A more common complication is failure to seat the crown at the original cementation because of failure to relieve hydraulic pressure within the crown using a cementation vent (Figure 16.6). The resulting poor marginal fit and exposure of a large amount of cement lute may result in soft tissue inflammation because of the increased bacterial plaque retention. A vent also helps to reduce excess cement from being extruded at the crown margins, which can give rise to considerable inflammation, including soft tissue abscess and fistula formation. Plaque retention and development of inflammation may also be the initial sign of a loose abutment (see below).

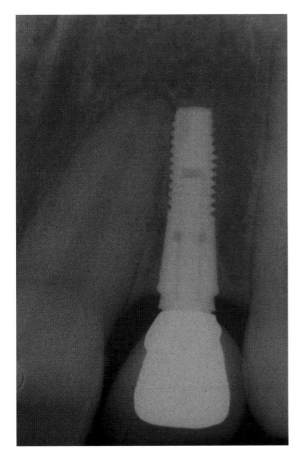

A

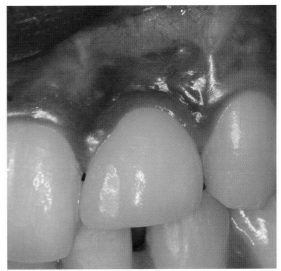

B

Figure 16.6

(A) Radiograph of an AstraTech single tooth implant where there has been failure to seat the cemented crown fully. A gap can be seen between the crown and abutment. This complication is largely avoided by adequate venting of the crown to allow excess cement to escape. (B) The clinical appearance of the case in (A), showing very good soft tissue health despite the unsatisfactory seating of the crown.

Fixed prostheses

The prostheses should be checked for signs of wear or breakage on a regular basis. Fixed restorations should have the cementation or screw fixation checked. This may include checking the screws that retain the prostheses (Figure 16.7) and those that retain the abutments (see below). The occlusion should be re-evaluated, particularly where there has been occlusal wear of the prostheses or coexisting natural dentition. It is not generally recommended to remove routinely the screw-retained bridge superstructures unless there is a suspicion that there is a problem with one of the implants/abutments. Fixed prostheses that have proved difficult to clean by the patient may require removal to allow adequate professional cleaning, which is easier with screw-retained fixed prostheses than cemented types.

The screws retaining a prosthesis to the abutment are often covered with a layer of restorative material, such as composite or glass ionomer, which may need replacing. Screws that are accessible should be checked to ensure that they have not loosened. This is more likely to occur in an ill-fitting prosthesis or where high loads have been applied.

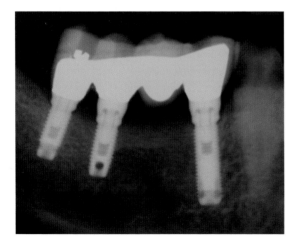

Figure 16.7

Radiograph of a posterior mandibular bridge. The loose bridge screw in the distal abutment is visible.

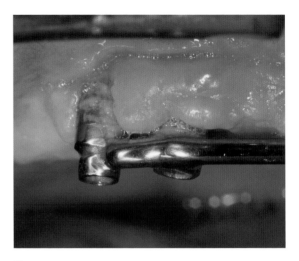

Figure 16.8

Implants joined by a bar used to support a maxillary denture. The oral hygiene is poor and the loading has been high, causing loss of osseointegration of the distal implant.

Removable prostheses (dealt with in detail in Chapter 17)

Removable prostheses need to be checked for retention and stability. In the case of prostheses with combined implant and mucosal support it is important to check that the implants are not suffering from overload caused by loss of mucosal support due to further ridge resorption (Figure 16.8). It has been suggested that removable prostheses often require more maintenance in the form of adjustment and replacement of retentive elements such as clips and 'ball retainers', compared with fixed prostheses.

Screw and abutment connections

Repeated chewing cycles may produce screw loosening, either at the bridge screw level or the abutment level. Most single tooth restorations have cemented crowns with no direct access to the abutment for screw tightening. Therefore, should this be required, removal of the crown is necessary. Abutment loosening

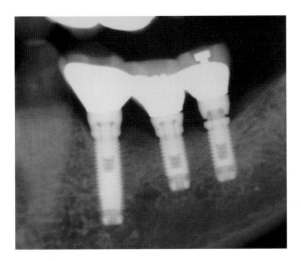

Figure 16.9

A radiograph of a posterior mandibular bridge on Brånemark implants, showing failure to seat the distal abutment (prior to completion of the bridge) and a loose bridge screw.

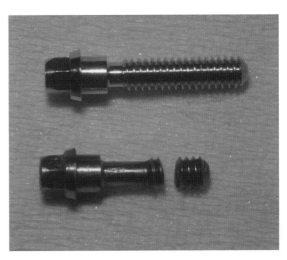

Figure 16.10

The lower screw is a retrieved fractured Brånemark abutment screw, compared with an intact screw above it. The fractured screw was removed from the case illustrated in Figure 16.12.

and development of a gap between abutment and implant will manifest as a loose prosthesis (Figure 16.9). This can even appear as though there has been failure at the implant level. Screw loosening can be prevented largely by attention to occlusal contacts and adequate tightening of the bridge and abutment screw, in the first place by using specifically designed torque wrenches/handpieces (see Chapters 13 and 14). Some implant systems, e.g. Nobel Biocare, suggest re-tightening of bridge screws 2 weeks after initial fitting of the bridge super-structure. The design of the abutment/implant interface may also reduce this complication. The internal abutment connection designs should produce a more stable joint than the flat top designs. Even with the latter design, the occurrence of screw loosening is low provided that the correct torque has been applied. Screw loosening is often an important sign of overload due to:

- poorly fitting prosthesis/non-passive fit
- poor design, e.g. overextension of a cantilever
- poor implant/crown ratio
- inadequate attention to occlusal contacts
- too few implants/teeth to establish an adequate occlusal table

- parafunctional activity

These factors require identification, correction and proper management to avoid this complication. Failure to deal with these problems, particularly in patients who exhibit parafunctional activities, may predispose to screw fracture (retention screws or abutment screws), which manifests as a loose prosthesis and may be detected radiographically (Figures 16.9 and 16.10). The fractured screws need to be removed and replaced. In many instances the fractured screw can be unwound by engaging the fractured surface with a sharp probe and moving the probe round in a counter-clockwise direction. Alternatively, a commercially designed retrieval kit may make this process easier. The screw then can be replaced and attention given to correct the cause of the problem in order to avoid a repeat of the problem and possibly ultimate failure of the implant. In some instances removal of the fractured screw proves to be impossible. Fractured screws are difficult to remove by drilling without causing considerable damage to the implant. This may make subsequent restoration impossible unless it is feasible to construct a custom-made post that can be cemented within the implant.

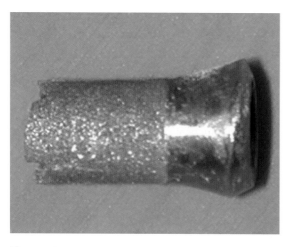

Figure 16.11

The top of a fractured Straumann implant. This hollow cylinder implant had progressively lost bone to the level where there were perforations in the implant cylinder, the level at which the implant fractured.

Implant fractures

Fortunately, fracture of an implant is rare. It is more likely to occur with:

* narrow diameter implants, particularly where the wall thickness is thin
* excessive load
* marginal bone loss that has progressed to the level of an inherent weakness of the implant (Figure 16.11), often the level where wall thickness is thin at the apical level of the abutment screw

Implant fracture is rarely retrievable, and requires either burying the fractured component beneath the mucosa or its removal (Figure 16.12). The latter can be difficult and traumatic, usually requiring surgical trephining that may leave a considerable defect in the jaw bone.

Soft-tissue evaluation and problems

The mucosa surrounding the implant abutments should appear free of superficial inflammation. Gentle pressure on the exterior surface of the soft tissue should not result in any bleeding or exudate and should produce minimal or no discomfort. Inflammation of the peri-implant mucosa has been termed 'peri-implant mucositis' to differentiate it from the more destructive lesion involving bone loss, so-called 'peri-implantitis'. Probing depths may be evaluated and will depend upon the thickness of the original mucosa, any overgrowth of soft tissue and any loss of attachment/marginal bone loss that

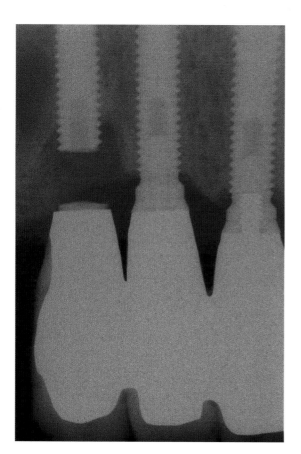

Figure 16.12

A radiograph of three Brånemark implants supporting a maxillary bridge that had been subjected to excessive loading. The anterior implant (right) had previously suffered a fractured abutment screw, the top half of which was removed and replaced with a gold screw (more radiopaque) but the apical part could not be removed. The distal implant (left) had a similar history that was followed by fracture of the implant at the level of the apex of the abutment screw. This latter situation usually requires removal or burial of the fractured implant.

may have occurred. Standard periodontal probes with a tip diameter of approximately 0.5 mm and a probing force of 25 g are recommended. Ideally probing depths should be relatively shallow (< 4 mm) with no or minimal bleeding. Studies have demonstrated that probing around implants is not dissimilar to probing around the natural dentition. In general the junctional epithelium is quite delicate and can be breached by the probe. The underlying connective tissue around implants is not connected by well-formed fibre bundles to the abutment/implant surface and forms parallel collagen fibre bundles. This offers less resistance to probing. In general the probe stops short of the bone margin by about 1 mm. If increased probing depths, soft tissue proliferation, copious bleeding, exudate or tenderness to pressure are found, the area should be examined radiographically (regardless of whether radiographic re-evaluation is scheduled) to determine whether there has been any loss of marginal bone or loss of osseointegration (see section on peri-implantitis). In these circumstances it may be advisable to dismantle a screw retained implant superstructure to allow adequate examination of individual abutments and implants.

Most inflammatory conditions can be corrected with attention to oral hygiene and professional cleaning. The latter is also considerably facilitated if the prosthesis can be dismantled and cleaned outside the mouth. However, there are a number of instances that may require surgical correction of the soft tissue problem:

* Soft-tissue overgrowth
* Soft-tissue deficiencies
* Persistent inflammation/infection
* Continuing bone loss (see peri-implantitis)

Soft-tissue overgrowth

Soft-tissue proliferation may occur around bridges with poorly designed embrasures and under supporting bars of implant dentures (see Chapter 17). It may require simple excision if there is adequate attached keratinized tissue apical to it, or an inverse bevel resection as used in periodontal surgery to thin out the excess

tissue but preserve the keratinized tissue to produce a zone of attached tissue around the abutment (see Figure 16.14).

Soft-tissue deficiencies

The transmucosal part of the implant restoration may emerge through non-keratinized mucosa, particularly in situations where there has been severe loss of bone, e.g. edentulous jaws. Non-keratinized mucosa looks redder and more delicate than keratinized tissue and may lack attachment to the underlying bone. This can give rise to soreness and compromised plaque control, particularly in implant denture cases. Persistent soreness and inflammation can be overcome by grafting keratinized mucosa to the site in a procedure that is the same as free gingival grafting using donor tissue from the palate. In other situations it may give rise to compromised aesthetics (Figures 16.13 and 16.14).

Persistent inflammation

Persistent inflammation or discomfort may arise due to poor implant positioning. It may require recontouring of the soft tissues to allow patient cleaning, and this may reveal the less than satisfactory aesthetics produced by poor planning and execution of treatment (Figure 16.14) In other more severe cases the only remedy may be to remove the implants or bury them permanently beneath the mucosa (Figure 16.15). Poorly designed or constructed protheses may need to be replaced, but in some cases this would also involve correction of the implant position. A compromise solution may therefore be sought.

Evaluation of marginal bone levels

It is important to establish baseline radiographs when the prosthesis is fitted. It would seem reasonable to radiograph annually for the first 3–5 years, then bi-annually up to 10 years in the absence of clinical signs or symptoms. In all

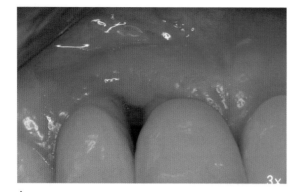

A

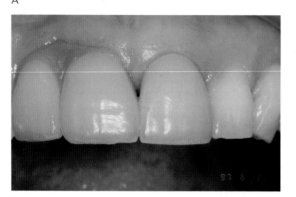

B

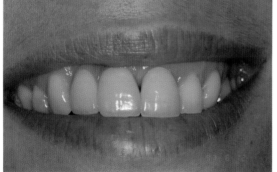

C

Figure 16.13

(A) The maxillary central and lateral incisors were replaced with single tooth implants. However, loss of interdental tissue has produced a very unaesthetic result. The soft tissue defect is difficult or impossible to correct surgically. (B) The crowns have been replaced with a splinted unit bearing a pink porcelain prosthetic 'interdental papilla'. (C) The improvement in aesthetics is shown with the patient smiling.

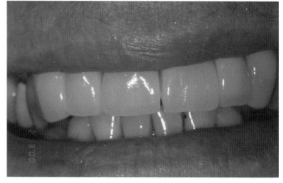

A

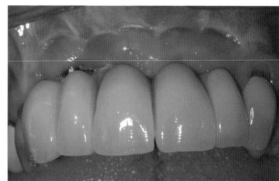

B

Figure 16.14

(A) This patient does not reveal the gingival margin when she smiles. (B) Retraction of the lips shows the unsatisfactory intraoral appearance of the receded soft tissue exposing the titanium abutments. The implants had been placed in the interdental zones and the patient had found it impossible to carry out adequate oral hygiene. Inflammation and soft tissue overgrowth had occurred, which required surgical resection resulting in this appearance.

cases every effort should be made to minimize distortion and produce comparable reproducible images to allow longitudinal assessment. Most implant systems report a small amount of bone loss in the first year following loading, followed by a steady state in subsequent years in the majority of implants. More marginal bone loss has been reported in patients who smoke. If progressive bone loss is detected, the clinician has to decide whether this is most likely due to excessive loading or bacteria-induced inflammation (peri-implantitis).

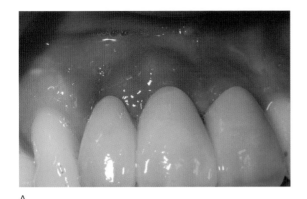

A

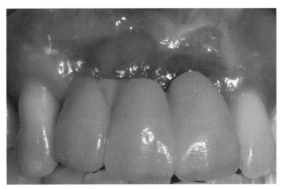

D

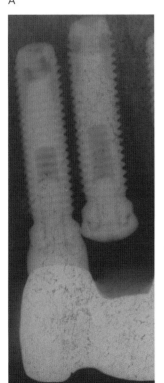

B

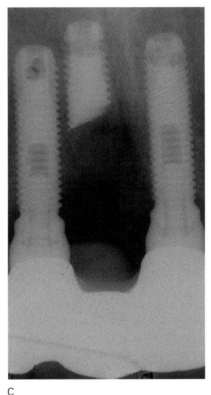

C

Figure 16.15

(A) Clinical appearance of a three-unit implant-supported bridge replacing the maxillary right lateral incisor and both central incisors. A small soft tissue abscess is visible at the right central incisor unit. Initially three implants had been inserted to replace each of the missing teeth as single units. (B) A radiograph of the bridge shows that there is a buried (unused/unconnected) implant beneath the right central incisor unit, in very close proximity to and in intraoral communication with the implant in the right lateral incisor region. This had led to a submucosal infection at the head of the buried implant. (C) The buried implant at the right central incisor site had been deemed to be unrestorable as an individual unit, and it proved impossible to remove simply in order to resolve the infection. Therefore, the coronal part of the implant was sectioned and removed, leaving the apical part *in situ*. (D) The healed result with resolution of the infection. The loss of soft tissue contour necessitated addition to the bridgework. The bridge was then remade. This problem could have been avoided by placement of only two implants in the limited space, rather than placing implants too close together to allow restoration.

Peri-implantitis

The incidence of peri-implantitis would appear to be low. A diagnosis of peri-implantitis means that an inflammatory lesion has caused obvious bone loss. Usually the marginal soft tissue will appear inflamed but this is not always the case because the lesion may be deep seated. Probing will suggest loss of marginal bone and radiographs will confirm this. It is quite possible that the bacteria implicated in periodontitis, such as *Porphyromonas gingivalis*, are also the major pathogens in peri-implantitis. There is therefore a possibility of colonization or infection of the implant surfaces from pre-existing periodontopathic bacteria. Therefore implants should not be placed in patients with untreated periodontal disease. The destruction of the supporting tissues

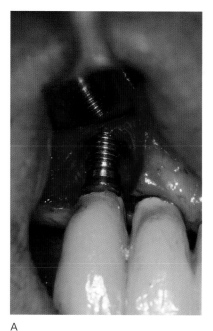
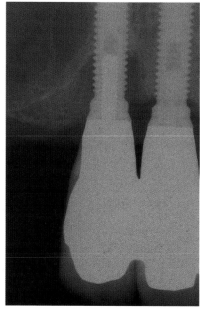

A   B

Figure 16.16

(A) A clinical photograph of a surgically exposed implant that has suffered from peri-implantitis. The inflammatory tissue has been removed to reveal bone loss that forms a circumferential gutter. (B) Radiograph of the lesion showing the wide saucerized pattern of bone loss typical of peri-implantitis.

of teeth and implants has many similarities but there are important differences due to the nature of the supporting tissues. This is particularly noticeable with the different patterns of tissue destruction observed. Peri-implantitis affects the entire circumference of the implant resulting in a 'gutter' of bone loss filled with inflammatory tissue extending to the bone surface (Figure 16.16). It would seem probable that destructive inflammatory lesions affecting both teeth and implants have stages in which the disease process is more rapid (burst phenomenon) followed by periods of relative quiescence.

Unfortunately there have been some very polarized views as to the incidence and nature of peri-implantitis. Some have contended that peri-implantitis only occurs at implants with rough surfaces that allow bacterial colonization. Conversely, bone loss at smoother implant surfaces was held to be due to overload. Clearly this simplistic distinction is false and unhelpful and is reminiscent of the debate about the importance of occlusal trauma in periodontitis. It must be conceded that the destruction of the marginal bone in a bacterially induced peri-implantitis may be difficult to differentiate from bone loss due to excessive forces. Moreover, the latter situation subsequently may be

prone to bacterially induced inflammation. It should be clear that any lesion giving rise to marked bone loss should be evaluated for both occlusal and bacterial factors and treated appropriately. Occlusal factors are more likely to be implicated in situations where there has been:

- a history of parafunction
- a history of breakages of the superstructure or retaining screws
- breakages or loosening of screws
- an angular/narrow pattern of bone loss
- too few implants placed to replace the missing teeth
- excessive cantilever extensions

Bacterially induced factors are more likely to be implicated where there is:

- poor oral hygiene
- retention of cement in the subgingival area
- macroscopic gaps between implant components subgingivally
- marked inflammation, exudation and proliferation of the soft tissue
- wide saucerized areas of marginal bone loss visible on radiographs

Management of peri-implantitis

Occlusal factors that could result in implant overload should be identified and corrected. Lesions that are thought to be due primarily to bacterial colonization or secondarily contaminated by bacteria are currently managed in a similar fashion to lesions of periodontitis around teeth, by gaining surgical access to the lesion. The keratinized mucosa should be preserved as much as possible, by employing an inverse bevel incision to separate it from the underlying inflammatory tissue. Following incision to bone, the soft tissue flaps should be elevated to expose normal adjacent bone. The inflammatory tissue surrounding the implant is readily removed (Figure 16.16A). The main difficulty is adequately disinfecting the implant surface. This is more readily accomplished on a relatively smooth surface but may be almost impossible on a very porous surface such as a hydroxyapatite coating. Therefore, rough surfaces require more extensive debridement than a smooth surface. Rougher surfaces may require removal of the contaminated layer with burs. Contaminated surfaces may be disinfected using a topical antiseptic such as chlorhexidine, detergents or topical antibiotics. Peri-implantitis lesions are not sufficiently common to have allowed comparison of different methods of cleaning. In many cases the soft tissue inflammation can be resolved and there may be some repair of the bone. Some clinicians attempt to regenerate the lost bone using techniques such as guided bone regeneration. In cases where regenerative techniques have been used and bone fill has occurred, most research has concluded that re-osseointegration is unlikely to occur.

Routine hygiene maintenance requirements

Single tooth restorations

An individual with a healthy dentition and a single tooth implant replacement should have the simplest maintenance requirements and few, if any, complications. The patient should be able to maintain the peri-implant soft and hard tissues in a state of health equivalent to that which exists around their natural teeth, almost without professional intervention (Figure 16.17). This can be achieved with routine toothbrushing and flossing. However, in some circumstances, the contour of the single tooth restoration is not ideal and instead of producing a smooth readily cleansable emergence profile, poor positioning of the implant may have resulted in a degree of ridge lapping. This will require modification of oral hygiene techniques to clean under the overhanging crown morphology, with dental tape or superfloss passed or threaded under the overhang. Single tooth restorations rarely have calculus formation on their highly glazed porcelain or polished gold surfaces. Professional scaling is not therefore normally required.

Fixed bridges and removable prostheses

In patients with more complex fixed prostheses, development of readily cleansable embrasure spaces by the technician considerably facilitates patients' oral hygiene. Difficulties occur with poor implant positioning, such as placement in embrasure spaces and implants placed too close together (Figures 16.14 and 16.15). The selection of abutments may have a considerable impact. Smooth titanium abutment surfaces are well tolerated by the soft tissues. With cemented restorations it is advisable to limit the subgingival extent of the cement junction to allow easier cementation, removal of excess cement and checking of marginal integrity.

Scaling of implant prostheses

Supragingival calculus deposition is most frequently seen in implants in the anterior mandible (often on implant denture abutments), in much the same pattern as natural teeth. Calculus should be removed from titanium abutments with instruments that will not damage the surface

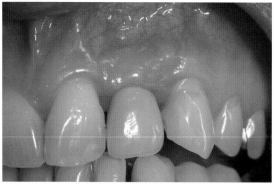

A

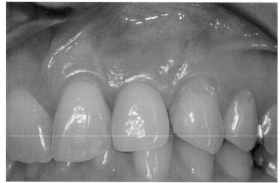

C

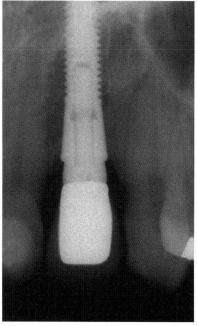

B

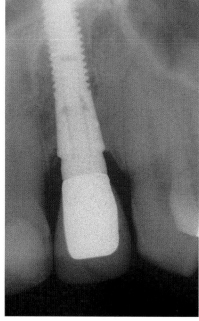

D

Figure 16.17

A series of photographs showing long-term maintenance of a single tooth implant restoration (AstraTech) replacing a maxillary lateral incisor. (A) Clinical appearance of the left lateral incisor unit at cementation. (B) Radiograph of the completed restoration at cementation. The bone levels are at the top of the implant. (C) The improvement of the soft tissue profile and excellent healthy appearance 6 years later. (D) Maintenance of bone levels at the top of the implant after 6 years.

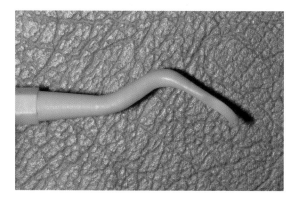

Figure 16.18

A plastic-tipped curette for scaling titanium abutments to avoid damage to them.

(Figure 16.18), therefore the instruments are usually made of plastic. In most cases where patients are treated with prostheses that have been optimized to produce good aesthetics, the abutments used are low profile with no exposure of titanium supragingivally and minimal exposure of the titanium surface subgingivally, so this problem does not arise. Ultrasonic instruments and steel-tipped instruments are contraindicated.

Conclusion

Ideally all patients should be in a recall/maintenance programme. This is particularly important in patients who have complex prostheses, where servicing requirements may be greater. Some patients fail to appreciate the importance of follow-up and complications may arise as a result.

Bibliography

Behr M, Lang R, Leibrock A, Rosentritt M, Handel G (1998). Complication rate with prosthodontic reconstruction on ITI and IMZ dental implants. *Clin Oral Implants Res* **9**: 51–8.

Bragger U (1998). Use of radiographs in evaluating success, stability and failure in implant dentistry. *Periodontol 2000* **4**: 77–88.

Carlsson B, Carlsson GE (1994). Prosthodontic complications in osseointegrated dental implant treatment. *Int J Oral Maxillofac Implants* **9**: 90–4.

Dharmar S (1997). Locating the mandibular canal in panoramic radiographs. *Int J Oral Maxillofac Implants* **12**: 113–7.

Eckert S, Wollan P (1998). Retrospective review of 1170 endosseous implants placed in partially edentulous jaws. *J Prosthet Dent* **79**: 415–21.

Ellegaard B, Baelum V, Karring T (1997). Implant therapy in periodontally compromised patients. *Clin Oral Implants Res* **8**: 180–8.

Ellen R (1998). Microbial colonization of the peri-implant environment and its longterm success of osseointegrated implants. *Int J Prosthodont* **11**: 443–51.

Esposito M, Hirsch JM, Lekholm U, Thomsen P (1998). Biological factors contributing to failures of osseointegrated oral implants: (I) Success criteria and epidemiology. *Eur J Oral Sci* **106**: 527–51.

Esposito M, Hirsch JM, Lekholm U, Thomsen P (1998). Biological factors contributing to failures of osseointegrated oral implants: (II) Etiopathogenesis. *Eur J Oral Sci* **106**: 721–64.

Esposito M, Hirsch JM, Lekholm U, Thomsen P (1999). Differential diagnosis and treatment strategies of biologic complications and failing oral implants. *Int J Oral Maxillofac Implants* **14**: 473–90.

Gunne J, Jemt T, Linden B (1994). Implant treatment in partially edentulous patients: a report on prostheses after 3 years. *Int J Prosthodont* **7**: 143–8.

Hammerle CH, Fourmosis I, Winkler JR, Weigel C, Bragger U, Lang NP (1995). Successful bone fill in late peri-implant defects using guided tissue regeneration. A short communication. *J Periodontol* **66**: 303–8.

Isidor F (1996). Loss of osseointegration caused by occlusal overload of oral implants. *Clin Oral Implants Res* **7**: 143–52.

Isidor F (1997). Histological evaluation of peri-implant bone at implants subjected to occlusal overload or plaque accumulation. *Clin Oral Implants Res* **8**: 1–9.

Jaffin R, Berman C (1991). The excessive loss of Brånemark fixtures in type IV bone. *J Periodontol* **62**: 2–4.

Jemt T, Lekholm U (1995). Implant treatment in the edentulous maxilla: a 5 year follow up report on patients with different degrees of jaw resorption. *Int J Oral Maxillofac Implants* **10**: 303–11.

Lekholm U, Sennerby L, Roos J, Becker W (1996). Soft tissue and marginal bone conditions at osseointegrated implants that have exposed threads: a 5 year retrospective study. *Int J Oral Maxillofac Implants* **11**: 599–604.

Levine RA, Clem DS, Wilson TG, Higginbottom F, Saunders SL (1997). A multicenter retrospective analysis of the ITI implant system used for single-tooth replacements: preliminary results at 6 or more months of loading. *Int J Oral Maxillofac Implants* **12**: 237–42.

Lindh T, Gunne J, Tillberg A, Molin M (1998). A meta analysis of implants in partial edentulism. *Clin Oral Implants Res* **9**: 80–90.

Lindquist LW, Carlsson GE, Jemt T (1996). A prospective 15 year follow up study of mandibular fixed prostheses supported by osseointegrated implants. *Clin Oral Implants Res* **7**: 329–36.

Mombelli A, Lang NP (1992). Antimicrobial treatment of peri-implant infections. *Clin Oral Implants Res* **3**: 162–8.

Persson LG, Ericsson I, Berglundh T, Lindhe J (1996). Guided bone regeneration in the treatment of peri-implantitis. *Clin Oral Implants Res* **7**: 366–72.

Rangert B, Krogh PH, Langer B, Van Roekel N (1995). Bending overload and implant fracture: a retrospective clinical analysis. *Int J Oral Maxillofac Implants* **10**: 326–34.

Sewerin IP, Gotfredsen K, Stoltze K (1997). Accuracy of radiographic diagnosis of peri-implant radiolucencies— an in vitro experiment. *Clin Oral Implants Res* **8**: 299–304.

van Steenberghe D (1989). A retrospective multicenter evaluation of the survival rate of osseointegrated fixtures supporting fixed partial prostheses in the treatment of partial edentulism. *J Prosthet Dent* **61**: 217–23.

van Steenberghe D, Klinge B, Linden U, Quirynen M, Herrmann I, Garpland C (1993). Periodontal indices around natural and titanium abutments: a longitudinal multicentre study. *J Periodontol* **64**: 538–41.

17
Implant dentures

Introduction

This chapter will describe prosthodontic complications and post-insertion maintenance of the completed implant dentures. Complications may occur before, during and after the prosthodontic phase of implant treatment; maintenance and repairs of the dentures and components will be required after the dentures are fitted. Various studies have shown different results for the maintenance requirements for implant dentures. Hemmings *et al.* (1994) concluded that implant dentures required less maintenance than fixed restorations, but others (Chan *et al.*, 1996; Watson and Davis, 1996; Watson *et al.*, 1997) have pointed out the necessity for replacement of clips, adjustments and remakes.

Complications before the prosthodontic phase of treatment

Placement of implants in an unplanned position

Implants may be inadvertently placed in an unplanned buccopalatal or buccolingual position, in an unplanned mesiodistal position, at an unplanned angulation or at an unplanned depth. Situations such as these are more likely when a stent is not available but may still occur even when a stent is used if there are unexpected findings during surgery.

Minor changes from the intended implant position or angulation usually can be accommodated within an overdenture, although an alternative attachment mechanism may have to be used, for instance, a smaller ball attachment may be needed (Figure 17.1). Some manufacturers provide a choice of sizes and these have been described in Chapter 6.

Greater deviations from the intended implant position will create an abnormal contour in the finished denture. This may be uncomfortable for the patient and may cause speech difficulties or even soft-tissue proliferation (Figures 17.2 and 17.3).

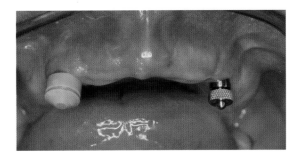

Figure 17.1

Maxillary implants placed too buccally. There is insufficient room for a Nobel Biocare standard ball attachment retention cap so a smaller 3i ball attachment is used instead. The figure shows a Nobel Biocare retention cap on the right implant and a 3i matrix on the left implant.

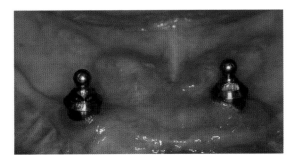

Figure 17.2

ITI/Straumann implants placed too superficially and the left implant placed too lingually. There is an unfavourable soft-tissue response around the left implant.

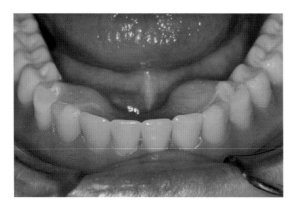

Figure 17.3

Completed denture has unfavourable contour owing to unplanned implant placement.

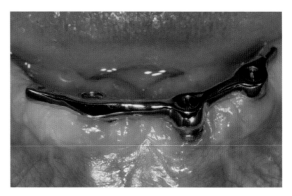

Figure 17.5

Nobel Biocare Macro-Ovoid bar on fixture head gold alloy cylinders enables a very low profile bar. The cast has been scraped to permit close adaptation. The blanching in the figure was evident only on immediate placement of the bar.

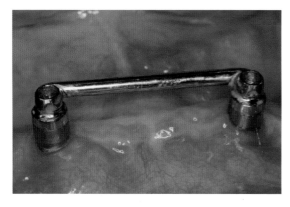

Figure 17.4

Superficial placement of Nobel Biocare implants. Round bar on 3-mm standard abutments is several millimetres away from the ridge. Labial inclination has also necessitated soldering the bar to the lingual surfaces of gold alloy cylinders to place clips in the thickest portion of the denture.

Where an implant has been placed in a position that is too superficial, there may be insufficient space for the prosthodontic components to be contained within the normal contour of the proposed denture. Even when there is sufficient bulk of acrylic resin, and a bar and clip system is planned, the resulting bar may be several millimetres away from the mucosa (Figure 17.4). Although this, in itself, is only critical when short implants are used and the leverage is increased under loading, the amount of

so-called dead space is increased and there may be tissue overgrowth beneath the bar.

Nobel Biocare have introduced fixture-head gold or titanium cylinders, originally designed to be used with a single-stage surgery implant where the external hex is superficial to the mucosa, to reduce the overall height of the supramucosal components. These cylinders fit directly onto the implant and can be reduced in height. They can be used instead of the abutment/gold cylinder system on a superficially placed implant to enable a bar to be placed close to the alveolar ridge mucosa (Figure 17.5).

A disadvantage of the one-piece ITI/Straumann implant is that no compensation is possible for an implant that has been placed in a position that is too superficial (Figure 17.2).

Where several implants have been placed too close together there may be insufficient space for clips between them. In such situations, cantilever extensions may be necessary but the clips are more likely to fracture or be pulled out of the resin.

Failure of integration of one or more implants

One or more implants may fail to integrate prior to the commencement of implant denture construction, leaving remaining implants in an unfavourable distribution. In the maxilla, a minimum of four implants ideally should be placed. If one or two should fail, an implant denture can still be made but the risks of overload are higher, particularly where there are opposing teeth in the mandible. If the remaining implants are unilateral, the stability of the implant denture will suffer.

In these situations, further implants should be placed to achieve the planned implant distribution. A transitional denture can be constructed but the risks of overloading the remaining implants must be considered.

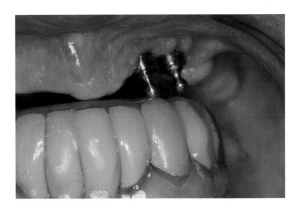

Figure 17.6

Two 3i ball attachments opposing natural teeth. A soft PVC mouthguard has been made for the mandibular teeth.

Failure of bone graft, preventing implant placement

If this happens, it is possible to repeat the procedure but, in our experience, the patients have usually decided to remain with a conventional denture. A new denture is usually required because of the inevitable change of contour of the residual ridge after the surgery and, more problematically, because of the change of sulcus elasticity due to scarring.

Complications during the prosthodontic phase of treatment

Complications include fracture of the existing denture after removal of acrylic resin to allow for the temporary soft lining, and loosening and damage to healing abutments. Existing cobalt–chromium-based dentures, even when widely cut away, are particularly hard on healing abutments, ball attachments or standard abutments that remain in the mouth during the prosthodontic phase of treatment. It is always preferable to have an acrylic-resin-based denture, especially as the soft lining materials adhere more securely.

Opposing teeth may damage healing abutments, standard abutments or ball attachments, particularly when a shearing or glancing contact is possible. This possibility must be taken into consideration during planning stages, even

to the extent of changing the retention system so that such contacts are vertical onto a flat surface away from a screw head. Where ball attachments are unavoidable, a soft PVC mouthguard can be made for night-time wear (Figure 17.6).

Where a bar and clip system is being used, it is advisable to try the bar in the mouth before the denture is finished. If the bar does not fit, it should be checked on the working cast. If it does not fit the working cast, it should be cut and resoldered, or remade, prior to trying it in the mouth again. If the bar fits the cast but not the mouth, the cast must be at fault and a new final impression will be required.

Dentures unable to be inserted over ball attachments

If one of the laboratory analogues was not inserted precisely into the impression, the error in the working cast may prevent the completed denture from being inserted. In such situations, retention caps can be removed and re-attached using autopolymerizing resin in an intraoral procedure, but the procedure is not easy. The relining/repairing procedure described later in Figures 17.21–17.35 is to be preferred.

Post-insertion complications and maintenance

Failure of integration of one or more implants

In common with most published studies, our experience has been that implant failure is very rare in the mandible. Some failures are seen in the maxilla, especially in smokers and where there have been opposing natural teeth. Where a bar is the retention system, the bar will need to be unscrewed to remove the failed implant and then sectioned to reduce its length (Figures 17.7 and 17.8), unless the failed implant is between two other quite close implants. The latter situation is quite unusual because most failures tend to be the most distal implants.

Fracture of ball attachment or implant

Fractures of ball attachments may occur when they oppose natural teeth. The remaining portion of the fractured ball attachment can be unscrewed with a dental explorer or the manufacturer may provide a 'rescue kit'. *In extremis*, the portion can be drilled out but it is difficult to avoid damaging the internal implant threads. The Nobel Biocare rescue kit comes with miniature taps to tidy up the internal thread and should probably be used whenever one of their damaged components is removed. Where an implant fails because of fracture, the denture may still be reasonably stable with a single remaining implant (Figures 17.9 and 17.10).

Fracture or wear of denture or components

Once implant dentures have been made, some patients appear to increase the force exerted upon the dentures during mastication or possibly parafunction. Although the implants may be able to withstand these forces, the prosthodontic components and the denture itself are more vulnerable. These increased forces may cause excessive wear of the occlusal surfaces of the

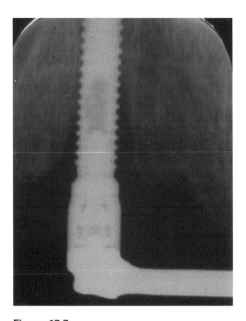

Figure 17.7

Radiograph of failed right maxillary implant supporting bar.

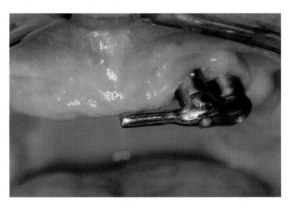

Figure 17.8

The bar has been sectioned near to remaining left maxillary implants leaving space for one clip.

teeth (Figure 17.11), perforation and fracture of denture base material (Figure 17.12), fracture of denture teeth (Figure 17.13), fracture of clips, dislodgement of clips from acrylic resin, wear and fracture of ball attachment matrices (Figure 17.14) and wear of bars. Components can be replaced using cold-cure acrylic resin as an intraoral procedure but extreme care is needed

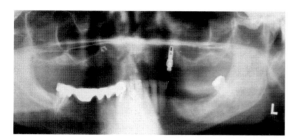

Figure 17.9

A dental panoramic tomograph (DPT) showing the apical portion of a fractured implant in the right maxillary canine region.

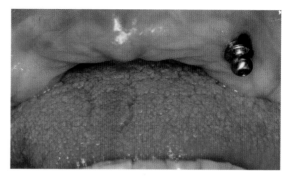

Figure 17.10

Implant in the right maxillary canine region has been removed, leaving one implant in the left canine region. The maxillary denture is still reasonably stable.

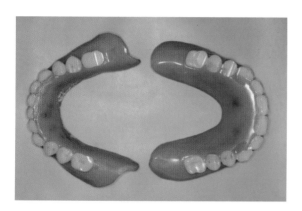

Figure 17.11

Excessive wear of denture teeth on implant dentures after 4 years of use.

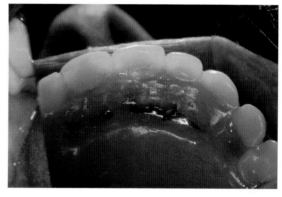

Figure 17.12

Perforation of denture base and exposure of clip retainers in maxillary denture opposed by crowned mandibular teeth.

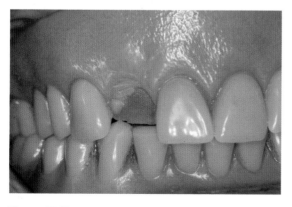

Figure 17.13

Fractured maxillary right lateral incisor of implant denture.

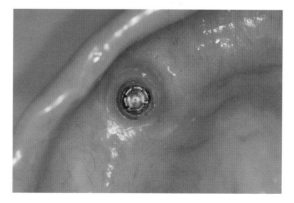

Figure 17.14

Fractured tines of Nobel Biocare gold alloy matrix for 2.25-mm ball attachment.

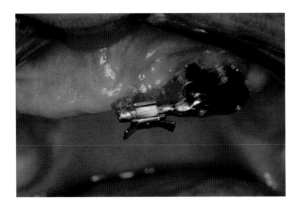

Figure 17.15

A Nobel Biocare clip has been positioned on round bar with spacer and wax used to block out bar.

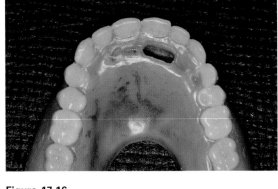

Figure 17.16

The old clip has been removed from maxillary denture and an access hole has been made through to the palatal surface of the denture.

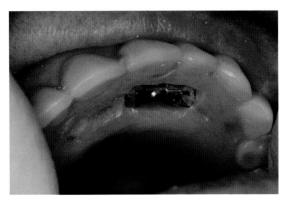

Figure 17.17

The hole is enlarged until the denture can be seated without disturbing the clip in place on the bar. Autopolymerizing resin is then fed through the hole to attach the retention elements of the clip to the denture. When this resin has set the denture can be removed from the mouth, additional resin is added around the clip and then this is polymerized under pressure for maximum strength.

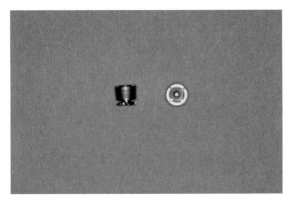

Figure 17.18

Titanium alloy matrix available from Nobel Biocare and ITI/Straumann. The removable cover can be unscrewed to replace the circlip.

(Figures 17.15–17.17). When replacing clips with such an intraoral procedure, it is helpful for some part of the denture to rest onto the bar complex so that the denture can be located accurately in the mouth. Some manufacturers' instructions have stated, however, that the denture should not rest on the gold cylinders. Alternatively, the components can be replaced using the relining procedure illustrated later (Figures 17.21–17.35).

The titanium alloy matrix available from Nobel Biocare and ITI/Staumann consists of three parts: a retention part that is embedded in the acrylic resin of the denture, a stainless-steel circlip and a removable cover for the circlip. If the circlip needs replacing, the cover can be unscrewed to

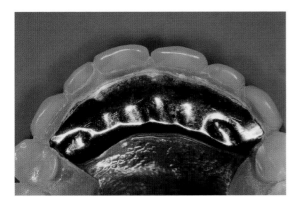

Figure 17.19

Cobalt–chromium alloy platform to oppose crowned mandibular teeth.

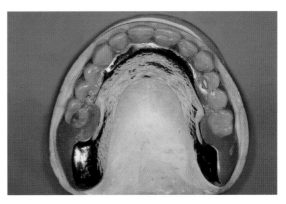

Figure 17.20

Cobalt–chromium alloy base for palateless maxillary implant denture.

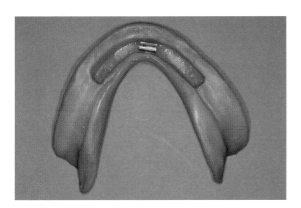

Figure 17.21

A mandibular denture in which the two distal clips had fractured from the resin.

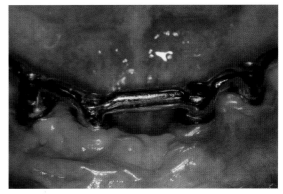

Figure 17.22

Nobel Biocare Macro-Ovoid bar retaining the denture shown in Figure 17.21.

allow replacement of the circlip without disturbing the retention part (Figure 17.18).

Cobalt–chromium alloy bases can be used to prevent excessive wear of acrylic resin, particularly when opposing crowned teeth (Figure 17.19) and also to prevent fracture of the base when this has been reduced in patients who have a strong gag reflex (Figure 17.20).

Continued bone resorption

Where there is evidence of continued bone resorption in the edentulous areas away from the implants, implant dentures can be relined using the relining procedure illustrated in Figures 17.21–17.35.

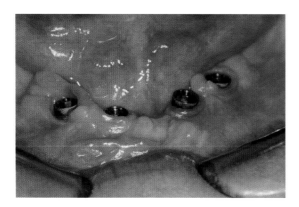

Figure 17.23

The bar is unscrewed from the standard abutments.

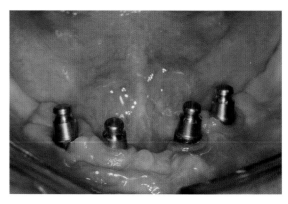

Figure 17.24

Bar impression copings are placed on the abutments. The bar impression copings are used because standard impression copings would require the pins to emerge through the denture teeth. If a ball attachment-retained denture is being relined, no impression copings are normally used (except for AstraTech, which have ball attachment impression copings).

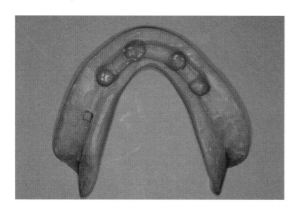

Figure 17.25

The remaining clip is removed, space is created for the impression copings and space is created for the impression material except for the stops marked. For a ball attachment-retained denture, space is created for the ball attachment (and coping if using an AstraTech ball attachment) and impression material.

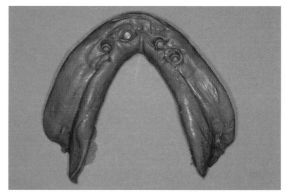

Figure 17.26

The impression is made using Impregum (Espe, D-8229 Seefeld, Germany) impression material. This material is sufficiently rigid to hold the prosthodontic components. The position of the denture is rehearsed before the impression is made and is checked while the impression is being made by reference to the opposing denture.

Overgrowth of mucosa under bar

Overgrowth of mucosa beneath a bar can be removed surgically if its presence causes discomfort or difficulty with cleaning.

Difficulty with speech

This is not uncommon with maxillary dentures where the palatal contour is bulky to accommodate a bar and clip system. If the patient cannot

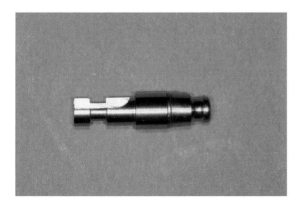

Figure 17.27

The bar impression copings are removed from the abutments and are attached to the abutment replicas.

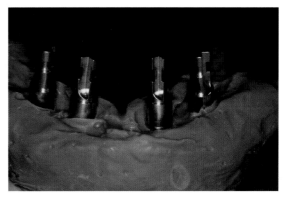

Figure 17.28

The impression copings, attached to the laboratory abutment replicas, are inserted into the impression. For a ball attachment-retained denture, ball attachment replicas are inserted into the impression.

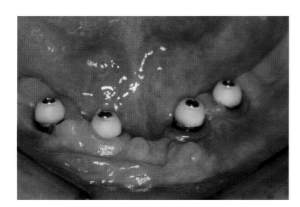

Figure 17.29

Plastic healing caps are attached to the standard abutments in the mouth to prevent food debris and calculus from entering the internal thread or to prevent damage from opposing teeth when present. Ball attachments require no such caps. If a previous denture is available, it can be modified to fit over the healing caps or ball attachments. The bar is retained for the laboratory procedure.

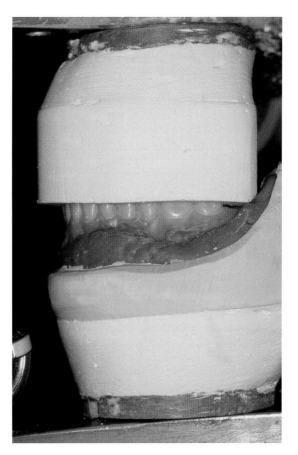

Figure 17.30

The impression is disinfected and boxed and the cast is poured. The cast is mounted on the lower member of an articulator and an overcast is attached to the upper member to record the position of the occlusal surfaces.

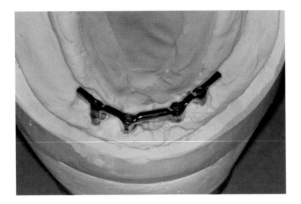

Figure 17.31

The denture is separated from the cast and the bar is attached to the laboratory replicas.

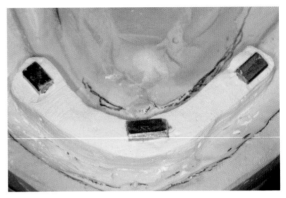

Figure 17.32

The new clips are positioned on the bar with appropriate spacers. The replicas, bar and clips are covered with plaster, except for the retention tags. In the Nobel Biocare system, the denture does not rest on any part of the bar assembly. With a ball attachment-retained denture, new retainers would be positioned on the replica and covered with plaster, except for the retention portion of the retainer. The titanium alloy matrix has a plastic insert so that the circlip and cover are not flasked.

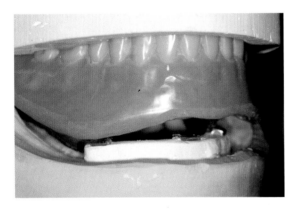

Figure 17.33

The impression material is removed from the denture base together with sufficient acrylic resin so that the denture can be positioned via the overcast without any part of the denture touching the clips or cast.

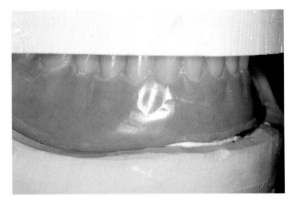

Figure 17.34

Once positioned, the borders of the denture are completed with wax. Then the cast is removed from the articulator complete with denture and flasked in the usual way. The new base is processed via a standard heat-curing method.

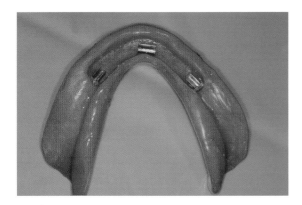

Figure 17.35

The relined denture showing the new clips. After the bar has been re-attached to the abutments, the denture is refitted preferably using a remount procedure to eliminate processing changes and errors in positioning the denture during the impression procedure.

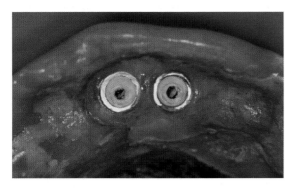

Figure 17.36

Two 3i O-rings that have deteriorated.

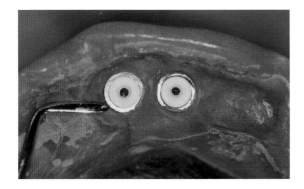

Figure 17.37

New 3i O-rings are easily placed with a suitable instrument.

get used to the new contour after several weeks, a different retention system such as ball attachments or magnets may have to be considered.

Maintenance schedule

After all normal post-insertion adjustments have been carried out and the patient is comfortable with the new implant dentures, the patient should be seen at least once per year for review (Mericske-Stern *et al*, 1994). The patient should be asked to make contact immediately if there are any sudden changes such as loosening of a bar or ball attachment or loosening of the dentures. The latter may indicate fracture of a clip or matrix, or deterioration of a rubber ring in a ball attachment retainer (Figures 17.36 and 17.37).

At the annual visit, dentures should be tested for stability on the mucosa and any rocking should be diagnosed, for example, bone resorption or wear or fracture of a prosthodontic component. Ball attachments should be checked for tightness using the appropriate screwdriver. Bars can be removed and individual abutments checked for tightness and implants checked for any mobility. With the bar off, any calculus can be removed easily from the abutments and from the bar itself with a plastic instrument. The ball attachment retainers in the dentures should be inspected for any fractures of the tines or deterioration of rubber rings. It is probably wise to change rubber rings at this visit, although the rings in Nobel Biocare standard ball attachment matrices seem to last for years. Clips in dentures should be checked for any fractures or looseness in the resin.

If any repairs or replacements of the denture components are required or the denture requires relining, the procedure illustrated in Figures 17.21–17.35 can be used. Alternatively, ball attachment retainers or clips can be replaced as an intraoral procedure, as mentioned earlier. Replacement of the intraoral prosthodontic components is usually a simple matter of unscrewing the worn part and replacing with a new part. If a new bar is needed, the illustrated procedure again can be used.

The implants themselves should be radiographed once per year using the same view (Batenburg *et al.*, 1998), otherwise any changes may not be detected. Where bone level changes are visible, overloading may be responsible and it may be worthwhile remounting the dentures and re-examining the lateral occlusion. The denture teeth can be adjusted to reduce the anterior guidance where necessary.

Bibliography

Batenburg RH, Meijer HJ, Geraets WG, vander Stelt PF (1998). Radiographic assessment of changes in marginal bone around endosseous implants supporting mandibular overdentures. *Dentomaxillofac Radiol* **27**: 221–4.

Chan MF, Johnston C, Howell RA (1996). A retrospective study of the maintenance requirements associated with implant stabilized mandibular overdentures. *Eur J Prosthodont Rest Dent* **4**: 39–43.

Hemmings KW, Schmitt A, Zarb GA (1994). Complications and maintenance requirements for fixed prostheses and overdentures in the edentulous mandible: a five year report. *Int J Oral Maxillofac Implants* **9**: 191–6.

Mericske-Stern R, Steinlin Schaffner T, Marti P, Geering AH (1994). Peri-implant mucosal aspects of ITI implants supporting overdentures. A five-year longitudinal study. *Clin Oral Implants Res* **5**: 9–18.

Watson RM, Davis D (1996). Follow up and maintenance of implant supported prostheses: a comparison of 20 complete mandibular dentures and 20 complete fixed cantilever prostheses. *Br Dent J* **181**: 321–7.

Watson RM, Jemt T, Chai J, Harnett J, Heath MR, Hutton JE, Johns RB, McKenna S, McNamara DC, van Steenberghe D, Taylor R, Herman I (1997). Prosthodontic treatment, patient response, and the need for maintenance of complete implant-supported overdentures: an appraisal of 5 years of prospective study. *Int J Prosthodont* **10**: 345–54.

Index

Page numbers in italics denote figure legends. Where there is a textual reference to the topic on the same page as a legend, italics have not been used.